The Research Report Series of the Institute for Social Research is composed of significant reports published at the completion of a research project. These reports are generally prepared by the principal research investigators and are directed to selected users of this information. Research Reports are intended as technical documents which provide rapid dissemination of new knowledge resulting from ISR research.

RESEARCH REPORT SERIES, INSTITUTE FOR SOCIAL RESEARCH

A Comparative Study of the Organization and Performance of Hospital Emergency Services

Selected Descriptive Findings and the Research Instruments

Basil S. Georgopoulos
and
Robert A. Cooke

with the assistance of

Linda M. Argote
Carl Goble
Cheryl Peck
Mark F. Peterson
Lorraine M. Uhlaner
N. Eser Uzun

Survey Research Center
Institute for Social Research
The University of Michigan

1980

ISR Code No. 9007

Library of Congress Cataloging in Publication Data:

Georgopoulos, Basil Spyros, 1926-
   A comparative study of the organization and performance of hospital emergency services.

   (Research report series - Institute for Social Research, the University of Michigan)
   Includes bibliographical references.
   1. Hospitals--Emergency service. 2. Hospitals--Emergency service--Evaluation. I. Cooke, Robert A., joint author. II. Title. III. Series: Michigan. University. Institute for Social Research. Research report series - Institute for Social Research, University of Michigan. [DNLM: 1. Emergency service, Hospital--Standards. 2. Emergency service, Hospital--Organ. WX215 G352c]
RA975.5.E5G46   362.1'8   80-13467
ISBN 0-87944-253-0

© 1980 by The University of Michigan, All Rights Reserved

Published in 1980 by:
The Institute for Social Research,
The University of Michigan, Ann Arbor, Michigan

6 5 4 3 2 1
Manufactured in the United States of America

ACKNOWLEDGMENTS

This is a research report about a comparative organizational study of hospital emergency services. The project is supported by Research Grant Number HS-02538 from the National Center for Health Services Research, OASH, U.S. Department of Health, Education and Welfare (now renamed Department of Health and Human Services).

The research is being conducted under the direction of Basil S. Georgopoulos, Ph.D., Program Director at the Institute for Social Research and Professor of Psychology, who is the principal investigator. Robert A. Cooke, Ph.D., Associate Research Scientist, is the study director. Linda M. Argote, Mark F. Peterson, Lorraine M. Uhlaner, and N. Eser Uzun served as graduate student research assistants until they completed their doctoral dissertations using data from the study. In the early stages, Barry A. Macy, Ph.D., also participated in the work. Carl Goble is the computer specialist on the project and Cheryl Peck is principal secretary and administrative assistant.

PREFACE

The present volume consists of three parts, as follows: Part I, an overview of the research; Part II, a special report of descriptive findings prepared for the use of the institutions which participated in the study; and Part III, the research instruments developed to collect the data.

The special report, Part II, includes selected preliminary findings from the project and was developed to provide feedback to the participating institutions. While it contains a variety of descriptive and evaluative findings about a great many variables of interest, it is neither a technical report nor the final product of the research. This special report does not directly specify any relationships among the variables investigated or test any particular hypotheses.

These latter tasks are the concern of the more detailed analyses of the data. Some of these analyses have just been finished and are reported in the doctoral dissertations written by the four students who served as research assistants on the project (Argote, 1979; Peterson, 1979; Uhlaner, 1980; Uzun, 1980).* The main analyses of the study, however, are still underway or are being planned for the coming year. When these remaining analyses are completed, the results will appear in technical publications and the final report of the project.

---

*Argote, L.M. "Input Uncertainty and Organizational Problem Solving in Hospital Emergency Service Units." Doctoral dissertation, The University of Michigan, 1979; Peterson, M.F. "Problem-appropriate Leadership in Hospital Emergency Units and Its Relation to Selected Organizational Variables." Doctoral dissertation, The University of Michigan, 1979; Uhlaner, L.M. "Management of the Coordination Problem in Hospital Emergency Units." Doctoral dissertation, The University of Michigan, 1980; Uzun, N.E. "A Study of Hospital Emergency Units Adapting to Their Social Environments: An Interorganizational Cooperation Perspective." Doctoral dissertation, The University of Michigan, 1980.

CONTENTS

Page

Acknowledgments v

Preface vii

List of Tables in Part II xiii

PART I – OVERVIEW OF THE RESEARCH 1

PART II – SPECIAL REPORT TO PARTICIPATING INSTITUTIONS 29

    Introduction

    Chapter

    1. SOME BASIC CHARACTERISTICS OF THE EMERGENCY UNITS
       IN THE STUDY 51

        The Physical Plant and Layout of Emergency Units
        Teaching affiliations, Training Programs, and
          Special Service Capabilities
         Patient Volume and "Emergency Service Definition"
         The Composition of Patient Inputs
         The Patients' Views of Their Problem
         Summary

    2. THE STAFF RESOURCES OF EMERGENCY UNITS 80

        Sufficiency, Acquisition, and Stability of Resources
        Access to On-Call Medical Specialists Within the Hospital
        Medical Staffing Pattern, Staff Size, and Physician
          Hours Worked
         Non-Medical Staffing Patterns
         Staff Capability for Different Levels of Patient Volume
         Summary

    3. CURRENT GOAL PRIORITIES, PROBLEMS, AND STRENGTHS . . . 114

        The Goal Priorities of Emergency Units
        Emergency Unit Strengths
        The Current Major Problems of Emergency Units
        Summary

    4. PERCEIVED LEADERSHIP EFFECTIVENESS AND THE INFLUENCE
       OF VARIOUS GROUPS 139

        Medical, Nursing, and Administrative Leadership
        The Influence of Key Groups
        Summary

Chapter	Page

5. WORK RELATIONS AND PROBLEM SOLVING WITHIN THE
   EMERGENCY UNIT. 157

   Overall Coordination of Staff Efforts and Activities
   Problem Solving Within the Emergency Units
   Work Relations Between Nurses and Physicians in
     the Units
   Tension Among Key Staff
   Summary

6. WORK RELATIONS WITH THE PARENT HOSPITAL 191

   Institutional Monitoring
   Relations with Hospital Administration
   Relations with Other Hospital Staff or Units
   Summary

7. RELATIONS WITH THE COMMUNITY. 208

   Information about Health Agencies and Extent
     of Inter-institutional Collaboration
   Work Contacts with Other Organizations and
     Patient Transfer Arrangements
   Overall Tension with the Community
   Work Contacts with Key Individuals from the
     Community
   Problem-Causing Aspects of the Community
   Summary

8. REPUTATION IN THE COMMUNITY AND PATIENT SATISFACTION. . . 236

   The Reputation and Responsiveness of Emergency Units
   Patient Satisfaction
   Summary

9. STAFF ATTITUDES AND SATISFACTION: SOCIAL EFFICIENCY. . . 258

   The Emergency Unit as a Place to Work
   Staff Identification with the Units
   Staff Perceptions of Certain Job Characteristics
   Staff Satisfaction with Financial and Non-Financial
     Rewards
   Summary

Chapter	Page

10. FINANCIAL ASPECTS AND ECONOMIC EFFICIENCY 277

    The Operating Budgets and Expenditures of
      Emergency Units
    Revenues in Relation to Costs and Expenditures
    Emergency Unit Service Charges
    Professional Staff Hours Worked in Relation to
      Patient Visits Processed
    Summary

11. CLINICAL EFFICIENCY: CARE PROCEDURES, STAFF
PERFORMANCE, AND QUALITY OF CARE 303

    The Appropriateness and Performance of
      Care Procedures
    Promptness of Medical Attention, Patient Waiting
      Time, and the Length of Patient Visits
    Assessment by Patients of Certain Aspects of
      Care Process and Outcome
    Patient Death Rates
    The Quality of Medical Management and Nursing
      Care for Patients with Certain Conditions
    The Quality of Overall Medical Care and Overall
      Nursing Care
    The Quality of Medical Care and Nursing Care as
      Compared to the Quality of Care in the Emergency
      Units of Other Hospitals
    Summary

Concluding Comments

Appendix

PART III - THE RESEARCH INSTRUMENTS. 383

    Introduction

    The Instruments

      Hospital Administrators' Interview
      Hospital Administrators' Questionnaire
      Emergency Unit Physicians' Interview
      Emergency Unit Physicians' Questionnaire
      Interview with Registered Nurses (RN's) in the Emergency Unit
      Questionnaire for Emergency Unit RN's
      Emergency Unit Supervising Nurse/Head Nurse Questionnaire

PART III (cont.)

    Interview for Selected Physicians in the Hospital
      (Outside the Emergency Unit)
    Interview with Respondents from the Community
    Interview for Full-Time LPN's (Licensed Practical Nurses)
      Working in the Emergency Unit
    Information from Administrative and Organizational Records
      (Staffing, Personnel, Census, and Financial Data)
    Questionnaire for Emergency Unit Patients

LIST OF TABLES IN PART II

Page

Introduction

Table 1. The Sample of Study Hospitals (Institutions Whose Emergency Units Were Studied) and the Population of Hospitals from Which it was Selected — 35

Table 2. Number of Individual Respondents Who Provided Data for the Study, Shown Separately for the Various Participating Groups of Respondents — 41

Chapter 1

Table 3. Number of Rooms and Beds in the Emergency Units (EU's) Studied — 53

Table 4. Adequacy of the Layout of Emergency Units as Reported by Registered Nurses (RNS) and Patients (PATS) — 55

Table 5. Emergency Units Operated by Hospitals with Medical Teaching Affiliations and Emergency Personnel Training Programs — 57

Table 6. Number of Institutions with Selected Special Facilities — 59

Table 7. Number of Patient Visits to the Emergency Units During the Most Recent Quarter and Most Recent Week — 61

Table 8. Patient Visits to the Emergency Units Studied in Relation to Hospital In-patient Admissions and In-patient Days for Most Recent Quarter — 63

Table 9. Percent of Patient Visits During the Most Recent Quarter That Were Scheduled in Advance or Involved Transfer — 66

Table 10. Percent of Patients Visiting the Emergency Units During the Most Recent Quarter Who Were Sent (by the EU) Elsewhere for Treatment — 68

Table 11. Percent of Patients Visiting the Emergency Units During the Most Recent Month Who Arrived by Ambulance — 71

Table 12. Percent of the Patients Visiting the Emergency Units "Over the Past Four Weeks" Who Arrived in a "Life-Threatening" Condition — 73

Table 13. Percent of the Patients Visiting the Emergency Unit Whose Problems Could Have Been Handled in a Doctor's Office, According to Physician Respondents — 75

	Page

Table 14. Emergency Unit Patients' Assessments of Their Particular Problems ... 77

Chapter 2

Table 15. Sufficiency of Emergency Unit Resources, as Evaluated by Hospital Administration Respondents (HAS) ... 83

Table 16. Sufficiency of Emergency Unit Resources, as Evaluated by the Physicians (MDS) Working in the Units ... 84

Table 17. The Relative Success of Emergency Units in Obtaining Requested Staff Resources, According to the Registered Nurses (RNS) ... 88

Table 18. Emergency Unit Staff Stability, as Assessed by the Supervising Nurses (SRNS) ... 90

Table 19. Physical Presence of Physicians and Registered Nurses in the Various Emergency Units at Different Times ... 92

Table 20. On-call Availability to the Emergency Units of Particular Medical Specialists ... 94

Table 21. Number of Emergency Units with Particular Medical Staffing Patterns, as Reported by the Chief Executive Officer of Each Hospital ... 97

Table 22. Number of Physicians Who Worked in the Emergency Unit and Physician Hours Worked During the Most Recent Week, Based on Data from Hospital Records (RECS) ... 100

Table 23. Number of Physician Hours Worked in the Emergency Unit During a Typical Week by the Physicians (MDS) Who Participated in the Study, Based on Their Own Reports ... 101

Table 24. Number of Budgeted Positions for Non-medical Personnel in the Emergency Units Studied, for Most Recent Quarter ... 104

Table 25. Number of Registered Nurses Who Worked in the Emergency Unit and Number of Hours Worked by Them During the Most Recent Week, Based on Data from Hospital Records (RECS) ... 106

Table 26. Number of Registered Nurse Hours Worked in the Emergency Unit During a Typical Week by the Registered Nurses (RNS) Who Participated in the Study, Based on Their Own Reports ... 107

Table 27. The Capability of Emergency Units for Handling a 10%-15% Increase in Patient Workload with Present Staff and at Current Levels of Care Quality ... 110

Page

Table 28. The Likely Effect on the Quality of Care of a 10%-15% Decrease in the Present Patient Workload of Emergency Units ... 112

Chapter 3

Table 29. Basic Goal Priorities of Emergency Units as Rank-Ordered by the Physicians (MDS) Who Work There ... 116

Table 30. Basic Goal Priorities of Emergency Units as Rank-Ordered by the Registered Nurses (RNS) Who Work There ... 117

Table 31. Basic Goal Priorities of Emergency Units as Perceived by Selected Respondents from the Community (CRS) ... 122

Table 32. The Most Important Strengths of Emergency Units, as Assessed by the Physicians (MDS) Who Work There ... 126

Table 33. The Most Important Strengths of Emergency Units, as Assessed by Selected Physicians (HMDS) in Their Respective Parent Hospitals ... 128

Table 34. The Most Important Strengths of Emergency Units, as Assessed by Hospital Administrator Respondents (HAS) ... 129

Table 35. The Current Major Problems of Emergency Units, as Assessed by the Physicians (MDS) Who Work There ... 133

Table 36. The Current Major Problems of Emergency Units, as Assessed by the Registered Nurses (RNS) Who Work There ... 134

Table 37. The Current Major Problems of Emergency Units, as Assessed by the Hospital Administrator Respondents (HAS) ... 136

Chapter 4

Table 38. Relative Effectiveness of the Medical Leadership of Emergency Units, as Assessed by Certain Groups of Respondents ... 141

Table 39. Relative Effectiveness of the Administrative and Nursing Leadership of Emergency Units, as Assessed by Certain Groups of Respondents ... 143

Table 40. The Influence of Various Groups on How the Emergency Units Operate, According to the Doctors (MDS) Who Work There ... 145

Table 41. The Influence of Various Groups on How the Emergency Units Operate, According to Hospital Administrator Respondents (HAS) ... 148

		Page
Table 42.	The Amount of Influence That Various Groups <u>Should Have</u> on How the Emergency Units Operate, According to Hospital Administrator Respondents (HAS)	151
Table 43.	The Amount of Influence That Various Groups <u>Should Have</u> on How the Emergency Units Operate, According to the Doctors (MDS) Who Work There	153

Chapter 5

Table 44.	Adequacy of the Overall Coordination of Staff Efforts in the Emergency Units, According to the Doctors (MDS) and Nurses (RNS) Who Work There	159
Table 45.	Extent to Which the Various People Who Work in the Emergency Units Take Into Account Each Other's Work Problems and Needs	162
Table 46.	Extent to Which the Various People Who Work in the Emergency Units Can Rely on the Performance of Co-Workers	164
Table 47.	Comparative Use of Different Types of Problem Solving in the Emergency Units, According to the Supervising Nurses (SRNS)	167
Table 48.	The Relative Effectiveness of Different Types of Problem Solving in the Emergency Units, According to the Doctors (MDS) Who Work There	170
Table 49.	Reliance by Emergency Unit Personnel on Certain Means for Insuring Proper Performance Contributions to the Work of the Unit According to Physicians (MDS)	174
Table 50.	Discretion Allowed and Help Provided by Physicians to the Nurses Working in Emergency Units, as Reported by the Nurses (RNS, LPNS)	176
Table 51.	Adequacy With Which Emergency Unit Physicians Explain Patient Needs to the Nurses, and the Adequacy of Joint Planning by Nurses and Physicians, as Reported by the Nurses (RNS)	179
Table 52.	Level of Mutual Understanding of Their Work Problems and Needs on the Part of the Doctors and Nurses Working in the Emergency Units	182
Table 53.	Tension Between Doctors and Nurses in the Emergency Units, as Reported by Certain Groups of Respondents	186
Table 54.	Tension Among Doctors Within the Emergency Unit, as Reported by Doctors and Other Respondents	188

Page

Chapter 6

    Table 55. Number of Institutions Having Emergency Department Committees and Formal Mechanisms for Monitoring the Work of the Emergency Unit 193

    Table 56. Hospital Administration's Understanding of the Work Problems and Needs of the Emergency Unit Staff 197

    Table 57. Tension Between Emergency Unit Staff and Hospital Administration 199

    Table 58. Tension Between Doctors in the Emergency Unit and Hospital Staff Outside the Unit 201

    Table 59. The Quality of the Work Contacts of Selected Hospital Physicians (HMDS) with the Emergency Unit 203

    Table 60. Adequacy with which Others in the Hospital Meet Emergency Unit Nurses' Requests for Services or Support, as Reported by the Nurses (RNS) 205

Chapter 7

    Table 61. Adequacy of Information Within the Institution About Outside Health Agencies and Regulatory Bodies 210

    Table 62. Extent of Institutional Collaboration with Other Hospitals or Emergency Units, as Reported by Hospital Administrator (HAS) and Supervising Nurse (SRNS) Respondents from Each Institution 212

    Table 63. Adequacy of the Work-Related Contacts of the Emergency Unit Staff with Relevant Organizations in the Community, According to Hospital Administrator (HAS) and Supervising Nurse (SRNS) Respondents 215

    Table 64. The Adequacy of Institutional Arrangements for Relevant Patient Transfers, as Reported by Physicians (MDS) Working in the Emergency Units 218

    Table 65. Tension Between Emergency Unit Staff and the Community Outside, as Reported by Certain Groups of Respondents 221

    Table 66. The Quality of Work Relations Between Selected Community Respondents (CRS) and Staff Working in the Emergency Unit, as Reported by CRS 223

    Table 67. Aspects of the Community Which Create Special Problems for the Emergency Unit, According to the Registered Nurses (RNS) Who Work in the Unit 228

		Page
Table 68.	Aspects of the Community Which Create Special Problems for the Emergency Unit, According to Hospital Administrator Respondents (HAS)	231
Table 69.	Aspects of the Community Which Tend to Create Problems or Difficulties for the Emergency Unit, According to the Selected Community Respondents (CRS) Associated with Each Unit	233

Chapter 8

Table 70.	The Emergency Unit's Reputation in the Community, as Perceived by Various Groups of Respondents	238
Table 71.	Adequacy with Which the Emergency Unit is Meeting Current Community Expectations, as Assessed by Various Groups of Respondents	241
Table 72.	Degree to Which the Community's Expectations about the Emergency Unit's Services are Realistic, According to Certain Groups of Respondents	244
Table 73.	Particular Aspects of Their Emergency Unit Visit that the Patients Found the Most Satisfactory	248
Table 74.	Staff's Understanding and Explanation to the Patients of Their Medical Problems	251
Table 75.	Patients' Assessments of the Care They Received from the Doctors and from the Nurses in the Emergency Unit	254

Chapter 9

Table 76.	Evaluation by the Staff of the Emergency Unit as a Place to Work	260
Table 77.	Staff Identification with Their Respective Emergency Units	263
Table 78.	Staff's Perception of Unreasonable Pressure for "Better Performance"	265
Table 79.	Inappropriateness of Work Responsibilities in the Emergency Unit, as Reported by the Nurses (RNS, LPNS)	268
Table 80.	Amount of Variety on the Job for Emergency Unit Nurses (RNS, LPNS)	270
Table 81.	Emergency Unit Staff Satisfaction with the Financial Rewards of Their Work	272
Table 82.	Emergency Unit Staff Satisfaction with the Non-Financial Rewards of Their Work	274

Chapter 10

		Page
Table 83.	The Emergency Unit's Operating Budget and Expenditures for the Most Recent Quarter	281
Table 84.	The Emergency Unit's Budget as a Percentage of the Hospital's Budget, For the Most Recent Quarter	283
Table 85.	Average Hospital Revenue Per Patient Visit to the Emergency Unit and Total Cost to the Hospital per Visit	285
Table 86.	Emergency Unit Revenues in Relation to Emergency Unit Expenditures During the Most Recent Quarter	289
Table 87.	Hospital Charges to Patients for Their Emergency Unit Visits (Exclusive of Physician Fees), for the Most Recent Quarter	292
Table 88.	Reaction to Patient Charges for Care in the Emergency Unit on the Part of Various Groups	295
Table 89.	Number of Patient Visits to the Emergency Unit in Relation to the Number of Hours Worked by the Registered Nurses (RNS) and by the Physicians (MDS) in the Unit	298

Chapter 11

Table 90.	Appropriateness of the Medical Treatment and Nursing Care Procedures Used in the Various Emergency Units, as Assessed by the Physicians (MDS) Who Work There	307
Table 91.	The Quality of Performance of the Medical Treatment and Nursing Care Procedures Used in Emergency Units, as Evaluated by the Registered Nurses (RNS) Who Work There	312
Table 92.	Percent of the Patients Visiting the Various Emergency Units Who Were Seen by a Doctor Within 15 Minutes After Arrival	316
Table 93.	Average Length (in Minutes) of Patient Visits to the Various Emergency Units in a Typical Day	318
Table 94.	Waiting Time After Arrival and the Total Length of Their Emergency Unit Visits, as Reported by Patients (PATS)	321
Table 95.	Assessment by Emergency Unit Patients (PATS) and Community Respondents (CRS) of Certain Aspects of Staff Competence	325
Table 96.	Percent of Emergency Unit Patients (PATS) Reporting that the Staff Could Have Done More for Them, and Percent Reporting Post-visit "Complications"	328
Table 97.	Death Rates per Thousand Patient Visits to the Various Emergency Units During the Most Recent Quarter	333

		Page
Table 98.	The Quality of Medical Management of Emergency Unit Patients in Selected Conditions, as Evaluated by the Physicians (MDS) Working in the Units	338
Table 99.	The Quality of Nursing Care Provided to Emergency Unit Patients in Selected Conditions, as Evaluated by the Registered Nurses (RNS) Working in the Units	340
Table 100.	The Quality of Overall Medical Care and Overall Nursing Care Provided in the Various Emergency Units, as Rated by Certain Nurse and Physician Respondents (Other Than the Performers in Each Case)	343
Table 101.	The Quality of Medical Care and Nursing Care in the Various Emergency Units Compared to the Quality of Care in the Units of Other Hospitals	348

Appendix

Table 102.	Length of Professional Experience for Selected Groups of Respondents	359
Table 103.	Length of Association with Their Respective Institutions for Selected Groups of Respondents	361
Table 104.	Length of Association with Their Respective Emergency Units for the Physicians (MDS) and Registered Nurses (RNS) Who Work There	363
Table 105.	The Length of Time Patient Respondents (PATS) Have Lived in the Communities in Which They are Currently Living	367
Table 106.	Percent of Respondents from Each Specified Group with the Sex and Age Characteristics Shown	369
Table 107.	Percent of Emergency Unit Patients (PATS) with Specified Levels of Formal Education	370
Table 108.	Percent of Patient Respondents (PATS) Reporting Particular Levels of Total Family Income	372
Table 109.	Percent of Patients (PATS) Giving Particular Reasons for Having "Chosen" to go to the Emergency Units to Which They Went for Care	374
Table 110.	Percent of Emergency Unit Patients (PATS) Indicating Particular Sources as Their "Usual" Sources for Medical Care	376
Table 111.	Selected Characteristics of the Population of the Cities (Towns) in Which the Study Hospitals are Located, Based on U.S. Census Data	377

PART I: OVERVIEW OF THE RESEARCH

PART I

OVERVIEW OF THE RESEARCH[1]

One important unanswered question in modern health services research is the question "What makes for an efficient and effective hospital emergency department or emergency unit (EU), and how can an EU improve its organization and problem-solving capabilities?" Answering this question presupposes research ability to assess the organizational effectiveness of hospital emergency units adequately and dependably. This is now a feasible task, although an extraordinarily difficult and complex one to accomplish. It requires both conceptual-theoretical sophistication and rigorous methodology.[2] It also requires comparative organizational analysis, i.e., cross-hospital comparisons or simultaneous study of a number of EU's. Above all, it requires an approach, or research model, which is suitable to understanding organizations such as EU's in all their complexity and capturing both their differences and similarities, along with their weaknesses and strengths.

This overview discusses such an approach. The research model that it describes is being used in a comparative organizational study of 30 hospital emergency units. Part II of the present report contains selected descriptive findings from this study, which is still in progress.

---

[1] The present overview in substantially the same form first appeared in Emergency Medical Services (Georgopoulos, B.S. "An Open-System Approach to Evaluating the Effectiveness of Hospital Emergency Departments," Emergency Medical Services, Vol. 7, No. 6, Nov.-Dec. 1978, pp. 118-129) and is used here with permission from that journal.

[2] Those interested in the underlying theoretical framework of this research see: Georgopoulos, B.S. and Cooke, R.A. "Conceptual-Theoretical Framework for the Organizational Study of Hospital Emergency Services," ISR Working Paper #8011, Ann Arbor: Institute for Social Research, The University of Michigan, 1979. Certain aspects of the framework are elaborated in the project's special task force reports on organizational adaptation, coordination, resource allocation, economic efficiency, and clinical efficiency (Georgopoulos, B.S., Cooke, R.A., and Associates, 1977).

The study encompasses a probability sample of voluntary hospitals -- the nongovernment, not-for-profit, short-stay general hospitals in the 100-500 bed range which are located in the states of Illinois, Indiana, Michigan, Minnesota, Ohio, and Wisconsin. It is relying on several independent sources of data, including organizational records (financial, personnel, and patient census records), interview and questionnaire data from staff and patients, patient records, and other sources of information. Nearly 1,500 individuals associated with the 30 institutions in the sample participated in the study as respondents. The data, reflecting several legitimate perspectives -- those of emergency unit nurses and physicians (i.e., the "performers"), medical "peers" and associates in the rest of the hospital, principal administrators, recent patients, and selected key respondents from the local community having contacts with each EU -- are now being analyzed.

Effectiveness is being assessed using multiple criteria. The principal criteria are: (1) *clinical efficiency*--quality of care and staff performance relative to available resources; (2) *economic(cost) efficiency*; (3) *social efficiency*--staff commitment to the unit and staff satisfaction with monetary and non-monetary "rewards"; (4) *patient satisfaction*; and (5) *responsiveness to community expectations*. Each of these criteria, in turn, is being assessed using a variety of measures which are based on data reflecting all of the above perspectives, as appropriate. The measures, it is believed, are such as to have *validity* within each EU (being meaningful to each institution) and *reliability* across EU's (having sufficient comparability from one EU to another).

In the research model, emergency units are viewed as a complex and specialized "subsystem" of the hospital, i.e., their parent organization. They are seen as work-performing and problem-solving subsystems which are not only engaged in "producing" special services but are also interacting with the outside community directly. Their overall effectiveness is a joint (though not equally weighted) outcome of clinical, economic, and social efficiency, and depends on their success in dealing with certain major organizational problems -- coordination and control of work efforts, availability and proper allocation of professional and other resources, maintenance of suitable work arrangements, resolution of strain and conflict, staff integration and involvement, and adaptation to the external environment. Data have, therefore, been obtained for the measurement of many important aspects in these problem areas as well as for the measurement of the above criteria of EU effectiveness (see Part III for the data collection instruments used).

One major objective of the research is to ascertain and understand the nature and sources of inter-hospital differences in emergency unit effectiveness (in its major aspects). Another key objective is to specify those organizational and social-psychological conditions which are likely to promote or impede the solution of work problems in the above areas and facilitate effective performance in an emergency department. A final objective is to test a number of specific hypotheses derived from organization theory and existing research literature on emergency medical services -- hypotheses that are likely to be both theoretically meaningful and pragmatically useful to those concerned with these important services.

Underlying Conceptual-Theoretical Rationale

The empirical data base about the organization, problems, and effectiveness of the dominant source of emergency medical care in this country -- the hospital emergency service -- is still at a relatively primitive state.

The problems and difficulties experienced by emergency departments are appreciated, at least from a practical standpoint and in terms of undesirable outcomes. However, they are inadequately understood in terms of their origins and correlates, and even more poorly understood in terms of their interrelationships and likely solution requirements. Especially missing is dependable knowledge about the factors and conditions (many of which potentially could be controlled by the system) which facilitate or hinder the effectiveness of emergency units in its major aspects -- the quality of care, economic and social efficiency, patient satisfaction, and responsiveness to community needs. Also missing is dependable knowledge about interinstitutional differences in EU effectiveness and their sources. There is a pressing need for high-quality organizational research that addresses these major problems. Most notably lacking is theory-based and methodologically rigorous research going beyond single case studies and tackling these problems on a scale that is commensurate with their magnitude and complexity. Comparative study designs, such as that of the present research, probably hold the greatest promise of success.

Superficially viewed, the emergency unit (department, room) in hospitals is an important and socially valued resource for patient care, a client-oriented facility with specialized personnel and equipment that provides certain professional services to the public. In less naive terms, the familiar hospital EU is a dynamic and complex organizational entity which, in order to do its work, must be able to deal with a variety of difficult problems -- internally, in relation to the parent hospital, and in relation to the external environment. These include problems of input and output as well as problems associated with internal structure and process, such as coordination of effort, resource allocation and control, and work relations and staff performance.

Conceptually, in the present study, the EU is viewed as a complex work-performing and problem-solving subsystem (of the hospital) that is functioning under constraints imposed by the nature of its work and work inputs, its relationships to the parent hospital, and the character of the external environment. Figure 1 provides a graphic representation of the place of the EU subsystem within its relevant organizational environment, showing (with arrows) the kinds of "external" relationships that are possible and should be kept in mind when considering the constraints under which an EU functions.

Figure 1. Place of the EU Subsystem in its Relevant Organization Environment

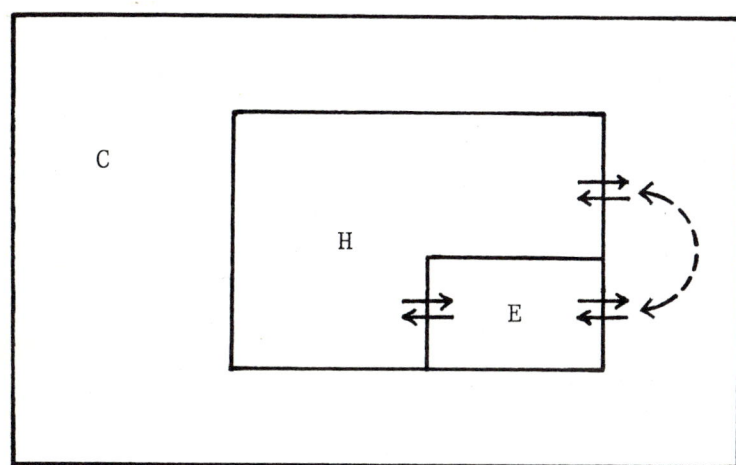

E: The EU subsystem

H: The parent hospital system

C: The outside community or relevant "super-system"

Solid arrows indicate direct relationships; dotted arrows indicate possible indirect relationships

The work inputs of EU's, though not all of an acute or immediate emergency kind, are on the whole non-uniform and relatively unpredictable (at least in the short-run and at the individual hospital level), while requiring immediate attention or rapid response by those who do the work -- doctors, nurses, and others. Performers must constantly deal with uncertainty, be able to tolerate ambiguity while being intolerant of error, and be ready to act promptly and properly. The work inputs also are of high social valuation, since they consist of human beings, and must be processed individually and with care to minimize risk in resolving the problem in each case.

The EU staff, which includes a variety of professional workers and specialists, intself tends to be heterogeneous and organizationally unstable, adding to the complexity and difficulties that apparently characterize the EU subsystem. Moreover, the organizational autonomy of the EU within the hospital is typically rather limited. For its resources, for example, an EU must depend on the hospital which controls it, and in carrying out its functions must observe constraints imposed by the hospital and by the external environment as well as by the nature of the work.

Equally important, in order to do its work, an EU must be able to make proper use of an advanced and intensive work technology, while having to rely a great deal on the timely cooperation, services, and facilities of other hospital units -- clinical, ancillary, and administrative support units. Under these circumstances, coordination of efforts and organizational rationality are exceedingly difficult to achieve and maintain, even in those cases where the environment within which the EU and its parent hospital operate may be only moderately complex or unstable.

Organizationally, therefore, though relatively small in size, the hospital EU constitutes one of the most complex and most problematic subsystems of the hospital. It is at once an "adaptive-boundary subsystem" -- one which deals directly with the external environment in the process of receiving patient inputs and in returning its output back to the community, and a "production subsystem" -- one which performs a significant portion of the hospital's work, by providing treatment and delivering medical and other professional services to incoming patients. As a consequence of this dual function, the EU must be responsive, and to an extent also accountable, both to its parent hospital system and to the outside community, maintaining proper relationships with both at all times. In addition, it must be relatively flexible internally because the workflow tends to be variable and uneven and the work-cycle short, with rapid patient turnover, while the unit is required to function on a continuous, 24-hour, basis and meet exogenous requirements over which it has little control.

The Present Study and Research Model

Hospital emergency units, in short, present a case of an interesting and complex type of organization. They also represent a socially salient component of the health services delivery system as well as an organizationally problematic subsystem of hospitals. Many of their operating problems and difficulties are generally appreciated. But the relevant data base on the organizational side is extremely weak, particularly with reference to present knowledge and understanding of interrelationships and likely solutions for the major problems of adaptation to the environment, internal coordination of effort, staffing and staff organization, resource allocation and utilization, and other problems affecting the clinical, economic, or social efficiency of emergency units.

In these important areas, only minimal research of a systematic or rigorous kind has heretofore been undertaken, and comparative research studying more than a few institutions simultaneously is almost totally lacking, as is research viewing EU's in systems terms. It is clear that the problems and difficulties encountered by this subsystem of hospitals and its members are not confined to any one hospital size category, any particular community environment, or any one region of the country. Yet, little is actually known on the basis of solid empirical evidence about the magnitude of the problems across hospitals that differ in size, location, affiliation and control, and other major characteristics, or about the relative effectiveness with which differently structured and functioning EU's are able to handle the problems.

The present research was undertaken to fill the gap. By comparing and contrasting a substantial number of emergency units from a probability sample of hospitals, the project will carefully assess many important aspects of the organizational situation of these units. Using an open-system theory perspective as its conceptual-theoretical base, it will both analyze the organization and evaluate the effectiveness of hospital EU's. It will then relate the observed differences on each major criterion of organizational effectiveness (clinical efficiency, social efficiency, economic efficiency, patient satisfaction, adaptiveness) to differences in organization patterns (e.g., staff composition and stability, goal priorities, resource availability and allocation, coordination and control) and organization problem solving. In this manner, the study will be able also to ascertain many of the sources and correlates of inter-institutional differences in EU effectiveness and identify specific variables which may facilitate it or impede it.

Major inter-institutional differences undoubtedly exist, both in organization patterns and organizational effectiveness, with some hospital EU's being able to do a much better job than others in dealing with the problems which they encounter and in providing health care services to their patients in a relatively efficient and effective manner. The magnitude, sources, and determinants of such important differences remain mostly unknown, partly because of their complexity and partly because of the paucity of relevant research.

To make matters worse, available organization theory is not too enlightening either as a guide to structuring and managing subsystems such as the hospital EU in ways that would facilitate problem-solving and promote organizational effectiveness or as a means for explaining differences in staff attitudes and work behavior in relation to effectiveness. Neither the so-called "organic" models, with their emphasis on participative decision-making and supportive human relations, nor the "mechanistic" models of organization, with their emphasis on bureaucratic prescriptions and centralized control, seem to fit the case or provide a satisfactory account for organizations such as the hospital EU subsystem. Some new theorizing, therefore, was also needed in order to develop a more adequate theoretical base, in addition to generating a better empirical data base than has been heretofore available. Our research was designed and carried out with both of these requirements in mind.

The basic conceptual-theoretical framework used draws heavily on the organization research model of Georgopoulos (1972). This is a problem-oriented model which, in its earlier versions, has guided the principal investigator's hospital studies (Georgopoulos and Mann, 1962; Georgopoulos and Wieland, 1964; Georgopoulos and Matejko, 1967; Georgopoulos and Christman, 1970). Most recently, the same model was used to analyze and review last decade's research output in the field of hospital organization (Georgopoulos, B.S., <u>Hospital Organization Research: Review and Sourcebook</u>, 1975). A comprehensive summary of the basic model may be found in Chapter 2 of <u>Organization Research on Health Institutions</u> (Georgopoulos, 1972).

Very briefly, according to the model, to "diagnose" the organizational state and assess the effectiveness of a complex organizational entity such as the hospital EU, it is important to consider not only available resources (particularly human resources) and *the work inputs in relation to output*, but also certain major intervening problems to which organizations must provide solutions if they are to survive and function effectively. Theoretically, organizational effectiveness is seen to reflect not only the *economic* and professional-technical or, in the present case, *clinical* efficiency, but also the *social* efficiency of a system, and to depend upon the relative success with which the system is able to provide solutions to a set of complex, on-going problems -- solutions which are never perfect and which are not always mutually reinforcing.

In more specific terms, internally, an organization must be able to: (a) *allocate* resources, authority, information, and rewards among various groups and members whose expectations may differ but whose work roles are interdependent; (b) *coordinate* the diverse activities and contributions of members, so that they function according to each other's work needs, and so that the efforts of all concerned are properly articulated (in time and space) to converge toward the solution of work problems and the attainment of organizational objectives; (c) *integrate* member aspirations and goals with group objectives and organizational goals; (d) *maintain* structural stability and orderly, if not entirely predictable, behavior patterns, along with sufficient flexibility to cope with complexity and uncertainty and respond to unanticipated stimuli; and (e) *deal with the tensions and strain* arising from the preceding, and also from relationships with the external environment. Further, external affairs problems also must be attended to continually in the organization's efforts to (f) *adapt* to instability, change, and uncertainty in the environment within which it functions and from which it obtains the requisite energy and resources in order to do its work. Successful problem solving in these key areas is hypothesized to account for much, if not most, of the variance in the economic, social, and clinical efficiency of hospital EU's.

The underlying assumption is that, controlling for the nature of the external environment as it bears upon the resources and patient inputs of hospital EU's, the overall effectiveness of this subsystem will be mainly a function of such things as: the nature of relationships between the EU and its parent hospital; available EU staff and other resources and supports, considering the volume and composition of the workload; EU structure, particularly task allocation and control structure, and staff organization and stability; EU goal priorities and prevailing definition/ scope of "emergency service" in the organization; and the nature of work relations and problem-solving practices within the unit. To the extent that emergency departments differ in these areas, they are expected also to differ in their clinical, economic, and social efficiency, and in patient satisfaction and responsiveness to community expectations -- i.e., in their effectiveness.

These different criteria of EU effectiveness are not expected to correlate highly, or even significantly, with one another in all cases (see Seashore, Indik, and Georgopoulos, 1960), and one useful contribution of the study will be to find out which of them correlate consistently and significantly and which do not. Similarly, the reliability of the different criterion measures is expected to vary, in some cases arguing for elimination of the measure from further consideration. For these reasons, although some overall indexes will be constructed (e.g., from the more specific measures of clinical efficiency, social efficiency, etc.) and used in the analyses, the several major criteria will be studied separately in relation to the various aspects of organization on which the research focuses.

Aspects of the EU Situation Investigated: The Principal Independent and Dependent Variables

The seven different classes of variables measured in order to accomplish the objectives of the research will now be briefly described, beginning with environmental variables. The overall patterns of relationships between the "independent" variables studied and the several criteria of EU effectiveness (or main "dependent" variables) that are expected by the model are graphically portrayed in Figure 2.

(1) <u>Community environment</u>. The most relevant aspects of the external environment pertain to issues of stability and complexity, including: urban-rural character; changes in public expectations about emergency care; number of family or primary care physicians in relation to the population; presence of other hospitals in the area; presence of BLS and ALS emergency systems in the community; existence of inter-institutional agreements (e.g., transfer protocols) among hospitals for emergency care and patient referral; and community knowledge and perceptions about an EU. Such variables as median family income, proportion of families below poverty level, school years completed, proportion of population in minority groups, population increase/decrease over time, and percent of workers working in county of residence also are being examined.

(2) <u>Parent hospital characteristics</u>. Since the hospital constitutes the immediate organizational environment within which an EU functions, as

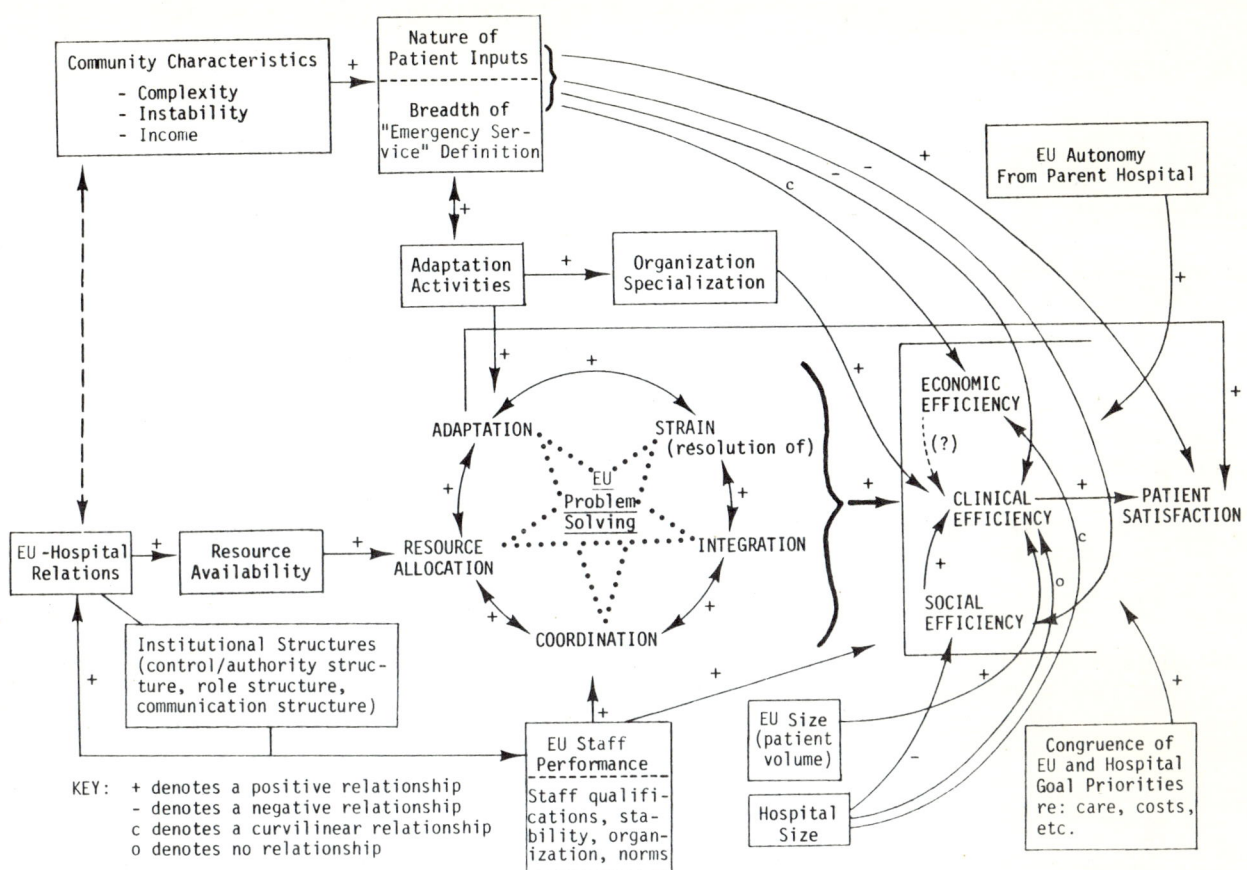

Figure 2. Expected Input-Internal Organization-Output Relationships for Hospital Emergency Units (EU's)

one among many subsystems, certain major characteristics of the hospital likewise are being studied, most as "control" or "moderator" variables. Included among these are hospital size, location, type of control, teaching affiliation, presence of medical and nursing training programs, and the hospital's goal priorities for the EU. Also included are: availability of medical resources and medical specialization, available facilities and services offered by the hospital, financial condition, research emphasis, presence of outpatient clinical facilities other than the emergency unit.

and current policies regarding allocation of resources to the EU and inter-institutional arrangements for emergency care.

(3) <u>EU-hospital relations</u>. Important aspects being considered in this area include: professional resources and financial resources allocated to the EU by the hospital (e.g., total EU expenditures by the hospital per patient visit in relation to the hospital's operating budget); EU success in obtaining requested resources or supports from its parent hospital; the relative organizational autonomy of the EU, and hospital control over the EU; monitoring of EU performance (quality control); responsiveness by other units (administrative, clinical, ancillary, and service units) to EU work needs or requests; adequacy of communication between these other relevant units and the EU, as perceived by both sides; the level of cooperation and support given to the EU by other hospital departments and by hospital and nursing administration (particularly as perceived by EU staff, since work interdependence is likely to be asymmetrical, with the EU being more dependent on the other units than the other way around); and other aspects.

(4) <u>EU goal priorities and "emergency service" definition</u>. The present study is concerned with both of these aspects. First, it will examine the relative importance, or rank-order, of selected relevant goals that may be differentially emphasized by hospital emergency units. These are: maintaining high standards of patient care; providing comprehensive emergency services; maintaining a good reputation in the community; maintaining a high level of patient satisfaction; minimizing waiting time; keeping the costs of the emergency service down; and improving working conditions for EU staff. Given the heterogeneity of inputs and uncertainty of work, EU goal priorities are particularly important to consider in relation to organizational effectiveness. EU staff agreement about priorities will

probably be found to facilitate problem-solving and organizational effectiveness, other things being equal. Furthermore, emphasis on economic goals will probably correlate with economic efficiency, while emphasis on community concerns will probably correlate with reputation in the community.

Second, the study will ascertain the *de facto* definition or scope of services offered by different hospital EU's and then relate the narrowness/breadth of "emergency service" definition to EU organization and effectiveness. The proportion of emergency-visit patients being admitted as in-patients (over a given period of time) is probably indicative of the relative breadth of emergency service definition at a hospital (a relatively high proportion, compared to other hospitals of the same type, would probably suggest a narrow definition, while a low proportion would suggest a broad definition). The ratio of emergency visits to the average daily in-patient census of the hospital, and to the number of inpatient days, provides additional measures. Breadth of definition is expected to be associated with most criteria of EU effectiveness, although the relationship is likely to be curvilinear in most cases (i.e., moderate breadth is expected to be associated with most criteria of EU effectiveness), and probably also with the nature of the external environment.

(5) <u>Available EU staff and other resources</u>. Principal variables in this area include: the number and composition (in terms of skills and specialties) of the medical and nursing staff working in the unit, full- as well as part-time; the number of professional hours worked (in relation to workload, e.g., total patient visits) by nurses and by physicians in the EU; type of assignment (regular vs. rotation schemes vs. contractual

arrangements for medical staff); access by the EU to medical specialists available within the hospital "on call"; patient transfer practices; medical and nursing leadership of the EU; and other staff characteristics. Other resources being studied are: financial resources (e.g., EU budget, personnel salaries, etc.); physical resources/facilities available; and information (about the rest of the hospital, the community, the patients, and various regulatory agencies). The key variables measured for each kind of resources are *availability*, *quantity*, *stability*, and *quality or adequacy*.

(6) <u>Work structure, work relations, and problem solving within the EU</u>. Staff size and composition (in terms of specialization, skills, and experience) are important aspects of organization, as are goal priorities and available resources. But, in addition, the work structure of the EU must be considered. The division of labor among the staff (who provides clinical and administrative leadership, who is responsible for what aspects of unit functioning, such as coordination with other services, the initial screening of patients, staff assigning, etc.) is, therefore, also being examined, as is the control structure. In particular, the amount of control/influence EU staff have over the work (e.g., how free they are to make patient care decisions according to their best judgment) and on how the EU operates, and the amount of authority that key staff (e.g., the head nurse) have considering their responsibilities, are expected to correlate with organizational effectiveness. In this connection, however, it is the "total amount of control" (see Tannenbaum, 1968) which the EU staff exercise, rather than how evenly the influence is distributed among them that is expected to be the crucial variable. Control over the allocation of resources is another important variable. Other structural

variables, such as formalization (specificity of job descriptions), routinization of work, and span of control (ratio of supervisory to non-supervisory staff) are probably less important in a subsystem such as the EU.

Regarding work relations and problem solving, communication and coordination variables are emphasized. Where work efforts are complexly interdependent and uncertainty is relatively high, programmed coordination, i.e., coordination based on formal programs or plans, is unlikely to be efficacious, in contrast to nonprogrammed coordination, or coordination based on feedback and informal adjustments on the part of performers (see Georgopoulos and Mann, 1962, chs. 6 and 7; Thompson, 1967; Longest, 1974; Hage, 1974). Preventive and promotive, in contrast to corrective or regulatory, coordination (Georgopoulos and Mann, 1962; Longest, 1974), in particular, are expected to be related to EU effectiveness. Promotive and preventive coordination are based upon, and achieved by, adequate task-centered communication about the work among performers; readiness on the part of collaborating staff to accomodate one another (this is the "adaptability" variable previously found by Mott, 1972, to correlate with organizational effectiveness in hospitals and other organizations); mutual understanding and complementarity of expectations between medical and nursing staff -- the extent to which they understand/appreciate each other's work problems and needs, are able to anticipate each other's work needs, and can rely on others to do their job right (Georgopoulos and Mann, 1962); and, generally, spontaneous adjustments and informal communication among staff (Hage, 1974).

The level of strain in the organization (work pressure, tensions, conflict, and friction experienced by the performers), particularly intergroup tension between doctors and nurses, and between EU staff and other collaborating hospital staff, constitutes another major variable. Strain may stem from unresolved problems or difficulties in any of the preceding areas, and is especially likely in organizational situations of relatively high complexity and uncertainty. In previous hospital studies, tension and other forms of strain (e.g., unreasonable pressure for better performance, as perceived by the worker) have been found to correlate positively with complexity (Wieland, 1965), and with staff instability and withdrawal or non-adaptive behavior (Lyons, 1967), but negatively with the adequacy of coordination (Georgopoulos and Mann, 1962; Wieland, 1965; Georgopoulos and Matejko, 1967; Smith, 1969). Strain is also likely to be symptomatic of low organizational integration -- staff dissatisfaction and low levels of member involvement and identification with the system.

(7) *EU effectiveness*. The concept of organizational effectiveness is a complex and multi-faceted concept. As earlier indicated, EU effectiveness is an outcome of economic, clinical, and social efficiency, and reflects the relative success with which an EU is able to deal with certain major problems, including adaptation to the environment and system maintenance problems, coordination and integration problems, resource acquisition and allocation problems, strain problems, and staff satisfaction problems. In short, the ability of an EU to achieve and maintain high levels of output, in terms of quantity, quality, cost, acceptability, and related aspects, given the resources at its disposal, and do so without incapacitating its resources and without undue strain for its members, is what organizational effectiveness entails. For useful discussions and critiques of the concept, as used in organizational research in the hospital field and other settings, see: Georgopoulos and Tannenbaum (1957); Georgopoulos and Mann (1962); Etzioni (1964); Katz and Kahn (1966);

Yuchtman and Seashore (1967); Georgopoulos and Matejko (1967); Price (1968, 1972); Ghorpade (1971); Mott (1972); and Georgopoulos (1972, 1975).

In this project, data have been obtained for assessing all of the major criteria of EU effectiveness -- clinical, economic, and social efficiency, and also patient satisfaction and responsiveness to community expectations. Relevant data, it will be recalled, have been collected from the medical and nursing staff working in each EU, from other key staff in the hospital, from organizational and patient records, from selected individuals in the outside community, and from EU patients. The principal criterion variables, for each major aspect of organizational effectiveness being studied, are as follows:

Economic or cost efficiency variables include: gross staff productivity measured by the ratio of work volume (total EU patient visits) to professional hours worked (by RN's, by MD's) during selected time periods; costs and charges for patient care per visit (hospital charges, and physician fees), since patients are likely to be reacting to charges rather than costs; personnel costs in relation to patient volume; revenues from EU patients; and total cost to the hospital per patient visit.

Social efficiency variables include: EU staff satisfaction with their work in the EU -- for physicians, nurses -- and with the hospital; staff satisfaction with personal goal-attainment (financial and non-financial); degree of personal identification with, or commitment to, the EU on the part of those working there; perceived professional autonomy and opportunity to exercise meaningful influence over the work and the operation of the EU on the part of the medical and nursing staff; staff consensus on goal priorities for the EU; and others.

Patient satisfaction. The main variable here is the level of satisfaction expressed by a group of patients visiting each EU for care -- overall satisfaction with the quality of care recieved, satisfaction with the doctor(s) and also the nurse(s) who took care of them, satisfaction with explanation of condition and with information received (e.g., for follow-up care), satisfaction with "waiting time," satisfaction with the charges (bill) for their emergency visit, and preference for using the same EU again should future need arise.

Responsiveness to external forces and community expectations. Important variables in this area include: responsiveness by the EU to community expectations regarding service, as evaluated by selected respondents from the community with knowledge about or contact with each EU (health department director, medical examiner, ambulance company personnel such as EMT's, police and fire department representatives, HSA and EMS people, and certain "most knowledgeable" persons in the community named by the chief executive officer of each hospital); overall appraisal by these community respondents of how good a job the EU is doing and how well it has been able to respond to changing community needs for emergency care; how satisfactory work relations are between many of these same respondents and the EU staff, as perceived by both; how well patient transfer arrangements with other institutions are working out; and the adequacy of knowledge/information that EU staff have about the community and about relevant health agencies and regulatory bodies.

Clinical efficiency. The principal criterion measures for which data have been obtained in this area (mainly from interviews and questionnaires and from hospital and patient records) include: perceived quality of overall, medical, and nursing care provided by the EU (as assessed by emergency unit physicians and RN's, selected physicians from the rest of the hospital, and patients and community respondents); patient "waiting" and "processing" time; strengths and weaknesses concerning the quality of care or service provided, mentioned spontaneously by respondents from the several groups which participated in the research; patient complaints, complications, and death rates; the quality of the emergency visit records of recent patients; excellence of performance by medical and nursing staff (including measures such as the proportion of MD's and of RN's in the EU who "are doing outstanding or excellent work consistently"); the extent to which medical treatment and nursing care procedures are "appropriate" from the standpoint of enabling the staff to provide "care of the highest quality possible," "at the lowest cost possible," and "as promptly as it should be provided," and "how well performed" the same procedures are; the quality of medical management and nursing care for patients in selected conditions (certain "quasi-tracer" conditions); and the quality of care compared to care in other hospital EU's. In addition, of course, patient satisfaction may be found to be indicative of clinical efficiency, but for well-known reasons it cannot be assumed that this in fact will be the case.

Some of the clinical efficiency measures are patterned after similar scales previously used in hospital research and found to (a) yield good reliability and (b) correlate with measures of quality based on either outside peer judgment or data from medical records (Georgopoulos and Mann, 1962; Denton, 1967; Neuhauser, 1971; Payne and Lyons, 1972). (For a critique and assessment of the usefulness of measures of this kind, see Price, 1972.) Moreover, both simple and "adjusted" measures of clinical efficiency are being studied.

Three kinds of adjustors are involved, as follows: (a) variables concerning workload composition/patient case-mix (measured with data from hospital records), such as the proportion of EU patients who arrived by ambulance, the proportion of patients sent directly by the emergency unit to one of the intensive care units and/or operating rooms of the hospital, and the proportion of EU patients who were admitted as inpatients; (b) control variables such as hospital size and urban-rural location; and (c) estimated severity indicators obtained from data provided by doctors and nurses (e.g., percent of patients arriving in a "life-threatening condition," percent considered "seriously ill or seriously injured").

The various criterion measures were examined for reliability and then intercorrelated to determine which measures (under each major criterion) can be legitimately incorporated into a more encompassing index of effectiveness. Uncorrelated, but reliable, measures will be retained and studied separately.

The research design makes it possible, of course, to correlate each independent variable with each criterion variable, whether the latter is treated separately or as a component of some more inclusive index. It also makes it possible to study the relationship between the independent and dependent variables, both on a simple zero-order basis and controlling for such things as hospital size or community environment. Inter-hospital differences in EU effectiveness, whatever the specific criterion, will be examined in relation to certain "control" or "moderator" variables to ascertain the extent to which each major difference could be attributed to the characteristics of parent hospitals and/or the nature of the community environment. If hospital size and environmental complexity are found to correlate significantly with EU effectiveness, for example, then they will be controlled for when analyzing the relationships between EU organization and organizational problem solving (the independent variables) and EU effectiveness in its various aspects (the main dependent variables).

References

Denton, J. C., et al. Predicting judged quality of patient care in general hospitals. *Health Services Research*, 1967, 2, 26-33.

Etzioni, A. *Modern organizations*. Englewood Cliffs, N. J.: Prentice-Hall, 1964.

Georgopoulos, B. S. *Hospital organization research: review and sourcebook*. Philadelphia, Pa.: W. B. Saunders Co., 1975.

Georgopoulos, B. S. (Ed.) *Organization research on health institutions*. Ann Arbor, Mich.: The University of Michigan, Institute for Social Research, 1972.

Georgopoulos, B. S. and Christman, L. The clinical nurse specialist: a role model. *American Journal of Nursing*, 1970, 70, 1030-1039.

Georgopoulos, B. S. and Mann, F. C. *The community general hospital*. New York: Macmillan, 1962.

Georgopoulos, B. S. and Matejko, A. The American general hospital as a complex social system. *Health Services Research*, 1967, 2, 76-112.

Georgopoulos, B. S. and Tannenbaum, A. S. A study of organizational effectiveness. *American Sociological Review*, 1957, 22, 534-540.

Georgopoulos, B. S. and Wieland, G. F. *Nationwide study of coordination and patient care in voluntary hospitals*. Ann Arbor, Mich.: The University of Michigan, Institute for Social Research, 1964.

Ghorpade, J. *Assessment of organizational effectiveness: issues, analysis, and readings*. Pacific Palisades: Goodyear Publishing Co., 1971.

Hage, J. *Communication and organizational control: cybernetics in health and welfare settings*. New York: Wiley-Interscience, 1974.

Katz, D. and Kahn, R. L. *The social psychology of organizations*. New York: Wiley, 1966. (Also 1978, revised edition.)

Longest, B. Relationships between coordination, efficiency, and quality of care in general hospitals. *Hospital Administration*, 1974, 19, 65-86.

Lyons, T. F. A study of social-psychological variables as they relate to turnover, propensity to leave, and absenteeism among hospital staff nurses. Doctoral dissertation, The University of Michigan, 1967.

Mott, P. E. *The characteristics of effective organizations*. New York: Harper and Row, 1972.

Neuhauser, D. *The relationship of administrative activities and hospital performance.* Chicago, Ill.: University of Chicago, Center for Health Administration Studies, Research Series 28, 1971.

Payne, B. C. and Lyons, T. F. *Method of evaluating and improving medical care quality* (Vol. 1 - Episode of illness study; Vol. 2 - Office care study; Vol. 3 - Continuing education study). Ann Arbor, Mich.: The University of Michigan, 1972. (Research Contract HSM 110-70-69, Health Services and Mental Health Administration, USPHS.)

Price, J. L. *Organizational effectiveness: an inventory of propositions.* Homewood, Ill.: Irwin-Dorsy, 1968.

Price, J. L. The study of organizational effectiveness. *The Sociological Quarterly*, Winter 1972, *13*, 3-15 (and Spring 1973, *14*, 271-278).

Seashore, S. E., Indik, B. P., and Georgopoulos, B. S. Relationships among criteria of job performance. *Journal of Applied Psychology*, 1960, *44*, 195-202.

Smith, C. G. Coordination and decision-making in mental hospitals. Research report, University of Wisconsin, 1969.

Tannenbaum, A. S. (Ed.) *Control in organizations.* New York: McGraw-Hill, 1968.

Thompson, J. D. *Organizations in action.* New York: McGraw-Hill, 1967.

Wieland, G. F. Complexity and coordination in organizations. Doctoral dissertation, The University of Michigan, 1965.

Yuchtman, E. and Seashore, S. E. A system resource approach to organizational effectiveness. *Americal Sociological Review*, 1967, *32*, 891-903.

PART II: SPECIAL REPORT TO PARTICIPATING INSTITUTIONS

PART II

SPECIAL REPORT TO PARTICIPATING INSTITUTIONS

Introduction

This is the first report of results from a comparative organizational study of hospital emergency services. It is a special feedback report initially addressed to the institutions which participated in the study. The research focuses on the emergency units (departments, rooms) of general hospitals in HEW Region V. The emergency units (EU's) of 30 institutions, and a total of nearly 1,500 individuals associated with them, have provided the data. Part III in the present volume contains the research instruments used to collect the data.

The overall purpose of the study is to analyze the organization and evaluate the effectiveness of hospital emergency units. One objective is to describe the organizational situation of EU's (including resources, goal priorities, problems, and strengths) and specify the main differences and similarities in how these important care delivery units operate. A related objective is to identify those organizational factors and social-psychological conditions which are likely to promote (or impede) the solution of work problems in the unit and facilitate effectiveness of performance. A final research objective is to examine and understand the nature and sources of inter-hospital differences in emergency unit effectiveness. The present report is mainly concerned with the first of these objectives, while also providing preliminary but essential data for pursuing the other two.

The ultimate purpose of the research is to generate and make available dependable knowledge about the organization and effectiveness of hospital emergency services. The underlying question is, "What makes for an efficient and effective emergency unit (EU), and how can an EU improve its organization and problem-solving capabilities?" It is this basic question that is being addressed by the present study.

Here, some of the descriptive findings of the study are summarized. Based upon the data provided by the various hospitals and individual respondents involved, results are presented on each of the following main topics: basic characteristics of the emergency units studied; current goal priorities, problems, and strengths; leadership effectiveness and the influence of various groups on how the unit operates; work relations and problem solving within the unit; work relations with the parent hospital; relations with the community; emergency unit reputation and patient satisfaction; staff attitudes and satisfaction, or "social efficiency"; financial aspects and economic efficiency; and, finally, clinical efficiency -- care procedures, staff performance, and quality of care. (Certain background information about the respondents and local populations is also included.) The results on each of these topics are presented for the 30 participating hospital EU's combined, and results for each of the participating hospitals were reported back to each EU. In many of the tables, the space where the individual result was filled in remains.

The sample of hospitals whose emergency units were studied is briefly discussed next, followed by a discussion of the respondents who provided the data. Then, the organization of this report is described, as is the form in which the results are presented.

The Study Sample

The research has been designed to compare and contrast, in a methodologically rigorous manner, the EU's of a cross-sectional sample of hospitals on a large number of variables in the above areas. Its main concern is to investigate the relationships among these variables. The focus of the study is on the hospital emergency unit, or department, as a work-performing and problem-solving subsystem of the hospital, and not on any particular groups or individuals as such. Since the "unit" of description and analysis is the hospital EU itself as an organizational entity, the sample of the study consists not of individuals but of institutions. It consists of the emergency units of the 30 hospitals which participated in the research.

Hospitals were selected statistically, on a random basis, from the population of 436 eligible institutions in HEW Region V. They were selected to constitute a "stratified random sample" representing the non-government, not-for-profit, short-stay general hospitals in the size range of 100-499 beds. Based upon both technical considerations and reasons of economy, the sample was designed to consist of a maximum of 44 hospitals (or 10% of the eligible population), with no provisions for replacing institutions unable to participate. This maximum number made allowance for an expected 10%-20% sample attrition due to non-cooperation.

At the same time, the sample was designed to represent, in proportion to their numbers in the population, all of the following subgroups of institutions: (a) "small" (100-199 beds), "medium" (200-299 beds), and "large" (300-499 beds) hospitals; (b) hospitals in urban areas and in non-urban areas; and (c) church operated as well as not church operated hospitals. Ideally, a minimum of 10 sample hospitals were desired for each of these "strata" or subgroupings. Additionally, hospitals were to be selected into the sample in proportion to the number of eligible institutions located in each different state within Region V. Finally, eligible hospitals (within each stratum) were to have an equal chance (probability) of being selected for study.

The objective of these requirements was to achieve reasonably adequate coverage of important subgroups of hospitals as well as of the total eligible hospital population, and to make possible statistical generalization of the relationships found among the variables studied to the population of institutions represented by the sample. The actual sample selection procedures were carried out, according to the requirements specified above, by the Sampling Section of the Survey Research Center.

Table 1 shows the selected study sample, in relation to the hospital population and population strata from which it was drawn. It also shows the number of hospitals from the sample which cooperated in the study, by providing the necessary data and allowing their relevant staff members to complete interviews and/or questionnaires for the research. Overall, 68% of the hospitals in the original sample, or a total of 30 institutions, participated in the project. These constitute the "effective sample" of the study. The hospital cooperation rate achieved is considerably higher than that of recent hospital studies with probability sample designs and data requirements approaching those of the present study. It is considered satisfactory for the research.

The 44 hospitals which were actually selected into the sample were distributed as follows in terms of the stratification characteristics outlined above: (a) 17 were small, 13 were of medium size, and 14 were large hospitals; (b) 31 were from SMSA, or urban areas, and 13 from non-SMSA communities; and (c) 16 were church operated (including 14 Catholic) while 28 were not church operated (including 3 osteopathic) hospitals. Clearly, in terms of these important characteristics, the distribution of sample hospitals reflects that of the larger population very well. By state, 14 of the sample hospitals are located in Illinois, 10 in Ohio, 7 in Michigan, 6 in Wisconsin, 4 in Indiana, and 3 in Minnesota.

A total of 33 of the hospitals in the original sample agreed, after intensive negotiations, to participate in the research (an additional 4 were willing to participate but not until some time in the spring of 1978, and

TABLE 1. THE SAMPLE OF STUDY HOSPITALS (INSTITUTIONS WHOSE EMERGENCY UNITS WERE STUDIED) AND THE POPULATION OF HOSPITALS FROM WHICH IT WAS SELECTED[a]

Hospital Grouping (Strata) Used for Sample Selection	Number of Eligible Hospitals in Population	Number of Hospitals Selected into the Sample	Number of Hospitals Which Cooperated and Were Studied	Sample Hospital Cooperation Rate
ALL GROUPINGS COMBINED:	436	44	30	68%
Size Strata				
Small Hospitals (100-199 beds)	165	17	14	82%
Medium-Size Hospitals (200-299 beds)	129	13	9	69%
Large Hospitals (300-499 beds)	142	14	7	50%
Location Strata[b]				
Hospitals in SMSA (urban) Areas	312	31	21	68%
Hospitals in non-SMSA Areas	124	13	9	69%
Control Strata				
Church Operated Hospitals	140	16	9	56%
Not Church Operated Hospitals	296	28	21	75%

[a] The hospitals involved are all non-government, not-for-profit institutions. They are short-stay general hospitals which are located in HEW Region V (Illinois, Indiana, Michigan, Minnesota, Ohio, Wisconsin), and whose size falls within the 100-499 bed range. The listing of the eligible population of hospitals from which the sample was drawn was obtained from the 1976 AHA <u>Guide to the Health Care Field</u>.

[b] In the sampling process, hospitals were selected separately by state in which located as well as on the basis of SMSA (Standard Metropolitan Statistical Area) vs. non-SMSA location.

this was too late for the project). Three of these, however, retracted as fieldwork was about to begin due to various internal problems. Thus, the total number of sample hospitals which actually cooperated and provided the required data turned out to be 30. Of these, 14, 9, and 7, respectively, are small, medium, and large hospitals; 21 are from urban (SMSA) communities and 9 from non-SMSA communities; and 9 are church operated (including 7 Catholic) while 21 (including 3 osteopathic) are not.

Overall, the distribution of the "effective sample" (i.e., of the 30 institutions actually studied) is quite satisfactory and, for some of the strata, closer to the distribution of the population than is the original sample. The effective sample of 30 hospitals/hospital EU's is equivalent to 7% of the eligible hospital population (a maximum of 10% was initially planned). Proportionately, more of the small, and fewer of the large, hospitals in the original sample cooperated (it should be noted, however, that the size of "small" hospitals in the present study is no smaller than 100 beds, ranging between 100-199 beds). And, similarly, fewer of the church operated than of the not church operated institutions cooperated. The smallest rate of cooperation achieved, as is evident from Table 1, involves the large church operated hospitals; and, accordingly, such institutions are the least well represented ones in the study. With this particular exception, the effective study sample represents the population and population strata from which it was selected remarkably well.[*]

---

[*] The effect of the relatively low cooperation rate on the part of the large church operated hospitals upon the relationships among the variables in which the research is interested will be estimated by special analyses when the relationships are ascertained. Based on preliminary estimates, it is not expected to be consequential. Furthermore, "sampling errors" already have been computed for a considerable number of variables representing the different kinds of variables measured by the study, and the computations yielded excellent results. For the large majority of the variables, the sampling error is smaller than it would be for a "simple random sample" of the same size as the effective sample of the study (this reflects gains from the stratification used to select the sample).

The results included in this report are shown both for the 30 participating institutions combined and separately for the institutions in each of the above stratification groupings (i.e., separately by hospital size category, by location in urban and non-urban areas, and by type of control). In addition, they are separately shown for certain other important groupings, as follows: (a) for hospitals with and without medical teaching affiliations; (b) for hospitals with and without emergency personnel training programs; and (c) for hospitals whose emergency units have a low, a medium, or a high patient volume -- correspondingly, fewer than 10,000 patient visits a year, 10,000 to 20,000 visits, and more than 20,000 visits. (When, however, the findings are shown for the patient volume groupings they are not also shown for the hospital size groupings.) These special groupings have been added because of their likely high interest to various institutions and readers of the report, and because preliminary interpretation of differences shown by some of the findings suggests that these "analytical groupings" may be very important to understanding the results of the study (and often more revealing than the sample stratification groupings).

Sources of Data and the Respondents

The present study is relying on several independent sources of data. These include: (a) organizational and administrative records about financial, staffing, and patient census characteristics; (b) interviews and questionnaires completed by seven different groups of respondents associated with the hospitals and emergency units studied; (c) the emergency visit records of recent patients, who also completed a mailed questionnaire for the study; and (d) certain supplementary sources, including the AHA Guide Issue(s) to the Health Care Field, observations by the field staff who collected the data in the various institutions, and U.S. Census reports. Most of the data were obtained from the first two of the above sources.

A set of twelve different, but coordinated, data collection instruments (forms) had to be developed in order to obtain the required information. The various instruments were first constructed and then pretested and revised. Then, the relevant data from the participating hospitals and emergency units were collected on location by specially trained professional interviewers from the Institute for Social Research, under research staff supervision. (Each of the 30 hospitals was scheduled for a seven-day period during which the fieldwork was carried out.) The relevant data from all hospitals and respondents, except patients, were collected during the last three months of 1977; and the questionnaire data from recent patients were obtained by mail during the period of November 1977-January 1978. Therefore, the research findings and the data on which they are based depict the situation then prevailing in the institutions studied.

Identical data collection instruments and procedures were used in all of the hospitals, and each participating group of respondents completed the same instrument (personal interview and/or questionnaire form) across hospitals. The seven groups of respondents participating in the study are as follows:

1. Emergency unit physicians (MDS): all physicians (doctors of medicine or osteopathy), including the medical director of the unit, working in the emergency unit during the seven-day period in which the data were collected from each particular hospital.

2. Emergency unit registered nurses (RNS): all full-time and part-time registered nurses working in the emergency unit during the seven-day data collection period, including the head nurse(s) or supervising nurses (SRNS) involved.

3. Emergency unit licensed practical nurses (LPNS): all licensed practical nurses working full-time in the emergency unit during the same period.

4. <u>Selected hospital physicians</u> (HMDS): relevant key physicians in the parent hospital who had knowledge of, but did not work in, the emergency unit, including the chief or president of the medical staff and chairman of the medical executive committee; the chairman of the emergency department/room committee (if any); the chief pathologist and chief radiologist of the hospital; the chairman of the trauma committee (if any); intensive care unit physicians; the chairman of the medical audit or peer review committee; the hospital's director of medical education; and the heads of the four major inpatient services -- medicine, surgery, pediatrics, and obstetrics/gynecology. (Obviously, one individual respondent often held more than one of the specified positions.)

5. <u>Hospital administrators</u> (HAS): The chief executive officer of each hospital, the next highest administrative official (if any) of the hospital responsible for the emergency unit, and the hospital's director of nursing.

6. <u>Selected community respondents</u> (CRS): selected individuals from the community having work contacts with, or special knowledge about, each hospital's emergency unit, including the local health department director or his/her designate; sheriff department, police department, and fire department representatives; the coroner or medical examiner; health systems agency (HSA) and emergency medical system (EMS) representatives, if any; ambulance company personnel (e.g., emergency medical technicians); and up to three additional individuals named by the chief executive officer of each hospital (when interviewed) as the "most knowledgeable individuals in the community outside the hospital concerning the emergency unit" (these often overlapped with other specified community respondents).

7. <u>Emergency unit patients</u> (PATS): all patients over 15 years of age visiting the emergency unit for care at any time from 8:00 a.m. Friday until 12:00 p.m. Saturday of the week during which each particular hospital was scheduled for on-site data collection, excluding those who were unable to, or who preferred not to, sign a consent form to participate in the research. Subsequently, within approximately three weeks after their emergency visits, these patients were contacted by the research staff and asked to complete a mail questionnaire for the study. (Copies of their emergency visit medical records already had been obtained, with their consent, from each participating institution.)

The capital-letter <u>initials</u> enclosed in parentheses after each designated group of respondents are used throughout this report, both in the tables and in the discussion which accompanies them, in order to conveniently identify the specific sources of data on which the findings are based in each case. In this connection, the designation "(RECS)" is similarly used, where appropriate, to identify organizational records as the source of those data which the hospitals supplied from their various records. The report contains findings based on the data provided by every one of the above groups of respondents. Not all of the information collected from each group, however, is summarized in the report. Some of the data were collected for special analysis purposes and are therefore excluded (the results of these forthcoming analyses will, of course, be included in the final report of the study).

The hospital administrators (HAS), emergency unit physicians (MDS), and registered nurses (RNS) involved completed both personal interviews and questionnaires for the study. The supervising nurses (SRNS) from the various emergency units completed a special questionnaire-type instrument in addition to the forms completed by the RNS. The licensed practical nurses (LPNS) involved completed a personal interview only. The selected physicians (HMDS) from the parent hospitals completed personal interviews, as did the selected community respondents (CRS) associated with each institution. And the patients (PATS) completed a mailed questionnaire, as pointed out earlier. The numbers of respondents from each group who provided data for the study are presented in Table 2.

A grand total of 1,446 persons associated with the 30 hospitals/emergency units studied are involved, as follows: 248 MDS, 278 RNS, 47 LPNS (nine of the hospitals had no full-time LPNS working in their emergency units), 215 HMDS, 68 HAS, 202 CRS, and 388 PATS (two of the hospitals did not allow patient participation in the study). A few additional persons, not included here, also were interviewed at the request of some of the hospitals on "special" or "courtesy" grounds. Thus, on the average, a total of nearly 50 persons per hospital participated in the study as respondents. The specific numbers of respondents associated with the various hospital strata (groupings) discussed earlier also are shown in Table 2.

TABLE 2. NUMBER OF INDIVIDUAL RESPONDENTS WHO PROVIDED DATA FOR THE STUDY, SHOWN SEPARATELY FOR THE VARIOUS PARTICIPATING GROUPS OF RESPONDENTS

Hospital/Emergency Units (EU's) Involved	Number of Respondents, by Group[a]							
	MDS	RNS	LPNS	HMDS	HAS	CRS	PATS	Total
ALL INSTITUTIONS IN THE STUDY SAMPLE (N=30 Hospitals/ Hospital EU's)	248	278	47	215	68	202	388	1446
YOUR INSTITUTION								
Hospitals of:								
Small Size (n=14)	106	111	17	80	28	95	182	619
Medium Size (n=9)	79	92	13	71	20	59	122	456
Large Size (n=7)	63	75	17	64	20	48	84	371
Hospitals/EU's Located in:								
SMSA (urban) Areas (n=21)	176	203	39	158	50	135	256	1017
Non-SMSA Areas (n=9)	72	75	8	57	18	67	132	429
Hospitals/EU's That Are:								
Church Operated (n=9)	94	80	9	48	20	60	53	364
Not Church Operated/ Osteopathic (n=3)	18	28	7	25	6	17	45	146
Not Church Operated/ Other (n=18)	136	170	31	142	42	125	290	936
Hospitals with EU's Having:								
Low Patient Volume (n=10)	97	83	8	47	21	70	79	405
Medium Pat. Volume (n=10)	72	77	17	85	21	57	112	441
High Patient Volume (n=10)	79	118	22	83	26	75	197	600
Hospitals Having:								
Medical Teaching Affiliations (n=17)	131	159	35	142	42	112	240	861
No Medical Teaching Affiliations (n=13)	117	119	12	73	26	90	148	585
Hospitals Having:								
Emergency Personnel Training Programs (n=15)	126	154	24	110	37	107	204	762
No Training Programs (n=15)	122	124	23	105	31	95	184	684

[a] MDS, RNS, and LPNS respectively designate the physicians, registered nurses, and full-time licensed practical nurses working in the various emergency units. HMDS designates selected physicians from the parent hospital, and HAS designates hospital administrators. CRS designates selected community respondents, and PATS designates patient respondents. (Two institutions did not allow patient participation, and nine of them had no full-time LPNS in their emergency units.)

The overall <u>response rate</u> achieved by the study for the collectivity of persons, other than patients, from the 30 hospitals who were eligible to participate as respondents turns out to be 94.4% -- an exceptionally high response rate. (If patients are combined with the other groups, the corresponding rate turns out to be 87.5%.) Across individual hospitals, the overall response rate ranges from 79% to 100%, with ten of the study hospitals showing a rate of 100%. The 79% figure signifies the lowest attained response rate for any one hospital; the next lowest rate is 86%. In fact, for 27 of the 30 cooperating hospitals the attained rate exceeds the 90% level.

In the case of emergency unit patients (PATS), from whom data were collected by mailed questionnaire, the overall response rate for the 28 institutions which allowed patient participation is 73%. Though lower than that of the other participating groups, this too is a good response rate, particularly when compared to either mailed questionnaire surveys of adult populations or other studies in the health services field involving former hospital patients. The corresponding response rates attained (for all study hospitals combined) for the other groups of respondents are as follows: for MDS, 90%; for RNS, 97%; for LPNS, 100%; for HMDS, 92%; for HAS, 100%; and for CRS, 95%. These are all excellent response rates.

Organization of the Special Feedback Report (Part II)

The findings selected for inclusion in this report are based on, and summarize, the data obtained from the sources and respondents discussed in the preceding section. They cover all of the major areas studied, roughly in proportion to the volume of available data in each case, in a way that takes into account the multiple perspectives contributed by the various groups of respondents. For purposes of reporting, the findings have been organized into a series of relatively self-contained but inter-related chapters.

Each chapter deals with several specific topics and presents the results about one of the major areas with which the research is concerned. Some of the items included in a particular chapter, however, may be highly relevant to the material presented in one or more of the other chapters as well. In part, the allocation of specific items into separate chapters was a matter of convenience and represents an attempt to bring together, in a logical manner, various inter-related findings for purposes of examination and ease of reference. Relationships among items reported in different chapters, of course, also exist. Therefore, the various chapters should not be regarded as independent of one another.

The arrangement of the chapters themselves also represents an attempt to enhance the logical order of presentation. The first three chapters focus on the structural characteristics and goal-priorities of the emergency units and on the nature of their organizational "inputs," including patient workload and available staff resources. The next several chapters (chapters 4-7) focus on internal organizational processes, work relations (within the unit, with the parent hospital, and with the community), and problem solving within the emergency units. And the remaining four chapters focus on important aspects of the "output" of the units -- on outcomes such as patient satisfaction, "social efficiency" or staff satisfaction, economic efficiency, and clinical efficiency. An appendix at the end of Part II provides background information about the respondents. Finally, Part III contains the research instruments developed to collect the data for the study.

The main areas and sub-areas about which findings are reported, in order of their presentation, are as follows:

<u>Some basic characteristics of the emergency units in the study</u> (including numbers of treatment rooms and beds, quality of layout, teaching affiliations and training programs, comprehensiveness of service, and patient composition).

The staff resources of emergency units (including sufficiency of resources, medical staffing patterns, specialists on call, nursing staff, professional staff hours worked, and staff stability).

Current goal priorities, problems, and strengths (as assessed by the staff of the units, others in the hospital, and outside "observers").

Perceived leadership effectiveness and the influence of various groups on how the unit operates (including the effectiveness of medical nursing, and administrative leadership, and the influence attributed to, and desired for, particular groups).

Work relations and problem solving within the emergency unit (including the adequacy of coordination of efforts, ways in which problems are solved, mutual understanding of work problems and needs by medical and nursing staff, and tension levels among the staff).

Work relations with the parent hospital (including the adequacy with which others in the hospital meet the emergency unit's requests for services or support, hospital administration's understanding, and provisions for monitoring the work or performance of the unit).

Relations with the community (including collaboration with other institutions, patient transfer arrangements, community characteristics "causing" problems for the emergency unit, and the quality of work contacts with various agencies and police, fire department, and ambulance personnel).

Emergency unit reputation and patient satisfaction (including the unit's reputation in the community, success in meeting community expectations, and patients' satisfaction with the care received and with other aspects of their emergency visit).

Staff attitudes and satisfaction: social efficiency (including commitment to the emergency unit by nurses and physicians, the unit as a place to work, and staff satisfaction with the financial and non-financial "rewards" of their work).

Financial aspects and economic efficiency (including the unit's operating budget and expenditures, revenues per patient visit, ratio of revenues to expenditures, patient charges, reactions to charges, and other aspects).

Clinical efficiency: care procedures, staff performance, and quality of care (including the appropriateness and performance of care procedures, the quality of patient management and nursing care for selected patient conditions, patient waiting time and patient "complaints" and death rates, the quality of overall medical care and nursing care, and other aspects).

Form of Presentation of Results

Each chapter, corresponding to one of the above major areas, contains a series of tables along with related discussion. Some of the tables summarize different findings based on the data provided by a single group of respondents (e.g., RNS) or a particular source such as hospital records (RECS). Other tables summarize findings derived from the answers of two or more groups of respondents (e.g., MDS, RNS, and HAS) to a particular item, such as a question about the work of the unit or about patient care. In the tables and the text which accompanies them, it will be recalled, the various groups of respondents are identified by the capital-letter initials assigned to designate them earlier. Moreover, whenever more than 10% of the respondents from a particular group did not answer (for any reason) the question involved, the nonresponse rate is indicated in the table. The item itself, along with the response alternatives provided, also is incorporated into the table. Finally, comments on the computations used to derive the findings are frequently also included, as necessary.

The report contains more than 100 tables. In general, the various tables are presented in the simplest form possible in order to facilitate examination of the findings. And although a few of them may be fairly complex in format, all have been carefully constructed with the interests of potential readers in mind. The majority of tables show results based on data from/about all of the 30 hospitals, or emergency units (EU's), participating in the study. In some cases, however, the total number involved is smaller than 30 because the necessary data had not been provided or were not available in all institutions. (Pertinent examples include data from patients, which were not collected in the case of two hospitals, and certain information supplied from hospital records.) Each table in the report, therefore, shows the total number of hospitals or EU's involved (or, if more appropriate, the number of respondents involved, as in the tables included in the Appendix). The number of hospital EU's involved whenever the 30 institutions are subdivided according to characteristics such as size, location, etc., is also indicated.

Results for individual hospitals and EU's are not being published in order to protect the anonymity of cooperating institutions. Similary, no findings are presented that could possibly violate the confidentiality of individual respondents who have provided data for the study. (To protect the persons involved, results from the data provided by hospital administrators and supervising nurses were not shown in the findings reported to individual hospitals.) In cases where data was excluded for reasons of confidentiality, the "missing" findings are indicated by "--" in the table.

In most of the tables, the results are presented in the form of mean scores, or averages, in the form of percentages or mean percentages, or in the form of frequencies (i.e., numbers of cases). For some of the variables measured, however, some other form of presentation (e.g., ratios instead of percentages, monetary values, and rates per 1000 cases) had to be used. Most of the data are summarized in the form of average scores, or means, or in the form of percentages and frequencies. These forms of presentation were chosen as the most appropriate for the kinds of findings included in the present report and as the most useful for making comparisons across hospital groupings.

Typically, the majority of questions asked of the various respondents were answered in terms of five-point scales (or similar scales) -- i.e., scales providing five response alternatives ordered from "high" to "low," from "excellent" to "poor," "favorable"/"satisfactory" to "unfavorable"/"unsatisfactory" -- or in some comparable manner. Some specific examples of scales used are:

(a) "1" excellent, "2" very good, "3" good, "4" fair, "5" poor; (b) "1" completely adequate, "2" very adequate, "3" fairly adequate, "4" not so adequate, "5" not adequate at all; and (c) "1" to a very great extent, "2" to a great extent, "3" to a fair extent, "4" to a small extent, "5" to a very small extent or not at all. Scales such as these make it possible to average the answers of any group of respondents to a particular item and obtain a mean score, or a mean, for the group. Mean scores of this kind, in turn, may be averaged for any number of respondent groups, for any number of hospitals, etc.

In a great many cases, the reported results were obtained by averaging the answers of respondents from each group involved, separately for each individual hospital, to questions involving five-point scales of the above kinds. In this manner, for each item or question used, a single mean score was obtained for each particular group of respondents and each particular hospital. Theoretically, these mean scores may range from 1.00 (when all individuals in a group answered by choosing response alternative "1") to 5.00 (when all chose alternative "5"). The vast majority of them, however, actually fall somewhere between 1.00 and 5.00.

The meaning of a particular mean score depends on the specific scale used. Thus, for example, a mean score of 2.00 on a scale ranging from "1" excellent to "5" poor (as shown above) corresponds exactly to "very good" while a mean score of 3.00 corresponds to "good." Similarly, a score of 2.50 would indicate the half-way mark between "very good" and "good," one of 3.50 would indicate the half-way mark between "good" and "fair," while one of 2.80 would indicate an almost "good" but not exactly "good" situation.

In addition, of course, the meaning of a particular mean score depends on how favorably or unfavorably that score compares to others in a particular series -- e.g., how the mean score from the answers of RNS in one hospital to a given item compares to the corresponding scores obtained for the other hospitals in the study. In this connection, however, the tables in the report do not show the separate mean scores of all the participating institutions. Instead, they show (1) the _average_ of the individual hospital means, i.e., the mean of the hospital means or the overall mean score for all of the hospitals, and (2) the _range_ of the individual hospital means (the range being defined by the _lowest_ mean score achieved by any one of the 30 hospitals in the study, at the one extreme, and the _highest_ score achieved, at the other extreme).

The closer a particular hospital's score is to the average of hospital means, the less its situation differs from the "average situation" prevailing in the 30 hospitals or (less accurately) from the situation of the "average hospital." (This "average" situation, of course, may be "good" or it may be "poor," or perhaps "fair," depending on the scale value of the particular average mean score.) Conversely, the further a particular hospital's mean score deviates from the average of hospital means, the more its situation differs from that of the "average hospital" in the study. In addition, the closer a particular hospital's score approaches one of the two extremes of the _range_ of hospital mean scores (shown for a particular item), whether it is the favorable or the unfavorable end of the range, the greater the likelihood (and also the confidence) that this hospital differs significantly -- either in a positive or in a negative direction -- from the rest.*

---

*Since this is not a technical report, results of statistical tests of significance are not included. However, such tests were performed in examining differences in scores between groupings of hospitals (according to size, location, etc.). Differences which were found to be "statistically significant" are high-lighted in the discussion which accompanies each table, but without presenting the test results themselves or... (continued on the following page)

In summary, for most of the findings, each table in the report first presents an overall mean score for all of the hospitals, or hospital EU's, in the study sample. This is the mean of the individual hospital means (in most cases, of the 30 hospital means). Next, directly below each overall mean score, the corresponding range of individual hospital means is shown. The range is enclosed in parentheses. The rest of the table presents the mean scores for each of the various "stratification groupings" and "analytical groupings" of hospitals/EU's described earlier. In this connection, however, it should be noted that when findings are shown for institutions grouped according to hospital size (number of beds) they are not also shown for institutions grouped according to emergency unit patient volume, and vice versa. Because hospital size and EU patient volume correlate positively (though far from perfectly), only one of them is used in each table -- the one which is more meaningful in terms of the subject matter or the one which discriminates more, i.e., shows more differences between groups of emergency units. (When meaningfulness and discriminability are about the same for both groupings, the grouping which appears in adjacent tables is used.) This method of presentation was chosen because some of the variables measured in the study appear to be related to patient volume but not to hospital size, and vice versa, or are more strongly related to one than to the other.

Finally, it should be remembered that the reported results are based on data which depict the situation in the various institutions as it existed

---

* (continued from preceding page) ...related technical details. The differences discussed may be of considerable practical interest to many readers of this report. From the standpoint of the research, however, differences between particular hospital groupings are of less interest than the variability among the 30 hospitals in the study sample, i.e., than the differences among all 30 individual hospitals. Most of the forthcoming analyses of the study will be concerned with the matter of these inter-hospital or inter-institutional differences and with the relationships among the variables investigated.

during the period in which the data were collected. Significant changes may have occurred since then in some of the participating institutions.

Chapter 1

SOME BASIC CHARACTERISTICS OF THE EMERGENCY UNITS IN THE STUDY

This chapter is concerned with the overall situation of emergency units (EU's), presenting findings on certain basic characteristics of these facilities and their patients. These include: (1) the physical plant and layout of the units; (2) medical teaching affiliations, training programs for emergency personnel, and special service capabilities; (3) patient volume and breadth of "emergency service definition"; (4) the composition of patient inputs in terms of selected "case-mix" variables; and (5) the patients' views of their medical problems. Most of the findings deal with the nature of each unit's "inputs" and are based on information supplied from hospital records.

Characteristics such as those considered in this chapter may have important implications for the work requirements of the units, for successful problem solving, and for organizational effectiveness. An emergency unit receiving a high percentage of patients with critical or "life-threatening" problems persistently, for example, must perform more complex tasks than one with a low percentage of such patients. The clinical and coordinative activities required in the former case may be substantially different than those in the latter case. This, in turn, could suggest the need for differential work procedures and/or staffing arrangements. Identical procedures and staffing patterns would not be equally appropriate in the two cases from the standpoint of clinical efficiency, economic efficiency, or staff satisfaction.

Generally, emergency units have little direct control over their patient inputs. To a certain extent, however, the nature of a unit's inputs over the long run might be affected by the behavior and performance of the unit. An EU which is doing excellent work consistently may come to be "preferred" by a particular population of patients or by referring agencies and individuals in the community. Equally important, an EU which has developed explicit arrangements (e.g., patient transfer or referral agreements) with other health care institutions and relevant agencies in the community in effect is exercising some control over the variability of its patient work load. Whether or not this is the case, of course, may be less important than differences in workload associated with the nature of patient inputs received by the various emergency units. Such differences are one concern of the study, both in their own right and in relation to the organizational characteristics of emergency units.

The Physical Plant and Layout of Emergency Units

The first table in this chapter, Table 3, shows the number of rooms and beds in the various emergency units. On the average, the 30 EU's in the study have 4.4 treatment rooms each. The specific number varies greatly across individual EU's, however, from a low of 1 to a high of 15. In addition to their treatment rooms, the same emergency units have an average of 2.2 "other" rooms (for individual EU's this number ranges from 0 to 10). The average number of beds per EU is 6.9, ranging from a minimum of 0 to a maximum of 25.

As might be expected, the number of treatment rooms, other rooms, and beds in the emergency units increases as the size of the parent hospitals increases. Furthermore, EU's in urban areas generally have more treatment rooms, other rooms, and beds than those in non-urban areas. The same is true (and somewhat also more pronounced) for units operated by hospitals having medical teaching affiliations and/or training programs for emergency personnel, compared to their counterparts in hospitals lacking such affiliations or programs.

TABLE 3. NUMBER OF ROOMS AND BEDS IN THE EMERGENCY UNITS (EU'S) STUDIED[a]

		Number of		
Hospital Emergency Units (EU's) Involved		Treatment Rooms	Other Rooms	Beds
ALL EU'S IN THE STUDY SAMPLE (N=30 Hospital EU's)	*Mean:* *Range:*	4.4 (1-15)	2.2 (0-10)	6.9 (0-25)
EU's in:				
Small Hospitals (n=14)		3.2	1.2	3.9
Medium Hospitals (n=9)		3.9	1.6	6.7
Large Hospitals (n=7)		7.3	5.5	13.3
EU's in:				
Church Operated Hospitals (n=9)		4.9	2.6	6.9
Osteopathic Hospitals (n=3)		3.7	1.0	3.7
All Other Hospitals (n=18)		4.2	2.2	7.5
EU's Located in:				
SMSA (urban) Areas (n=21)		4.9	2.5	8.0
Non-SMSA Areas (n=9)		3.1	1.4	4.3
EU's in Hospitals Having:				
Medical Teaching Affiliations (n=17)		5.6	2.8	9.2
No Medical Teaching Affiliations (n=13)		2.7	1.5	4.0
EU's in Hospitals Having:				
Emergency Personnel Training Programs (n=15)		5.4	2.9	8.9
No Training Programs (n=15)		3.3	1.5	5.0

[a]Based on data from hospital records (RECS).

Concerning the layout of emergency units, registered nurses (RNS) and patients (PATS) who participated in the study were asked their views. Table 4 presents the findings from these data. On the average, registered nurses consider the layout of their respective units only "fairly adequate." The overall mean score for the 30 EU's in the study is 2.92 (1.00 would signify "completely adequate" layout and 5.00 would signify "not adequate at all"). Across individual EU's, however, the scores range very widely, from 1.83 (indicating very satisfactory layout) to 4.60 (indicating unsatisfactory layout). Apparently, some of the units have problems in this area.

Patients evaluate the layout of the units more favorably than do the nurses. Inter-unit variability in this respect is much smaller according to the data from patients by comparison to the data from registered nurses.

For the various groupings of emergency units included in Table 4, the pattern of evaluations by RNS and PATS is fairly similar. Both groups evaluate the layout slightly more favorably in emergency units with a high, in contrast to medium, patient volume. The same is true concerning EU's in non-urban as contrasted to urban areas, and also for EU's in church operated hospitals compared to other hospitals. The results show no differences in the adequacy of emergency unit layout between institutions which have and those which do not have medical teaching affiliations or emergency personnel training programs (whether the data from RNS or the data from PATS are considered).

Teaching Affiliations, Training Programs, and Special Service Capabilities

Although not related to the adequacy of emergency unit layout, medical teaching affiliation is related to a great many other variables measured in the study, as is evident throughout this report. The same applies regarding training programs for emergency personnel (technicians, nurses, physicians).

TABLE 4. ADEQUACY OF THE LAYOUT OF EMERGENCY UNITS AS REPORTED BY
REGISTERED NURSES (RNS) AND PATIENTS (PATS)

Hospital Emergency Units (EU's) Involved		Level of Adequacy According to	
		RNS[a]	PATS[b]
ALL EU'S IN THE STUDY SAMPLE (N=30 Hospital EU's)	Mean: Range:	2.92 (1.83-4.60)	2.05 (1.33-3.00)
YOUR HOSPITAL'S EU			
EU's with:			
Low Patient Volume (n=10)		2.80	2.02
Medium Pat. Volume (n=10)		3.18	2.16
High Patient Volume (n=10)		2.77	1.95
EU's in:			
Church Operated Hospitals (n=9)		3.00	1.99
Osteopathic Hospitals (n=3)		2.57	2.09
All Other Hospitals (n=18)		2.93	2.07
EU's Located in:			
SMSA (urban) Areas (n=21)		3.04	2.14
Non-SMSA Areas (n=9)		2.63	1.85
EU's in Hospitals Having:			
Medical Teaching Affiliations (n=17)		2.97	1.97
No Medical Teaching Affiliations (n=13)		2.84	2.16
EU's in Hospitals Having:			
Emergency Personnel Training Programs (n=15)		2.90	1.89
No Training Programs (n=15)		2.93	2.18

[a] The question asked of RNS was: "Considering what this emergency unit needs to provide high quality care to its patients at reasonable cost, how adequate would you say is the quality of... the layout of the emergency unit facility?" The response alternatives were: (1) Completely adequate, (2) very adequate, (3) fairly adequate, (4) not so adequate, (5) not adequate at all. Thus, the lower the mean scores shown, the better the layout of the EU's involved.

[b] The question asked of PATS was: "All other things aside, how satisfactory would you say was the physical plant and layout of the emergency room that you visited?" The response alternatives were: (1) Extremely satisfactory, (2) very satisfactory, (3) fairly satisfactory, (4) not so satisfactory, (5) not satisfactory at all. Thus, the lower the mean scores shown, the better the physical plant and layout of the EU's involved.

For this reason, the 30 institutions in the study have been grouped according to whether or not they have such teaching affiliations, and also such training programs, and the resulting groupings are used in the report to summarize some of the findings.

Table 5 shows the number of EU's operated by hospitals having and not having (a) medical teaching affiliation(s) of any kind, and (b) training program(s) for emergency service personnel of any kind. As reported by the chief executive officer of each institution, 17 of the hospitals involved have some teaching affiliations while the other 13 do not. The numbers of hospitals which have training programs also are indicated in Table 5, separately by type of personnel involved. For all types of emergency personnel considered together (not shown in Table 5), half of the hospitals have some kind of training program while the other half (15 in each case) do not. Most such programs are for technicians, only three institutions reporting similar training programs for either emergency nurses or emergency physicians.

Medical teaching affiliations are more prevalent in hospitals whose emergency units have a medium or high, as opposed to low, patient volume. They are also more prevalent in hospitals which are not church operated, and in hospitals located in urban compared to non-urban areas. Training programs for emergency technicians, which are the most numerous of all the training programs reported for emergency personnel, are most often found in hospitals whose emergency units have a high patient volume, and in hospitals which are located in urban areas.

Data were also obtained about the "comprehensiveness" of services offered by the various emergency units and about special service capabilities. Regarding the former, according to the chief executive officer of each hospital, six of the 30 EU's in the study offer "comprehensive" services, while an additional

TABLE 5. EMERGENCY UNITS OPERATED BY HOSPITALS WITH MEDICAL TEACHING AFFILIATIONS AND EMERGENCY PERSONNEL TRAINING PROGRAMS[a]

Hospital Emergency Units (EU's) Involved		Number of the Hospitals With			
		Medical Teaching Affiliation(s)	EMT Training Program(s)	Emergency Nurse Training Program(s)	Emergency Physician Training Program(s)
ALL EU'S IN THE STUDY SAMPLE (N=30 Hospital EU's)	n: %:	17 (56.7%)	14 (46.7%)	3 (10.3%)[b]	3 (10.3%)[b]
EU's with:					
Low Patient Volume (n=10)		2	4	1	1
Medium Pat. Volume (n=10)		8	2	0	0
High Patient Volume (n=10)		7	8	2	2
EU's in:					
Church Operated Hospitals (n=9)		3	5	0	1
Osteopathic Hospitals (n=3)		2	1	0	0
All Other Hospitals (n=18)		12	8	3	2
EU's Located in:					
SMSA (urban) Areas (n=21)		14	10	3	3
Non-SMSA Areas (n=9)		3	4	0	0
EU's in Hospitals Having:					
Medical Teaching Affiliations (n=17)		17	9	1	1
No Medical Teaching Affiliations (n=13)		0	5	2	2
EU's in Hospitals Having:					
Emergency Personnel Training Programs (n=15)		9	14	3	3
No Training Programs (n=15)		8	0	0	0

[a] According to data obtained from the chief executive officer of each hospital.

[b] In these cases, the percentage figures are based on a total N of 29 hospital EU's, and not on an N of 30, because of incomplete information from one of the hospitals.

14 offer "nearly comprehensive" services. The remaining ten units (or one-third of all the EU's) offer less comprehensive services or just "basic" services. Institutions with medical teaching affiliations and large, compared to other, institutions are more likely to have emergency units offering comprehensive or nearly comprehensive services. (The findings about comprehensiveness of service are not reported in any of the tables.)

Information about the prevalence of selected emergency service capabilities in the institutions studied is presented in Table 6. Briefly, half of the hospitals report having a poison control or substance abuse center or unit. Such facilities are more likely to be found in hospitals whose emergency units have a high patient volume, as opposed to medium or low volume, and in not church operated (excluding osteopathic) institutions. They are also somewhat more prevalent in hospitals having emergency personnel training programs.

Nearly half of the hospitals (47%) similarly report having a trauma center or unit. The likelihood of having this kind of service facility increases as the patient volume of emergency units increases. It is also higher for hospitals with medical teaching affiliations than for hospitals without such affiliations. Table 6 also shows that one-third of the institutions in the study sample, but half of those whose emergency units have a high patient volume, report having a mental health center or unit.

Concerning special service capabilities, moreover, the physicians (MDS) and registered nurses (RNS) working in the various EU's were asked whether their respective unit specialized in, or concentrates on, the treatment of any particular kinds of patients. The results (not included in any of the tables) show that only 12% of the physicians, from all institutions combined, responded affirmatively to this question. Those responding affirmatively, moreover, are scattered among 22 different EU's. In fact, only one of the 30

TABLE 6. NUMBER OF INSTITUTIONS WITH SELECTED SPECIAL FACILITIES[a]

	Number of Institutions With a		
Hospital Emergency Units (EU's) Involved	Poison Control or Substance Abuse Center or Unit	Trauma Center or Unit	Mental Health Center or Unit
ALL EU'S IN THE STUDY SAMPLE (N=30 Hospital EU's)	n: 15 %: (50.0%)	14 (46.7%)	10 (33.3%)
EU's with:			
Low Patient Volume (n=10)	4	2	3
Medium Pat. Volume (n=10)	3	5	2
High Patient Volume (n=10)	8	7	5
EU's in:			
Church Operated Hospitals (n=9)	3	3	3
Osteopathic Hospitals (n=3)	0	0	0
All Other Hospitals (n=18)	12	11	7
EU's Located in:			
SMSA (urban) Areas (n=21)	11	9	7
Non-SMSA Areas (n=9)	4	5	3
EU's in Hospitals Having:			
Medical Teaching Affiliations (n=17)	9	9	6
No Medical Teaching Affiliations (n=13)	6	5	4
EU's in Hospitals Having:			
Emergency Personnel Training Programs (n=15)	9	6	6
No Training Programs (n=15)	6	8	4

[a] Based on data from hospital records (RECS). The figures shown represent the number of hospitals having the indicated special facility located either within the emergency unit or within the hospital.

units is considered by at least half of the physicians who work there as specializing in the treatment of some particular kind of patients.

Similarly, only 17% of all the registered nurses in the study indicate that their respective units "specialize." Again, these particular respondents are scattered among 21 different EU's, and only one unit is considered to specialize by half or more of its registered nurses. Incidentally, types of patients most frequently mentioned by MDS or RNS as those on which the emergency unit concentrates (when it does) are cardiac, trauma, and orthopedic cases. Overall, however, the data indicate little "specialization in treating particular kinds of patients" on the part of the emergency units studied. Apparently, with few if any exceptions, emergency units are like a "microcosm" of the entire hospital in this respect, reflecting the great variety of patient types and conditions treated and focusing more on comprehensiveness of service than on special treatment capabilities.

Patient Volume and "Emergency Service Definition"

The number of patient visits to the emergency units studied during the "most recent quarter," and "most recent week," for which information was available at the time of data collection in each hospital is shown in Table 7. For the quarter, the average number of patient visits per EU approaches 5,000, ranging across units from a low of 655 to a high of nearly 12,000 visits. As might be expected, on the average, the number of patient visits to the various emergency units increases as the size of the parent hospitals increases. The number of visits per EU also is larger for institutions in urban than non-urban areas, and institutions with either teaching affiliations or training programs (compared to the remaining institutions in each case). The number is smaller for church operated than for other institutions, but this is

TABLE 7. NUMBER OF PATIENT VISITS TO THE EMERGENCY UNITS
DURING THE MOST RECENT QUARTER AND MOST RECENT WEEK[a]

Hospital Emergency Units (EU's) Involved		Number of Patients During	
		Most Recent Quarter	Most Recent Week
ALL EU'S IN THE STUDY SAMPLE (N=30 Hospital EU's)	Mean: Range:	4801 (655-11,847)	348 (87-877)
YOUR HOSPITAL'S EU			
EU's in:			
Small Hospitals (n=14)		3200	244
Medium Hospitals (n=9)		4846	326
Large Hospitals (n=7)		7953	571
EU's in:			
Church Operated Hospitals (n=9)		3426	302
Osteopathic Hospitals (n=3)		3847	239
All Other Hospitals (n=18)		5572	392
EU's Located in:			
SMSA (urban) Areas (n=21)		5240	361
Non-SMSA Areas (n=9)		3650	319
EU's in Hospitals Having:			
Medical Teaching Affiliations (n=17)		6110	422
No Medical Teaching Affiliations (n=13)		2947	243
EU's in Hospitals Having:			
Emergency Personnel Training Programs (n=15)		5827	455
No Training Programs (n=15)		3702	249

[a] Based on data from hospital records (RECS). For the EU's belonging to each grouping included in the table, the numbers of patient visits have been averaged and the obtained means are shown.

probably due to the low cooperation rate in the study on the part of large church-operated hospitals.

While mere numbers of visits may be indicative of total patient volume, and possibly also of gross staff work load, they are not very instructive about the nature of the work load. Two emergency units may have an identical number of patient visits, but vastly different work requirements. One of them, for example, may have an unusually high proportion of patients who (because of the seriousness of their condition) require admission to the hospital as in-patients, while the other may have an unusually high proportion of "walk-in" or "primary care" patients who could have been treated just as well in a doctor's office instead of the emergency unit.

The work requirements would be less complex in the latter unit. The latter type of situation, moreover, in effect, would be indicative of a rather broad definition of "emergency" service while the former would be indicative of a relatively narrow, or stricter, definition. The breadth of prevailing service definition in emergency units, in turn, may have important implications for required resources, staffing, and performance. For these reasons, patient visits to the emergency units have been examined in relation to each hospital's in-patient admissions and in-patient days (and also in relation to certain other variables discussed in other parts of the report). The results are presented in Table 8.

Considering first all of the EU's in the study sample, the results show that, on the average, for every in-patient admission to the hospital there are 2.36 patient visits to the institution's emergency unit. (The higher this ratio, the broader the prevailing *de facto* definition of "emergency" service.) But, this ratio differs very greatly from hospital to hospital, ranging across institutions from a low of only 0.52 to a high of 5.30 (the latter indicates

TABLE 8. PATIENT VISITS TO THE EMERGENCY UNITS STUDIED IN RELATION TO HOSPITAL IN-PATIENT ADMISSIONS AND IN-PATIENT DAYS FOR MOST RECENT QUARTER[a]

Hospital Emergency Units (EU's) Involved		Ratio of EU Visits to	
		Hospital In-Patient Admissions	Hospital In-patient Days
ALL EU'S IN THE STUDY SAMPLE (N=30 Hospital EU's)	*Mean:* *Range:*	2.36 (0.52-5.30)	0.37 (0.09-0.94)
YOUR HOSPITAL'S EU			
EU's in:			
Small Hospitals (n=14)		2.51	0.42
Medium Hospitals (n=9)		2.31	0.33
Large Hospitals (n=7)		2.11	0.30
EU's in:			
Church Operated Hospitals (n=9)		1.76	0.28
Osteopathic Hospitals (n=3)		2.72	0.38
All Other Hospitals (n=18)		2.53	0.40
EU's Located in:			
SMSA (urban) Areas (n=21)		2.32	0.35
Non-SMSA Areas (n=9)		2.45	0.41
EU's in Hospitals Having:			
Medical Teaching Affiliations (n=17)		2.42	0.37
No Medical Teaching Affiliations (n=13)		2.26	0.37
EU's in Hospitals Having:			
Emergency Personnel Training Programs (n=15)		2.26	0.34
No Training Programs (n=15)		2.48	0.40

[a] Based on data from hospital records (RECS). Ratios were first computed separately for each EU and then averaged for the EU's involved in each grouping. They were computed by dividing the number of patient visits to the EU by the number of hospital in-patient admissions for one of the ratios and the number of in-patient days for the other.

ten times as many emergency visits per in-patient admission to the hospital compared to the former). The implications of this finding for the economic, clinical, and social efficiency of emergency units will be an important subject in some of the forthcoming special analyses of the research.

Considering next the various groupings of EU's, the results indicate a higher average ratio (broader service definition) for the emergency units of small hospitals than for the units of large hospitals (medium-size hospitals occupying an intermediate position in this respect). A similar pattern emerges when comparing the hospitals which are not church operated (including the few osteopathic institutions) to the church operated hospitals in the study; the latter have a narrower "emergency service" definition than the former. The groupings according to location, teaching affiliation, and training programs do not show any appreciable differences in the ratio of emergency visits to in-patient admissions.

Finally, if the ratio of EU patient visits to hospital in-patient days (instead of admissions) is examined, based on the data in Table 8, the patterns of findings are almost identical to the patterns just discussed for the ratio of patient visits to in-patient admissions.

The Composition of Patient In-puts

The remaining tables in this chapter present findings about various aspects of the patient in-put in the different emergency units, including such aspects as the proportion of patient visits resulting from transfers, the proportion of patient visits scheduled in advance, the proportion of patients who were sent to an intensive care unit or operating room by the emergency unit, the proportion of patients who arrived by ambulance, also in "life-threatening" condition, and other important aspects.

Table 9 shows the percent of patient visits to the emergency units during the most recent quarter which (a) were scheduled in advance, (b) involved transfers from outside the hospital, and (c) involved transfers from other parts of the parent hospital in each case.

The results show that, on the average, nearly 6% of the patient visits to the emergency units in the study during the most recent quarter were scheduled in advance. Across individual EU's, the figure ranges from 0% to 38%, indicating major differences in this respect. Interestingly, the emergency units of the large hospitals in the study had no patient visits scheduled in advance. At the other extreme, the medium-size hospital EU's had 10% of their patient visits scheduled in advance (for small hospital EU's the figure is half as large). The groupings of institutions by location, teaching affiliation, and training programs, on the other hand, show no substantial differences on this variable.

The percent of patient visits to the various emergency units that were transfers from outside the parent hospital in each case is extremely small, averaging less than 1% for the 30 EU's. Such transfers are somewhat more prevalent for the emergency units of non-urban hospitals and church operated hospitals than for any of the other groupings. Across individual EU's the relevant percentage figures range from 0% to 3.1%.

In contrast, transfers into the emergency units from other parts of the parent hospitals are much more frequent. On the average, during the most recent quarter, 4.2% of the patient visits to each EU were transfers of this kind, the figure ranging from 0% to a high of almost 51% across individual emergency units. Osteopathic institutions, in particular, had a high proportion of such transfers. The other not church operated institutions, however, do not differ from those which are church operated with respect to this kind

TABLE 9. PERCENT OF PATIENT VISITS DURING THE MOST RECENT QUARTER THAT WERE SCHEDULED IN ADVANCE OR INVOLVED TRANSFER[a]

Hospital Emergency Units (EU's) Involved		Percent of Visits Per EU That Were		
		Scheduled in Advance	Transfers from Other Parts of the Hospital	Transfers from Outside the Hospital
ALL EU'S IN THE STUDY SAMPLE (N=30 Hospital EU's)[b]	Mean%: Range:	5.6% (0%-38.1%)	4.2% (0%-50.9%)	0.6% (0%-3.1%)
YOUR HOSPITAL'S EU				
EU's in:				
Small Hospitals (n=14)		5.5	6.6	0.8
Medium Hospitals (n=9)		10.1	2.6	0.6
Large Hospitals (n=7)		0.0	0.6	0.0
EU's in:				
Church Operated Hospitals (n=9)		4.7	1.6	1.0
Osteopathic Hospitals (n=3)		0.6	27.1	0.0
All Other Hospitals (n=18)		7.0	1.7	0.2
EU's Located in:				
SMSA (urban) Areas (n=21)		5.6	5.6	0.2
Non-SMSA Areas (n=9)		5.4	1.7	1.3
EU's in Hospitals Having:				
Medical Teaching Affiliations (n=17)		4.5	1.7	0.8
No Medical Teaching Affiliations (n=13)		6.4	6.7	0.6
EU's in Hospitals Having:				
Emergency Personnel Training Programs (n=15)		5.9	1.6	0.6
No Training Programs (n=15)		5.2	7.4	0.7

[a] Based on data from hospital records (RECS). Percentage figures were first computed separately for each EU and then averaged for the EU's involved in each grouping. They were computed by dividing the number of patient visits scheduled in advance (and, similarly, the number involving transfer) by the total number of visits during the quarter.

[b] Of the 30 EU's in the sample, ten could not provide data concerning visits scheduled in advance or visits involving transfer from other parts of the hospital, and eighteen could not provide data for visits involving transfers from outside the hospital. The percentages shown in each case were computed for those EU's which were able to provide the data.

of transfers (both groups averaging less than 2%). Other findings indicate that the transfers in question are more prevalent for emergency units in small than in large hospitals, in hospitals which do not have medical teaching affiliations or training programs, and in hospitals located in urban compared to non-urban areas. The significance of transfers to the staff and to the operations and effectiveness of emergency units will be ascertained when the detailed analyses of the study are completed in the coming year.

The composition of patient inputs can be examined not only in terms of the entry characteristics discussed above but also in terms of treatment process requirements, which may reflect the relative seriousness of condition of the patients visiting the various emergency units. Table 10 presents the findings from four relevant measures, respectively showing the percent of EU patients who were sent (for treatment) by each emergency unit to: (a) one of its parent hospital's intensive care units; (b) the operating room; (c) some other in-patient service of the hospital; and (d) some other hospital outside.

On the average, for all of the 30 EU's in the study for which the necessary data were available (see Table 10), the results show that 2.2% of all the patients visiting the EU during the most recent quarter were sent by the EU to one of the hospital's intensive care units for treatment. The inter-hospital range on this measure is very considerable, from 0.3% to 12.6%. The higher the percentage figure, the greater the apparent severity of condition of the patients visiting an emergency unit (assuming, of course, that the patients sent to an ICU indeed required intensive medical care).

Proportionately more of the patients visiting the emergency units of large than either small or medium-size hospitals were sent to an ICU. A similar pattern is evident for institutions located in urban compared to non-urban areas, for institutions with vs. without medical teaching affiliations, and

TABLE 10. PERCENT OF PATIENTS VISITING THE EMERGENCY UNITS DURING THE MOST RECENT QUARTER WHO WERE SENT (BY THE EU) ELSEWHERE FOR TREATMENT[a]

Hospital Emergency Units (EU's) Involved		Percent of Patients Per EU Who Were Sent to			
		One of the Hospital's ICU's	One of the Hospital's OR's	Some Other Part of the Hospital	Some Other Hospital Outside
ALL EU'S IN THE STUDY SAMPLE (N=30 Hospital EU's)[a]	Mean%:	2.2%	0.6%	17.0%	1.1%
	Range:	(0.3%-12.6%)	(0%-2.4%)	(4.0%-97.3%)	(0%-5.6%)
YOUR HOSPITAL'S EU					
EU's in:					
Small Hospitals (n=14)		1.8	0.5	19.0	1.6
Medium Hospitals (n=9)		1.4	0.9	9.4	0.5
Large Hospitals (n=7)		3.6	0.3	20.6	0.5
EU's in:					
Church Operated Hospitals (n=9)		1.6	0.4	22.5	1.6
Osteopathic Hospitals (n=3)		1.2	0.7	6.6	0.6
All Other Hospitals (n=18)		2.7	0.7	16.6	0.9
EU's Located in:					
SMSA (urban) Areas (n=21)		2.4	0.6	18.7	0.9
Non-SMSA Areas (n=9)		1.7	0.5	11.9	1.4
EU's in Hospitals Having:					
Medical Teaching Affiliations (n=17)		2.6	0.7	21.5	0.5
No Medical Teaching Affiliations (n=13)		1.6	0.5	10.9	1.5
EU's in Hospitals Having:					
Emergency Personnel Training Programs (n=15)		1.6	0.7	15.8	1.1
No Training Programs (n=15)		2.8	0.5	18.3	1.1

[a] Based on data from hospital records (RECS). Percentage figures were first computed separately for each EU and then averaged for the EU's involved in each grouping. Of the 30 EU's in the sample, six could not provide data concerning EU patients sent to an ICU and ten could not provide data concerning patients sent to the OR. Similarly, six of the EU's could not provide data about patients sent to other parts of the hospital for treatment. And finally, eleven of the EU's could not provide data about the number of their patients sent to some other hospital for treatment. The percentages shown in each case were computed for those EU's which were able to provide the data.

for institutions lacking emergency personnel training programs compared to those having such programs.

The percent of patients visiting the EU's who were sent to an operating room is very small, only 0.6% on the average. And the range across institutions is likewise small (0% to 2.4%), as might be expected. Consequently, the data do not differentiate one group of emergency units from another when the various groupings are examined.

The percent of EU patients sent to some other hospital for treatment also is rather small, averaging 1.1% for all of the EU's in the study for which data are available. The inter-institutional range on this variable is moderate, namely 0%-5.6%. The higher the figure, the lower the overall capability of a unit (and/or of its parent hospital) to treat its patients without having to refer some of them elsewhere. It is also possible, of course, that EU's refer patients elsewhere in the best interests of the patient or because more appropriate treatment facilities are available in other institutions. This, however, still would not explain the differential rates of such referrals indicated by the data for the emergency units studied.

Finally, Table 10 shows the percent of patients visiting the various emergency units who were sent to some part of its parent hospital, other than an ICU or an OR, for treatment. In this case, the average percentage figures for all of the EU's for which data are available is rather substantial, specifically 17%, and the range across individual emergency units is extremely large, from 4% to 97%, suggesting very great differences on this variable from one unit to another. These are very interesting and unanticipated findings.

The meaning and significance of this variability are not clear at this stage of the research. (Whether or not, for example, this finding reflects great differences in patient composition, differences in emergency unit staff practices, or attempts by some of the hospitals to increase in-patient admissions and/or occupancy rates by admitting a considerable proportion of the patients who visit their emergency units can not be determined from the data.) What is clear is that the apparent capability (and/or, perhaps, desire) of emergency units to treat their patients within the unit and without having to send them to some other part of the hospital varies widely. For some reason or another, moreover, the emergency units in medium-size hospitals, osteopathic hospitals, hospitals in non-urban areas, and hospitals not having medical teaching affiliations send a smaller proportion of their patients to some other part of the hospital for treatment than is the case of the emergency units in the other groupings for which data are presented in Table 10.

Other results, presented in Table 11, probably reflect the composition of patient in-puts more clearly and more directly than the findings just discussed. The results in question concern the proportion of patients visiting the various emergency units who arrived by ambulance. Other things being equal, it is probably fair to assume that the higher this proportion the greater the average severity of condition exhibited by in-coming patients.

The data about ambulance arrivals were obtained from the physicians and registered nurses working in each unit and, where available, from institutional records. The results summarize both kinds of data. For the 30 EU's in the study considered as an aggregate, the physicians estimate than on the average 15% of the patients visiting their respective units during the most recent month (preceding data collection) arrived by ambulance. Across emergency units this figure ranges from 5% to 41%, indicating considerable inter-unit variability. The corresponding findings from the data provided by the registered nurses (whose estimates are slightly but consistently higher than the estimates provided by physicians) are similar, the average percentage figure in this

TABLE 11. PERCENT OF PATIENTS VISITING THE EMERGENCY UNITS DURING THE MOST RECENT MONTH WHO ARRIVED BY AMBULANCE[a]

Hospital Emergency Units (EU's) Involved		Percent Arriving by Ambulance, According to		
		MDS	RNS	RECS[b]
ALL EU'S IN THE STUDY SAMPLE (N=30 Hospital EU's)	Mean%:	15.3%	17.5%	9.4%
	Range:	(5.1%-41.0%)	(6.3%-32.0%)	(1.5%-29.4%)
YOUR HOSPITAL'S EU				
EU's in:				
Small Hospitals (n=14)		14.0	16.3	8.6
Medium Hospitals (n=9)		13.6	16.0	6.1
Large Hospitals (n=7)		19.9	21.8	14.1
EU's in:				
Church Operated Hospitals (n=9)		14.8	16.3	12.2
Osteopathic Hospitals (n=3)		12.7	13.9	2.8
All Other Hospitals (n=18)		15.9	18.7	8.8
EU's Located in:				
SMSA (urban) Areas (n=21)		16.7	18.7	10.3
Non-SMSA Areas (n=9)		11.9	14.7	7.7
EU's in Hospitals Having:				
Medical Teaching Affiliations (n=17)		16.3	16.6	9.5
No Medical Teaching Affiliations (n=13)		13.9	18.7	9.2
EU's in Hospitals Having:				
Emergency Personnel Training Programs (n=15)		14.3	17.3	11.7
No Training Programs (n=15)		16.2	17.7	7.2

[a] Based both on direct percentage estimates provided by MDS and RNS and on data from hospital records (RECS).

[b] The percentages in this column were first computed (dividing number of ambulance arrivals by total patient visits to the EU) separately for each EU and then averaged for the EU's involved in each grouping. Data from hospital records about ambulance arrivals were available for nineteen of the EU's in the sample.

case being 17.5% and the range being 6%-32%. According to the data from hospital records (available for 19 of the 30 EU's in the study sample), the proportion of patients arriving by ambulance during "the most recent month" is smaller than that estimated by either the physicians or the registered nurses. Specifically, on the average, 9.4% of the patients arrived by ambulance according to these data, the figure ranging across emergency units from 1.5% to 29.4%.

Overall, regardless of the specific source of data, the findings show considerable inter-unit variability on this measure (as for most other measures examined in this chapter). Moreover, the general pattern of findings for the various groupings of EU's is substantially the same according to the data from both MDS and RNS. Briefly, the emergency units of the large hospitals and of hospitals in the urban areas show the highest rates of ambulance arrivals. The data from hospital records are consistent with this findings. (For some additional but less clear cut differences, see Table 11.)

Still another general indicator of the relative severity of condition characterizing the patients visiting the various emergency units is presented in Table 12. This measure is based on the responses of physicians (MDS), registered nurses (RNS) and hospital administrators (HAS) from the institutions studied to the following question: "Over the past four weeks, about what percent of the patients visiting this emergency unit arrived in what you would judge to be a 'life-threatening' condition?"

The estimates provided by MDS are generally somewhat smaller than those provided by RNS, which in turn are somewhat smaller than those provided by HAS. According to the MDS, an average of 6.4% of the patients in their respective emergency units arrived in a "life-threatening" condition. Across units the average ranges from 2.7% to 16.7%, indicating considerable

TABLE 12. PERCENT OF THE PATIENTS VISITING THE EMERGENCY UNITS "OVER THE PAST FOUR WEEKS" WHO ARRIVED IN A "LIFE-THREATENING" CONDITION[a]

		Percent of Patients Arriving in Life-threatening Condition, According to		
Hospital Emergency Units (EU's) Involved		MDS	RNS	HAS
ALL EU'S IN THE STUDY SAMPLE (N=30 Hospital EU's)	*Mean%:* *Range:*	6.4% (2.7%-16.7%)	8.8% (3.2%-16.1%)	9.5% (2.0%-25.0%)
YOUR HOSPITAL'S EU				--
EU's with:				
Low Patient Volume (n=10)		5.5	6.0	9.7
Medium Pat. Volume (n=10)		6.8	9.9	8.3
High Patient Volume (n=10)		7.0	10.5	10.6
EU's in:				
Church Operated Hospitals (n=9)		6.1	7.6	10.4
Osteopathic Hospitals (n=3)		8.0	7.7	8.2
All Other Hospitals (n=18)		6.3	9.6	9.3
EU's Located in:				
SMSA (urban) Areas (n=21)		6.5	8.7	9.0
Non-SMSA Areas (n=9)		6.3	9.1	10.6
EU's in Hospitals Having:				
Medical Teaching Affiliations (n=17)		7.3	8.9	8.8
No Medical Teaching Affiliations (n=13)		5.2	8.7	10.4
EU's in Hospitals Having:				
Emergency Personnel Training Programs (n=15)		7.3	8.8	11.1
No Training Programs (n=15)		5.6	8.8	8.0

[a] Based on direct percentage estimates by MDS, RNS, and HAS from each institution. More than 90% of the RNS, 89% of the MDS, and 79% of the HAS provided these estimates.

variability. According to the data from RNS, the average for the 30 units is 8.8% and the range is 3.2% to 16.1%. The corresponding figures according to the data from HAS are 9.5% and 2.0% to 25.0%, respectively.

Considering next particular groupings of emergency units, the results show that a larger proportion of the patients visiting emergency units with a high patient volume arrived in a "life-threatening" condition, compared to patients in emergency units with a low or medium volume. MDS, RNS, and HAS are all in agreement in this respect, although the differences are small and the proportions associated with high, medium, and low patient volume units vary somewhat depending upon the specific source of data. The data from MDS also indicate that emergency units in hospitals with medical teaching affiliations and emergency personnel training programs receive a somewhat higher proportion of patients in life-threatening condition than do units in hospitals without such programs and affiliations. The data from RNS do not show any differences in this connection.

Perhaps at the other extreme of the spectrum, in contrast to patients arriving in life-threatening condition, are those patients whose medical problems should, or at least could, have been handled in a doctor's office instead of the emergency unit. Relevant data were, therefore, obtained also about the proportion of patients falling into the latter category (sometimes referred to as "primary care" patients or "walk-in" patients). These were provided by (a) the physicians (MDS) working in each emergency unit and (b) selected key physicians from the rest of the hospital (HMDS) in each case. The results are presented in Table 13.

First, it is clear that, according to both MDS and HMDS, the majority of patients visiting the various emergency units (over the past four weeks) "should have gone to a private physician or had a problem that could have been

TABLE 13. PERCENT OF THE PATIENTS VISITING THE EMERGENCY UNIT WHOSE PROBLEMS COULD HAVE BEEN HANDLED IN A DOCTOR'S OFFICE, ACCORDING TO PHYSICIAN RESPONDENTS[a]

		Percent According to	
Hospital Emergency Units (EU's) Involved		MDS	HMDS
ALL EU'S IN THE STUDY SAMPLE (N=30 Hospital EU's)	*Mean%:* *Range:*	55.9% (36.0%-77.0%)	51.8% (28.3%-75.0%)
YOUR HOSPITAL'S EU			
EU's with:			
Low Patient Volume (n=10)		55.9	55.2
Medium Pat. Volume (n=10)		54.8	47.0
High Patient Volume (n=10)		57.1	53.4
EU's in:			
Church Operated Hospitals (n=9)		53.5	60.3
Osteopathic Hospitals (n=3)		54.7	50.6
All Other Hospitals (n=18)		57.4	47.9
EU's Located in:			
SMSA (urban) Areas (n=21)		54.7	49.8
Non-SMSA Areas (n=9)		59.0	56.5
EU's in Hospitals Having:			
Medical Teaching Affiliations (n=17)		56.5	48.1
No Medical Teaching Affiliations (n=13)		55.2	56.8
EU's in Hospitals Having:			
Emergency Personnel Training Programs (n=15)		54.1	51.6
No Training Programs (n=15)		57.8	52.1

[a] Based on direct percentage estimates provided by MDS and HMDS from each institution. The question asked of MDS was: "About what percent of the patients visiting this emergency unit over the past four weeks would you estimate should have gone to a private physician or had a problem that could have been handled in a doctor's office instead of the emergency unit?" The question asked of the HMDS was: "Please think of all the patients visiting this emergency unit who have come to your attention in the past six months or so. About what percent of them would you estimate should have gone to a private physician or had a problem that could have been handled in a doctor's office instead of the emergency unit?" The nonresponse rate was less than 10% in the case of MDS and 16.7% in the case of HMDS.

handled in a doctor's office instead of the emergency unit." The average percentage of such patients for the 30 emergency units in the study turns out to be 56% based on the estimates given by MDS and 52% based on the estimates given by HMDS. Across individual emergency units, the figure ranges from a low of only 36% to a high of 77% in the former case and from 28% to 75% in the latter.

The percent of patients in question is higher for emergency units in non-urban, compared to urban, areas, according to both MDS and HMDS. (Some other differences based on data from the latter are not supported by the data from the former.) Generally, however, the important point is that a very large proportion of the patients who visit hospital emergency units for care are not considered entirely appropriate or "emergency" cases by physicians. The meaning and significance of these findings, of course, remain to be established in further analyses of the data (and also of the data discussed earlier in this chapter concerning the breadth of "emergency service definition" prevailing in the various emergency units).

The Patients' Views of Their Problems

Finally, certain findings about how the patients themselves assess their medical problems are presented in Table 14. These are based on the answers of the participating patient respondents (PATS) to two questions: (a) "How sure were you of what was wrong with you before you arrived at the emergency room?" and (b) "How important was it for you to have received immediate medical attention?"

On the average, the patients from the various emergency units indicate that they had a fairly good idea about what was wrong with them prior to arriving at the unit. (The overall mean score is 2.40, with 2.00 on the

TABLE 14. EMERGENCY UNIT PATIENTS' ASSESSMENTS
OF THEIR PARTICULAR MEDICAL PROBLEMS

Hospital Emergency Units (EU's) Involved		Patients' Responses to	
		"How sure were you of what was wrong with you before you arrived at the emergency room?"[a]	"How important was it for you to have received immediate medical attention?"[b]
ALL EU'S IN THE STUDY SAMPLE (N=30 Hospital EU's)	*Mean:*	2.40	2.49
	Range:	(1.00-3.86)	(1.75-4.00)
YOUR HOSPITAL'S EU			
EU's with:			
Low Patient Volume (n=10)		2.09	2.73
Medium Pat. Volume (n=10)		2.65	2.45
High Patient Volume (n=10)		2.44	2.30
EU's in:			
Church Operated Hospitals (n=9)		2.06	2.87
Osteopathic Hospitals (n=3)		2.56	2.22
All Other Hospitals (n=18)		2.53	2.37
EU's Located in:			
SMSA (urban) Areas (n=21)		2.47	2.52
Non-SMSA Areas (n=9)		2.25	2.43
EU's in Hospitals Having:			
Medical Teaching Affiliations (n=17)		2.67	2.32
No Medical Teaching Affiliations (n=13)		2.04	2.72
EU's in Hospitals Having:			
Emergency Personnel Training Programs (n=15)		2.41	2.47
No Training Programs (n=15)		2.39	2.52

[a] The response alternatives for this question were: (1) Yes, I knew exactly what was wrong, (2) I had a very good idea, (3) I had a fair idea, (4) I had only a vague idea, and (5) No, I did not know what was wrong. Thus, the lower the response, the more certain the patient was about his or her problem.

[b] The response alternatives for this question were: (1) It was extremely important, (2) it was very important, (3) it was fairly important, (4) it was not so important, (5) it was not important at all. Thus, the lower the response, the more urgent the patient thought his or her condition was.

scale corresponding to "a very good idea.") At the same time, there are considerable differences across individual emergency units, the patients of some units indicating much more definitive or much less certain knowledge of their problems than the average score of all the emergency units would suggest. (The relevant means range from 1.00 to 3.86.) Patients in emergency units with low patient volume were more sure, on the average, than their counterparts in medium volume units, with the patients in high volume units occupying an intermediate position. Similarly, patients in church operated units were more sure than those in other institutions. On the other hand, patients in the emergency units of hospitals with medical teaching affiliations were considerably less sure in the knowledge of their problems than were their counterparts in institutions lacking such affiliations.

The average importance, according to the patients, "to have received immediate medical attention" was fairly high to high. The overall mean for all the participating units is 2.49 -- midway between 2.00, which corresponds to "it was very important" to have received immediate attention, and 3.00, which corresponds to "it was fairly important." Again, however, the means range widely, from 1.75 to 4.00, across emergency units, suggesting considerable inter-unit differences on this variable.

Further, the results in Table 14 show that patients visiting the emergency units of institutions with medical affiliations felt it was more important to have received immediate attention than did their counterparts in other institutions. The opposite is true of patients in low volume units, compared to other emergency units, and patients in church operated units, compared to other emergency units. These findings show a reversed pattern when compared to the results about the knowledge which patients had of their problems. It, therefore, appears that the less sure were the patients of a unit about what was wrong with them, the more important they felt it was for them to have received immediate medical attention -- a perfectly rational pattern.

Summary

This chapter presented research findings about some of the general characteristics of the emergency units and their patients. The results indicate substantial differences among individual units and groups of units (based on such things as patient volume, parent hospital size, location, and teaching affiliations), both with respect to the organizational characteristics of the units and the composition of their patient "inputs." Since this is the first chapter of findings, the particular differences revealed by the data were discussed in considerable detail. Some of the most interesting findings concern such things as: the ratio of emergency visits to each hospital's inpatient admissions and inpatient days (suggestive of the relative breadth of "emergency service definition" prevailing in the various emergency units); the percent of patients arriving by ambulance, also in a "life-threatening" condition; the proportion of patients sent to an ICU or another part of the hospital for treatment; the percent of patients who "should have gone to a private physician or whose problems could have been handled in a doctor's office instead of the emergency unit"; and the views of patients about their medical problems. Other findings involve characteristics of the emergency facilities themselves, such as physical plant and layout, affiliations, training programs, and others. The next chapter focuses on the staff resources of the emergency units studied.

Chapter 2

THE STAFF RESOURCES OF EMERGENCY UNITS

In the preceding chapter, findings were presented about certain characteristics of the emergency units and their patient inputs. At least of equal importance are the staff resources available in the various EU's, the subject of the present chapter. Successful unit functioning requires, among other things, adequate staffing, in terms of both quantity and skills. The size, quality, and stability of the staff can greatly facilitate, or hinder, the clinical, economic, and social efficiency of a unit. The availability of sufficient numbers of physicians and registered nurses, in particular, may be a major determinant of organizational effectiveness.

The present chapter focuses on these and other aspects of the staff resources of the emergency units studied. First, it presents certain findings about staff sufficiency, success in obtaining staff to work in the unit, and staff stability. Second, it considers the presence/absence of physicians and registered nurses in the unit, on a 24-hour basis, and the unit's access to various medical specialists within the hospital on an on-call basis. Third, it reviews the medical staffing patterns and the numbers of physicians and physician hours worked in the various units. Fourth, it examines the corresponding characteristics of the nursing staff. And, finally, it presents certain findings about the likely effects of patient volume changes on the staff's work capability or performance.

Most of the results, like those in Chapter 1, are based on data supplied from hospital records (RECS). The balance of the findings, mainly those concerning the sufficiency, stability, and work capability of the staff, are based on interview and questionnaire data from relevant groups of respondents. These latter kinds of data depict the "perceived" staff situation in the various emergency units. Perceived adequacy of resources, however, may reflect not only availability but also the efficiency of resource utilization in an organization. Accordingly, the results about staff sufficiency, stability, and capability should be interpreted in the light of other aspects of the emergency unit's situation that may reflect inefficient or inappropriate resource utilization. The results on economic and clinical efficiency, reported in Chapters 10 and 11 respectively, are especially relevant in this connection, and the reader would be in a better position to evaluate the adequacy of staff resources after examining those two chapters. In fact, a strong argument can be made that available staff resources may be properly evaluated only in the context of the clinical, economic, and social efficiency of a unit, and vice versa.

Sufficiency, Acquisition, and Stability of Resources

The first two tables in this chapter, Tables 15 and 16, respectively show how the hospital administrators (HAS) from the various institutions and the physicians (MDS) who work in the emergency units appraise the sufficiency of staff. They also show, for comparison purposes, how they appraise the sufficiency of the financial and physical resources of EU's. For both staff and these other resources, the respondents were asked to assess sufficiency "considering what the unit needs to provide high quality care to its patients at reasonable cost."

First, according to both administrators and physicians, the quantity of each of the four resources specified -- medical staffing, RN staffing, the unit's budget, and the unit's space and physical facilities -- on the average is at least "fairly sufficient," approaching the "very sufficient" level in some cases. Least sufficient of all, though still "fairly sufficient," according to both administrators and physicians are the physical facilities of emergency units. The two groups also agree, in effect, that second among the four resources in overall sufficiency is the RN staffing of the units, which is regarded almost as "very sufficient" by the HAS (with an overall mean score of 2.33) and midway between "very" and "fairly" sufficient by the MDS (with an overall mean score of 2.43).

The other two resources, however, are assessed differently by the two groups. Specifically, according to the administrators, the budget allocated to the unit is the most sufficient of all four resources, being regarded almost as "very" sufficient (with an overall mean score of 2.26), while according to the physicians the budget is much less adequate, being regarded only as "fairly" sufficient (with a mean score of 2.82) and at about the same level as physical facilities. In contrast, the medical staffing of emergency units is the most sufficient of the four resources according to the MDS, who regard it as "very" sufficient (the overall mean score is 2.15). The administrators assess medical staffing midway between "very" and "fairly" sufficient (the mean score being 2.45), and somewhat as less adequate than either the budget or the RN staffing of the units.

The above patterns, of course, are average patterns, and do not necessarily apply to individual emergency units. In fact, as the range of scores associated with each of the resources shows, there is extremely great variability across EU's in how the respondents assess the sufficiency of a given resource. This is particularly the case in the data from HAS (which, for every resource, show more inter-unit variability than the data from MDS), but even the data from MDS indicate large differences across units. Interestingly,

TABLE 15. SUFFICIENCY OF EMERGENCY UNIT RESOURCES, AS EVALUATED BY HOSPITAL ADMINISTRATION RESPONDENTS (HAS)[a]

Hospital Emergency Units (EU's) Involved		Sufficiency of			
		Medical Staffing of the EU	RN Staffing of the EU	The Budget Allocated to the EU	EU Space and Physical Facilities
ALL EU'S IN THE STUDY SAMPLE (N=30 Hospital EU's)	Mean: Range:	2.45 (1.50-5.00)	2.33 (1.00-4.00)	2.26 (1.00-3.00)	3.07 (1.50-5.00)
YOUR HOSPITAL'S EU		--	--	--	--
EU's with:					
Low Patient Volume (n=10)		2.87	2.17	2.35	3.02
Medium Pat. Volume (n=10)		2.30	2.75	2.43	3.12
High Patient Volume (n=10)		2.18	2.07	2.00	3.08
EU's in:					
Church Operated Hospitals (n=9)		3.09	2.24	2.33	3.06
Osteopathic Hospitals (n=3)		2.00	2.83	2.67	3.00
All Other Hospitals (n=18)		2.20	2.29	2.16	3.09
EU's Located in:					
SMSA (urban) Areas (n=21)		2.14	2.37	2.23	3.29
Non-SMSA Areas (n=9)		3.17	2.22	2.33	2.56
EU's in Hospitals Having:					
Medical Teaching Affiliations (n=17)		2.18	2.46	2.17	3.19
No Medical Teaching Affiliations (n=13)		2.81	2.15	2.38	2.92
EU's in Hospitals Having:					
Emergency Personnel Training Programs (n=15)		2.40	2.26	2.20	3.17
No Training Programs (n=15)		2.50	2.40	2.32	2.98

[a] Based on data from a multiple-part question: "Considering what this emergency unit needs to provide high quality care to its patients at reasonable cost, how sufficient would you say is the quantity (amount) of each of the following resources?" Among the resources specified were those included in the present table. The response alternatives were: (1) Completely sufficient, (2) very sufficient, (3) fairly sufficient, (4) not so sufficient, and (5) not sufficient at all. Thus, the lower the mean scores the more sufficient the quantity of the particular resource. Mean scores were first computed separately for each EU and then averaged for the EU's in the different categories.

TABLE 16. SUFFICIENCY OF EMERGENCY UNIT RESOURCES, AS EVALUATED BY THE PHYSICIANS (MDS) WORKING IN THE UNITS[a]

Hospital Emergency Units (EU's) Involved		Sufficiency of			
		Medical Staffing of the EU	RN Staffing of the EU	The Budget Allocated to the EU[b]	EU Space and Physical Facilities
ALL EU'S IN THE STUDY SAMPLE (N=30 Hospital EU's)	*Mean:* *Range:*	2.15 (1.20-3.50)	2.43 (1.50-3.25)	2.82 (2.17-3.33)	2.95 (1.33-4.44)
YOUR HOSPITAL'S EU					
EU's with:					
Low Patient Volume (n=10)		2.37	2.46	2.81	2.66
Medium Pat. Volume (n=10)		1.95	2.31	2.72	3.11
High Patient Volume (n=10)		2.15	2.51	2.93	3.08
EU's in:					
Church Operated Hospitals (n=9)		2.46	2.66	3.01	3.04
Osteopathic Hospitals (n=3)		2.10	2.63	2.90	2.97
All Other Hospitals (n=18)		2.01	2.27	2.71	2.90
EU's Located in:					
SMSA (urban) Areas (n=21)		2.08	2.47	2.76	2.97
Non-SMSA Areas (n=9)		2.33	2.32	2.95	2.90
EU's in Hospitals Having:					
Medical Teaching Affiliations (N=17)		2.01	2.47	2.81	2.98
No Medical Teaching Affiliations (n=13)		2.34	2.37	2.83	2.90
EU's in Hospitals Having:					
Emergency Personnel Training Programs (n=15)		2.11	2.45	2.84	3.02
No Training Programs (n=15)		2.20	2.40	2.80	2.88

Table 16 Continues

TABLE 16
(Continued)

---

[a] Based on data from a multiple-part question: "Considering what this emergency unit needs to provide high quality care to its patients at reasonable cost, how sufficient would you say is the quantity (amount) of each of the following resources?" Among the resources specified were those included in the present table. The response alternatives were: (1) Completely sufficient, (2) very sufficient, (3) fairly sufficient, (4) not so sufficient, and (5) not sufficient at all. Thus, the lower the mean scores, the more sufficient the quantity of the particular resource. Mean scores were first computed separately for each EU and then averaged for the EU's in the different categories.

[b] Nearly 14% of the MDS were unable to respond to the question with reference to the budget.

the smallest variability according to both HAS and MDS involves the sufficiency of the budget, which apparently differs less from one unit to another than does the sufficiency of each of the other three resources (of which space and physical facilities are the most variable in terms of sufficiency). More important, of course, the variability across emergency units is very substantial for both medical and RN staffing, more so for the former, according to the data from both administrators and physicians, and especially the administrators.

Considering next the staff resources of the various groupings of EU's, it is clear from the results in Tables 15 and 16, that the quantity of medical staff in the units of hospitals which are not church operated is generally evaluated as more sufficient, by both HAS and MDS, than it is in the case of church operated hospitals. Similarly, the emergency units of hospitals with medical teaching affiliations also are seen to have, on the average, more sufficient medical staffing than do the units of hospitals lacking such affiliations, by both groups of respondents but especially the administrators. Interestingly, however, the latter have more sufficient RN staffing than do the former, based on the data from HAS (the difference is in the same direction but minimal according to the data from MDS). The same pattern emerges, moreover, with respect to both medical and RN staffing, when comparing the results for emergency units in urban and non-urban areas. Finally, with respect to patient volume, the results show that medical staffing is, on the average, regarded as least sufficient in emergency units with a low patient volume by both HAS and MDS (the two groups fail to agree, however, about the sufficiency of RN staffing as it relates to patient volume).

However sufficient the staff resources of an emergency unit may be at any particular time, it is also important for a unit to be able to obtain particular kinds of staff when needed. Findings concerning the relative success of emergency units in obtaining requested staff resources from their parent hospitals are presented in Table 17. The resources in question include doctors to work in the EU, doctors on call to the EU, and registered nurses for the EU. The results are based on data from the registered nurses (RNS) working in the various units.

For all the EU's in the study sample, the findings show that, on the average, emergency units are usually able to obtain "most" of what they request concerning each of the three kinds of staff resources specified. Overall success, in this respect, is about equal for doctors to work in the unit, doctors on call, and registered nurses. The results also show, however, that across individual units success varies considerably. Regarding doctors to work in the unit, some of the EU's are usually able to obtain "all or nearly all" of what they request while, at the other extreme, some other EU's are only able to obtain "about half" of what they request. The same pattern holds regarding requests for registered nurses. And for doctors on call, the differences across units are even more pronounced, some of the units being able to obtain "less than half" of what they request.

Although inter-unit variability (see the ranges of mean scores in Table 17) concerning success in obtaining each of the requested staff resources is very substantial, the differences from one grouping of emergency units to another (based on location, parent hospital size, etc.) are not. The data concerning requests for registered nurses, in particular, show practically no differences. Concerning requests for doctors to work in the unit, it appears that the units of osteopathic hospitals are the most successful while their counterparts in church operated hospitals are the least successful. The emergency units of large hospitals are usually more successful than those of small hospitals (those in medium-size hospitals occupy an intermediate

TABLE 17. THE RELATIVE SUCCESS OF EMERGENCY UNITS IN OBTAINING REQUESTED STAFF RESOURCES, ACCORDING TO THE REGISTERED NURSES (RNS)[a]

Hospital Emergency Units (EU's) Involved		Success in Obtaining		
		Doctors to Work in the EU	Doctors on-call to the EU[b]	Registered Nurses for the EU
ALL EU'S IN THE STUDY SAMPLE (N=30 Hospital EU's)	Mean:	1.89	1.95	1.93
	Range:	(1.00-3.00)	(1.17-4.00)	(1.00-2.83)
YOUR HOSPITAL'S EU				
EU's in:				
Small Hospitals (n=14)		1.92	2.21	1.93
Medium Hospitals (n=9)		1.96	1.81	2.05
Large Hospitals (n=7)		1.73	1.62	1.78
EU's in:				
Church Operated Hospitals (n=9)		2.11	2.19	1.96
Osteopathic Hospitals (n=3)		1.67	2.14	2.20
All Other Hospitals (n=18)		1.81	1.80	1.87
EU's Located in:				
SMSA (urban) Areas (n=21)		1.83	1.89	1.96
Non-SMSA Areas (n=9)		2.02	2.10	1.86
EU's in Hospitals Having:				
Medical Teaching Affiliations (n=17)		1.79	1.68	2.03
No Medical Teaching Affiliations (n=13)		2.02	2.30	1.80
EU's in Hospitals Having:				
Emergency Personnel Training Programs (n=15)		1.91	1.96	1.85
No Training Programs (n=15)		1.86	1.95	2.01

[a] The mean scores shown are based on data from the question: "Considering this emergency unit's requests to the hospital for resources of each of the following kinds, on the whole, how successful is the emergency unit in obtaining the requested resources?" The response alternatives were: "(1) Usually this unit obtains all or nearly all of what it requests, (2) most of what it requests, (3) about half of what it requests, and (4) less than half of what it requests." Accordingly, the <u>lower</u> the mean scores, the <u>greater</u> the success in obtaining the requested staff resources.

[b] For this item, 15% of the RNS did not know or could not answer.

position) concerning their requests for doctors on call. Units in hospitals which are not church operated (but excluding osteopathic institutions) are similarly more successful in this respect than are units in church operated hospitals. Finally, the emergency units of hospitals with medical teaching affiliations are usually more successful than those in hospitals without such affiliations in having their requests for doctors on call met.

The stability of staff resources is another important variable measured in the study. The data in this case were obtained from the supervising nurses (SRNS) in the various units, in response to the following question: "Considering both their quantity and quality (or adequacy), how stable over time would you say are the resources available to the emergency unit?" The question was asked about the physicians and about the nurses working in each unit. The results are summarized in Table 18.

On the average, the SRNS see the nursing staff of their respective units as "very stable" (the overall mean score is 2.14), but depending upon the particular unit the situation ranges from "extremely stable" to only "fairly stable." It is even more variable for medical staffing, ranging from "extremely stable" to "not so stable," although on the average the medical staff for all the EU's in the sample also is seen as almost "very stable" (the overall mean score is 2.34) by the supervising nurses. Generally, the medical staff of emergency units is regarded as more stable (a) in osteopathic hospitals than other institutions (the same tends to be true of the nursing staff), particularly in church operated institutions, (b) in units with a high patient volume compared to a medium or low volume, and (c) in units located in urban compared to other areas. The results show no comparable differences, for either the medical or the nursing staff, between institutions with and without medical teaching affiliations or institutions with and without emergency personnel training programs.

TABLE 18. EMERGENCY UNIT STAFF STABILITY, AS ASSESSED BY THE SUPERVISING NURSES (SRNS)[a]

Hospital Emergency Units (EU's) Involved		Mean Stability Level for Emergency Unit Physicians	Mean Stability Level for Emergency Unit Nurses
ALL EU'S IN THE STUDY SAMPLE (N=30 Hospital EU's)	Mean:	2.34	2.14
	Range:	(1.00-4.00)	(1.00-3.00)
YOUR HOSPITAL'S EU		--	--
EU's with:			
Low Patient Volume (n=10)		2.55	2.20
Medium Pat. Volume (n=10)		2.50	2.25
High Patient Volume (n=10)		1.97	1.97
EU's in:			
Church Operated Hospitals (n=9)		2.78	2.39
Osteopathic Hospitals (n=3)		1.67	1.83
All Other Hospitals (n=18)		2.23	2.06
EU's Located in:			
SMSA (urban) Areas (n=21)		2.25	2.13
Non-SMSA Areas (n=9)		2.56	2.17
EU's in Hospitals Having:			
Medical Teaching Affiliations (n=17)		2.24	2.24
No Medical Teaching Affiliations (n=13)		2.47	2.01
EU's in Hospitals Having:			
Emergency Personnel Training Programs (n=15)		2.28	2.11
No Training Programs (n=15)		2.40	2.17

[a] The results are based on data from the question: "Considering both their quantity and quality (or adequacy), how stable over time would you say are the resources available to the emergency unit?" The response alternatives were: (1) Extremely stable, (2) very stable, (3) fairly stable, (4) not so stable, and (5) not stable at all. Accordingly, the lower the mean scores shown, the more stable the staff over time.

Certain additional data concerning staff stability were provided by hospital administrators (HAS), who were asked to indicate how easy/difficult it is for their respective institutions to "recruit and maintain professional nursing staff for the emergency unit." (These data are not included in Table 18.) On the average, HAS indicated only some difficulty in this connection, reporting intermediately between "it is fairly easy" and "not as easy as it should be" (but closer to the latter). Overall, hospitals apparently do not experience substantial difficulty. As with the other measures, inter-unit variability is again very large. Some individual hospitals, in other words, experience considerable difficulty, while others do not, in recruiting and maintaining professional nursing staff for their emergency unit. The data show no appreciable differences, however, between one grouping of EU's and another.

A final measure concerning the stability, and possibly also adequacy, of the regular medical and nursing staff working in the various EU's deals with the physical presence of registered nurses and physicians in the unit on a 24-hour basis. The pertinent data, supplied from hospital records, are summarized in Table 19.

Exactly two-thirds of the hospitals in the study report having at least one RN physically present in their emergency unit at all times. All units with a high patient volume report this to be the case, compared to fewer than half of the units which have a low patient volume, and slightly more than half of the medium volume units. The large majority of institutions with teaching affiliations, and also training programs, likewise report having an RN physically present in the unit at all times, compared to just less than half of the institutions which do not have such affiliations or training programs. Similarly, fewer than half of the osteopathic and church operated

TABLE 19. PHYSICAL PRESENCE OF PHYSICIANS AND REGISTERED NURSES
IN THE VARIOUS EMERGENCY UNITS AT DIFFERENT TIMES[a]

Hospital Emergency Units (EU's) Involved	A doctor is physically present during the			An RN is physically present at all times
	Day Shift	Evening Shift	Night Shift	
ALL EU'S IN THE STUDY SAMPLE (N=30 Hospital EU's) n: %:	18 (60.0%)	19 (63.3%)	20 (66.7%)	20 (66.7%)
EU's with:				
Low Patient Volume (n=10)	2	2	2	4
Medium Pat. Volume (n=10)	6	7	8	6
High Patient Volume (n=10)	10	10	10	10
EU's in:				
Church Operated Hospitals (n=9)	3	3	3	4
Osteopathic Hospitals (n=3)	2	2	2	1
All Other Hospitals (n=18)	13	14	15	15
EU's Located in:				
SMSA (urban) Areas (n=21)	15	15	16	15
Non-SMSA Areas (n=9)	3	4	4	5
EU's in Hospitals Having:				
Medical Teaching Affiliations (n=17)	13	13	14	14
No Medical Teaching Affiliations (n=13)	5	6	6	6
EU's in Hospitals Having:				
Emergency Personnel Training Programs (n=15)	11	12	12	13
No Training Programs (n=15)	7	7	8	7

[a] Based on data from hospital records (RECS).

institutions have an RN physically present, compared to the large majority of the other hospitals. Finally, proportionately more of the institutions located in urban, compared to non-urban, areas have an RN physically present in their emergency unit at all times.

With only minor exceptions, the data concerning the physical presence of a physician in the unit show very similar patterns to those above concerning the presence of RN's. Of the 30 EU's in the study, 18, 19, and 20, respectively, report that a doctor is physically present in the unit during the day, evening, and night shifts. It is perhaps of some interest that the night shift is at least as well off, in this respect, as either of the other two shifts. Apart from this finding, the important thing to reiterate is that the patterns of physician presence in relation to the various groupings of emergency units are basically the same as those found for registered nurses, as discussed above. As with other measures, of course, for individual emergency units the patterns in question may differ considerably.

Access to On-Call Medical Specialists Within the Hospital

In addition to their "regular" medical and nursing staff, emergency units typically have access, on an on-call basis, to a variety of medical specialists who are on the hospital's staff. A complete understanding of EU staff resources, therefore, also requires information about each unit's access to such specialists. Accordingly, relevant data on this aspect were obtained from the hospital records supplied by each institution. These data are summarized in Table 20.

Of the ten different specialists about whom information was asked, a cardiologist from the parent hospital is available to the emergency unit on-call for 20 of the 30 EU's in the study (in one case the cardiologist is

TABLE 20. ON-CALL AVAILABILITY TO THE EMERGENCY UNITS
OF PARTICULAR MEDICAL SPECIALISTS[a]

Hospital Emergency Units (EU's) Involved		Cardio-logist	Obste-trician/ Gynecol-ogist	Pedia-trician	Psychia-trist	Oral Surgeon
Number of EU's With Designated Specialist On Call						
ALL EU'S IN THE STUDY SAMPLE (N=30 Hospital EU's)	n: %:	20 (66.7%)	16 (53.3%)	14 (46.7%)	14 (46.7%)	14 (46.7%)
EU's with:						
Low Patient Volume (n=10)		5	3	2	3	4
Medium Pat. Volume (n=10)		7	7	6	6	5
High Patient Volume (n=10)		8	6	6	5	5
EU's in:						
Church Operated Hospitals (n=9)		4	3	2	3	3
Osteopathic Hospitals (n=3)		2	1	1	0	1
All Other Hospitals (n=18)		14	12	11	11	10
EU's Located in:						
SMSA (urban) Areas (n=21)		13	11	11	8	9
Non-SMSA Areas (n=9)		7	5	3	6	5
EU's in Hospitals Having:						
Medical Teaching Affilia-tions (n=17)		12	10	10	9	9
No Medical Teaching Af-filiations (n=13)		8	6	4	5	5
EU's in Hospitals Having:						
Emergency Personnel Train-ing Programs (n=15)		9	8	6	6	6
No Training Programs (n=15)		11	8	8	8	8

Table 20 Continues

TABLE 20. (Cont.) ON-CALL AVAILABILITY TO THE EMERGENCY UNITS OF PARTICULAR MEDICAL SPECIALISTS[a]

		Number of EU's with Designated Specialist On Call				
Hospital Emergency Units (EU's) Involved		Ophthal-mologist	Ortho-pedist	Neuro-surgeon	Plastic surgeon	Burn Specialist
ALL EU'S IN THE STUDY SAMPLE (N=30 Hospital EU's)	n: %:	13 (43.3%)	13 (43.3%)	7 (23.3%)	5 (16.7%)	2 (6.7%)
EU's with:						
Low Patient Volume (n=10)		3	3	0	0	0
Medium Pat. Volume (n=10)		5	5	4	2	2
High Patient Volume (n=10)		5	5	3	3	0
EU's in:						
Church Operated Hospitals (n=9)		2	2	0	0	0
Osteopathic Hospitals (n=3)		1	2	1	0	0
All Other Hospitals (n=18)		10	9	6	5	2
EU's Located in:						
SMSA (urban) Areas (n=21)		9	9	7	5	2
Non-SMSA Areas (n=9)		4	4	0	0	0
EU's in Hospitals Having:						
Medical Teaching Affiliations (n=17)		8	8	6	4	2
No Medical Teaching Affiliations (n=13)		5	5	1	1	0
EU's in Hospitals Having:						
Emergency Personnel Training Programs (n=15)		6	6	4	3	0
No Training Programs (n=15)		7	7	3	2	2

[a] Based on data from hospital records (RECS). The data concern medical specialists only <u>within the parent hospital</u> who are on-call to the EU. Of all the medical specialists listed, however, one cardiologist, one oral surgeon, one orthopedist, and one psychiatrist were on duty within the EU of their respective hospitals rather than just on call.

working within the unit). Similarly an obstetrician or gynecologist is available on call for 16 of the units. Fourteen of the 30 EU's (not necessarily the same ones) have similar access to a pediatrician, to a psychiatrist (in one case a psychiatrist is working within the unit), and to an oral surgeon (again, in one case an oral surgeon is working within the unit). And 13 of them have similar access to an ophthalmologist, and to an orthopedist (in one case an orthopedist is working within the unit). At the other extreme, only 2, 5, and 7 of all the emergency units, respectively, have comparable access to a specialist in burn medicine, to a plastic surgeon, and to a neurosurgeon. These latter three specialists are only available to units which have a high or medium patient volume, in hospitals which are not church operated, and in hospitals located in urban areas.

It follows that the rest of the emergency units, in each case, apparently have no access on an on-call basis within their parent hospital to the designated medical specialist. Overall, as might be expected, on-call availability of the various medical specialists is more scarce for emergency units having a low patient volume than for other units; for the emergency units of hospitals which do not have medical teaching affiliations, compared to those which do; and for the emergency units of the church operated and osteopathic hospitals, compared to other hospitals in the study. (It should be remembered in this connection, however, that large church operated institutions are underrepresented among the institutions that cooperated in the research.)

Medical Staffing Pattern, Staff Size, and Physician Hours Worked

The distribution of emergency units with particular basic staffing patterns is portrayed in Table 21. The data were provided by the chief executive officer of each participating hospital. Very briefly, nine of the

TABLE 21. NUMBER OF EMERGENCY UNITS WITH PARTICULAR MEDICAL STAFFING PATTERNS, AS REPORTED BY THE CHIEF EXECUTIVE OFFICER OF EACH HOSPITAL[a]

Hospital Emergency Units (EU's) Involved		Basic Medical Staffing Pattern				
		Rotation of attending staff	Contract with hospital-based group	Contract with nonhospital-based group or corporation	Individual doctors on contract (full-time or part-time)	All other
ALL EU'S IN THE STUDY SAMPLE (N=30 Hospital EU's)	n:	7	5	9	4	5
	%:	(23%)	(17%)	(30%)	(13%)	(17%)
EU's with:						
Low Patient Volume (n=10)		5	0	3	0	2
Medium Pat. Volume (n=10)		2	0	3	3	2
High Patient Volume (n=10)		0	5	3	1	1
EU's in:						
Church Operated Hospitals (n=9)		4	2	0	1	2
Osteopathic Hospitals (n=3)		0	0	3	0	0
All Other Hospitals (n=18)		3	3	6	3	3
EU's Located in:						
SMSA (urban) Areas (n=21)		3	4	7	4	3
Non-SMSA Areas (n=9)		4	1	2	0	2
EU's in Hospitals Having:						
Medical Teaching Affiliations (n=17)		1	5	6	2	3
No Medical Teaching Affiliations (n=13)		6	0	3	2	2
EU's in Hospitals Having:						
Emergency Personnel Training Programs (n=15)		4	5	5	1	0
No Training Programs (n=15)		3	0	4	3	5

[a] For four of the 30 EU's in the study, the basic medical staffing pattern represented a modified version of one or another of the patterns shown here.

emergency units are reported as having a contractual arrangement with some non-hospital based group or corporation. Seven other units are staffed by rotating medical staff from their parent hospital. An additional five units have a contractual arrangement with a hospital-based group and four more are staffed with individual doctors (full- or part-time) on contract. The remaining five units report some other basic staffing pattern -- in most cases a modified version of one or another of the preceding patterns.

Examination of the various groupings of EU's shows a number of interesting differences in medical staffing patterns. Half of the units with a low patient volume, for example, rely on rotation of their parent hospital's attending staff, while none of the high-volume units uses this type of arrangement. The latter units tend to rely on contractual arrangements with either some hospital based group (none of the low-volume or medium-volume units uses this arrangement) or, less frequently, a non-hospital based group. The medium-volume units use all of the several staffing patterns, except the one noted, about equally.

Other findings show that the emergency units of church operated institutions use hospital staff rotation (but no contractual arrangements with non-hospital based groups -- the most common pattern for the total sample) more than do the units of other institutions. The units of hospitals with teaching affiliations most commonly use contractual arrangements either with non-hospital based or with hospital-based groups. Their counterparts in hospitals with no teaching affiliations use attending staff rotation more than any of the other staffing patterns. And the EU's of hospitals which have emergency personnel training programs predominantly use contractual group arrangements, while relatively few of the units in the rest of the hospitals do.

The next two tables, Tables 22 and 23, respectively summarizing data from hospital records (RECS) and from the physicians (MDS) working in the various EU's, present findings about medical staff size and physician hours worked. They both deal with the same variables, but one relies on information from records while the other relies on information from physicians. More specifically, they both show: (a) the average number of physicians working in the units whether full- or part-time; (b) the total number of hours worked within the units by these physicians; and (c) the average number of hours worked per physician. As usual, results are shown for the total sample of EU's as well as for the various groupings of EU's used in the present report.

It will be noted that the medical staffing data from hospital records (Table 22) are about the "most recent week" prior to fieldwork for which the information was available at each institution, and that five of the 30 hospitals were unable to supply relevant information. The parallel data provided by physicians (Table 23), on the other hand, were obtained from those particular physicians (MDS) who were working in each emergency unit during the week of fieldwork; and, the work hours reported by these physicians refer to an "ordinary" week. Consequently, findings in the two tables are not completely comparable in a strict sense. In spite of the differences between the two tables concerning the total number of EU's, the particular physicians to whom the data pertain, and the relevant time frames involved, the findings in the two tables are still very similar.

First, for the 25 EU's for which data were available from records, Table 22 shows that the average number of physicians working in the various units was 7.8 per unit (the number ranges from a low of 1 to a high of 22 across individual EU's). During the "most recent week," these physicians

TABLE 22. NUMBER OF PHYSICIANS WHO WORKED IN THE EMERGENCY UNIT AND
PHYSICIAN HOURS WORKED DURING THE MOST RECENT WEEK,
BASED ON DATA FROM HOSPITAL RECORDS (RECS)[a]

Hospital Emergency Units (EU's) Involved		Number of Physicians[b]	Total Physician Hours Worked	Average Number of Hours per Physician
ALL EU'S IN THE STUDY SAMPLE (N=25 Hospital EU's)[a]	Mean: Range:	7.8 (1-22)	151 (25-252)	24.5 (3.9-48.0)
YOUR HOSPITAL'S EU				
EU's with:				
Low Patient Volume (n=7)		5.7	92	23.2
Medium Pat. Volume (n=8)		7.4	160	23.8
High Patient Volume (n=10)		9.7	185	25.8
EU's in:				
Church Operated Hospitals (n=7)		7.4	100	21.1
Osteopathic Hospitals (n=3)		6.0	164	29.4
All Other Hospitals (n=15)		8.4	172	25.0
EU's Located in:				
SMSA (urban) Areas (n=19)		8.9	158	21.9
Non-SMSA Areas (n=6)		4.5	130	32.6
EU's in Hospitals Having:				
Medical Teaching Affiliations (n=15)		8.5	171	27.0
No Medical Teaching Affiliations (n=10)		6.9	121	20.6
EU's in Hospitals Having:				
Emergency Personnel Training Programs (n=13)		8.9	162	22.1
No Training Programs (n=12)		6.7	139	27.0

[a] The numbers shown under each column were first computed separately for every EU and then averaged for the EU's involved in each grouping. Five of the 30 EU's in the study were unable to provide the necessary data.

[b] Includes the total number of individuals who worked, regardless of the number of hours that they worked.

TABLE 23. NUMBER OF PHYSICIAN HOURS WORKED IN THE EMERGENCY UNIT DURING A TYPICAL WEEK BY THE PHYSICIANS (MDS) WHO PARTICIPATED IN THE STUDY, BASED ON THEIR OWN REPORTS[a]

Hospital Emergency Units (EU's) Involved		Number of MDS[b]	Total Number of Hours Worked by MDS	Average Number of Hours Worked per Person
ALL EU'S IN THE STUDY SAMPLE (N=30 Hospital EU's)	Mean: Range:	6.8 (3-12)	124 (25-231)	21.1 (3.6-48.0)
YOUR HOSPITAL'S EU				
EU's with:				
Low Patient Volume (n=10)		7.6	89	12.7
Medium Pat. Volume (n=10)		6.1	128	23.1
High Patient Volume (n=10)		6.6	155	27.5
EU's in:				
Church Operated Hospitals (n=9)		7.7	81	11.5
Osteopathic Hospitals (n=3)		5.7	161	32.2
All Other Hospitals (n=18)		6.5	140	24.0
EU's Located in:				
SMSA (urban) Areas (n=21)		7.2	136	21.9
Non-SMSA Areas (n=9)		5.8	97	19.1
EU's in Hospitals Having:				
Medical Teaching Affiliations (n=17)		6.5	141	24.9
No Medical Teaching Affiliations (n=13)		7.2	101	16.2
EU's in Hospitals Having:				
Emergency Personnel Training Programs (n=15)		6.9	122	20.0
No Training Programs (n=15)		6.7	126	22.2

[a] The numbers shown under each column were first computed separately for every EU and then averaged for the EU's involved in each grouping. All are based on questionnaire data.

[b] Includes all MDS, regardless of the number of hours that they worked, who completed questionnaires for the study (which closely approaches the number of physicians working in the various EU's during the week of field work).

worked a combined total of 151 hours (the number ranges from 25 to 252 hours across units). And the average number of hours worked per physician is 24.5 (with an inter-unit range of 3.9 to 48.0). The corresponding numbers and ranges based on the self-reported data by the physicians working in the 30 emergency units during field work, as shown in Table 23, are: 6.8 (range 3-12), 124 (range 25-231), and 21.1 (range 3.6-48.0), respectively.

Obviously, there are large differences among individual emergency units in the number of physicians who work there, the total hours worked by them, and the average number of hours worked per physician. The number of hours worked per physician is highest, on the average, for units with a high patient volume and lowest for units with a low patient volume (the medium-volume units occupy an intermediate position), according to the data in both Table 22 and Table 23. Similarly, according to both sets of data, the average number of hours per physician is higher for the units of hospitals which are not church operated than for the units of church operated institutions. In addition, it is higher for the emergency units of hospitals with medical teaching affiliations than for their counterparts in hospitals without such affiliations.

Readers may wish to examine Tables 22 and 23 in greater detail. Even more important, they may wish to examine the findings about physician staffing (and also those about nurse staffing presented below) in the light of the results on economic efficiency and clinical efficiency, which are discussed in Chapters 10 and 11 of this report. Among other things, for example, Table 89 in Chapter 10, shows number of patient visits in relation to number of hours worked by doctors and by registered nurses in the various emergency units.

Non-Medical Staffing Patterns

Presented in this section are findings about the non-medical staffing of emergency units. These are analogous to the above findings about medical staffing. First, the numbers of budgeted positions for nurses and other unit personnel are considered (Table 24). Then, the numbers of registered nurses and registered nurse hours worked in the various units are examined, using data from hospital records (Table 25). Finally, comparable data reported by the registered nurses themselves are presented (Table 26) and discussed.

Table 24 shows the number of FTE positions budgeted in the various emergency units for registered nurses (including supervising nurses), licensed practical nurses, technicians, other non-medical personnel, and all of these groups combined. The data are from hospital records (RECS) for the "most recent quarter" in all cases. For all of the non-medical groups combined, Table 24 shows an average total of 13.3 budgeted FTE positions per emergency unit. Across individual units, however, this number varies widely, from a low of only 1.0 position to a high of 31.0 positions. Almost exactly half of these budgeted positions, or an average 6.6 per unit, are for registered nurses. An additional 2.8 positions are for licensed practical nurses. Of the remaining FTE budgeted positions, 1.1 are for technicians and 2.8 are for all other non-medical personnel working in the emergency unit.

For each of the groups involved, and all of them combined, the average total number of budgeted positions per unit is larger for units having a high patient volume (which average a total of 21.6 non-medical positions each) than for units having a medium patient volume (which average 12.4 positions) or a low patient volume (which average only 6.0 positions). The emergency units of hospitals in urban areas also average a larger number of FTE budgeted positions for non-medical staff than their counterparts in non-urban

TABLE 24. NUMBER OF BUDGETED POSITIONS FOR NON-MEDICAL PERSONNEL IN THE EMERGENCY UNITS STUDIED, FOR MOST RECENT QUARTER[a]

Hospital Emergency Units (EU's) Involved		FTE Budgeted Positions for				
		Registered Nurses	Licensed Practical Nurses	Technicians	All Other	TOTAL
ALL EU'S IN THE STUDY SAMPLE (N=30 Hospital EU's)	Mean:	6.6	2.8	1.1	2.8	13.3
	Range:	(2.5-14.3)	(0.0-10.8)	(0.0-7.4)	(0.0-11.5)	(1.0-31.0)
YOUR HOSPITAL'S EU						
EU's with:						
Low Patient Volume (n=10)		4.1	1.4	0.3	0.6	6.0
Medium Pat. Volume (n=10)		5.9	3.2	0.4	3.6	12.4
High Patient Volume (n=10)		10.0	4.0	2.7	4.7	21.6
EU's in:						
Church Operated Hospitals (n=9)		5.4	2.1	0.1	2.1	11.7
Osteopathic Hospitals (n=3)		5.0	3.0	0.0	4.0	11.0
All Other Hospitals (n=18)		7.7	3.2	2.0	3.0	14.6
EU's Located in:						
SMSA (urban) Areas (n=21)		7.0	3.0	1.1	3.3	15.1
Non-SMSA Areas (n=9)		5.6	2.3	1.1	1.7	9.2
EU's in Hospitals Having:						
Medical Teaching Affiliations (n=17)		8.3	3.7	1.3	4.1	15.9
No Medical Teaching Affiliations (n=13)		4.4	1.7	0.9	1.3	9.9
EU's in Hospitals Having:						
Emergency Personnel Training Programs (n=15)		7.9	2.9	1.4	3.1	15.8
No Training Programs (n=15)		5.1	2.7	0.9	2.5	10.9

[a] Based on data from hospital records (RECS). For all non-medical budgeted positions combined, shown under "TOTAL," data were available for all 30 hospital EU's. For each of the other four columns data were available for 27 of the 30 EU's.

areas (15.1 vs. 9.2 positions). The same pattern holds true for units in hospitals with teaching affiliations, and emergency personnel training programs, than for their counterparts in hospitals which do not have these characteristics. More important, perhaps, is the fact that all of these patterns hold true when considering registered nurse staffing separately. As pointed out earlier, the emergency units in the study average a total of 6.6 FTE budgeted positions for registered nurses (which accounts for half of all the budgeted positions for medical personnel). For individual emergency units, however, this number ranges from a low of 2.5 to a high of 14.3, indicating great inter-unit variability in highly skilled nurse staff resources.

The next two tables, Tables 25 and 26, based on data from hospital records (RECS) and from the registered nurses (RNS) working in the various EU's, respectively, show: the number of registered nurses working in the unit; the total number of hours worked by these nurses; and the average hours worked per RN. As with the parallel data about physicians that were discussed earlier, the information summarized in Table 25 pertains to the "most recent week," while the information in Table 26 was provided by the registered nurses who were actually working in each unit during the week in which the fieldwork was scheduled and whose reported work hours are about a "typical week."

The findings in the two tables are remarkably alike (and more similar than was the case for the corresponding findings about physicians earlier), in spite of the different data sources and time frames involved, indicating strong validity both for the data from records and for the questionnaire data provided by registered nurse respondents. The results in Table 25 show that the average number of RN's working in the emergency units during the "most recent week" was 8.9 per unit, ranging across units from a low of 4 to a high of 16 (indicative of a four-fold variation). These nurses worked a combined

TABLE 25. NUMBER OF REGISTERED NURSES WHO WORKED IN THE EMERGENCY UNIT AND NUMBER OF HOURS WORKED BY THEM DURING THE MOST RECENT WEEK, BASED ON DATA FROM HOSPITAL RECORDS (RECS)[a]

Hospital Emergency Units (EU's) Involved		Number of Registered Nurses	Total Registered Nurse Hours Worked	Average Number of Hours per Registered Nurse[b]
ALL EU'S IN THE STUDY SAMPLE (N=30 Hospital EU's)	*Mean:* *Range:*	8.9 (4-16)	239 (104-568)	26.7 (10.6-36.0)
YOUR HOSPITAL'S EU				
EU's with:				
Low Patient Volume (n=10)		7.4	162	23.5
Medium Pat. Volume (n=10)		7.4	188	25.6
High Patient Volume (n=10)		12.0	367	31.0
EU's in:				
Church Operated Hospitals (n=9)		7.2	190	26.3
Osteopathic Hospitals (n=3)		8.0	192	23.6
All Other Hospitals (n=18)		9.9	271	27.4
EU's Located in:				
SMSA (urban) Areas (n=21)		9.8	260	26.7
Non-SMSA Areas (n=9)		7.0	189	26.7
EU's in Hospitals Having:				
Medical Teaching Affiliations (n=17)		9.6	277	28.5
No Medical Teaching Affiliations (n=13)		8.0	189	24.3
EU's in Hospitals Having:				
Emergency Personnel Training Programs (n=15)		10.1	297	28.5
No Training Programs (n=15)		7.7	181	24.8

[a] The numbers shown under each column were first computed separately for every EU and then averaged for the EU's involved in each grouping.

[b] Includes total number of persons who worked, whether full-time or part-time.

TABLE 26. NUMBER OF REGISTERED NURSE HOURS WORKED IN THE EMERGENCY UNIT
DURING A TYPICAL WEEK BY THE REGISTERED NURSES (RNS) WHO
PARTICIPATED IN THE STUDY, BASED ON THEIR OWN REPORTS[a]

		As Reported by RNS:		
Hospital Emergency Units (EU's) Involved		Number of RNS[b]	Total Number of Hours Worked by RNS	Average Number of Hours Worked per Person
ALL EU'S IN THE STUDY SAMPLE (N=30 Hospital EU's)	*Mean:* *Range:*	8.8 (4-17)	242 (102-512)	27.1 (17.1-37.3)
YOUR HOSPITAL'S EU				
EU's with:				
Low Patient Volume (n=10)		7.5	164	23.2
Medium Pat. Volume (n=10)		7.4	201	26.8
High Patient Volume (n=10)		11.6	361	31.4
EU's in:				
Church Operated Hospitals (n=9)		8.4	209	24.6
Osteopathic Hospitals (n=3)		9.3	220	23.0
All Other Hospitals (n=18)		8.9	262	29.1
EU's Located in:				
SMSA (urban) Areas (n=21)		9.1	253	27.4
Non-SMSA Areas (n=9)		8.2	215	26.4
EU's in Hospitals Having:				
Medical Teaching Affiliations (n=17)		9.1	272	29.6
No Medical Teaching Affiliations (n=13)		8.5	202	23.9
EU's in Hospitals Having:				
Emergency Personnel Training Programs (n=15)		9.8	288	29.0
No Training Programs (n=15)		7.9	196	25.3

[a] The numbers shown under each column were first computed separately for every EU and then averaged for the EU's involved in each grouping. All are based on questionnaire data.

[b] Includes all RNS, whether working full-time or part-time, who completed questionnaires for the study (which is almost identical to the number of registered nurses working in the various EU's during the week of field work).

total of 239 hours during that week (the number ranges from 104 to 568). And the average number of hours worked per RN was 26.7, ranging across individual units from a low of 10.6 to a high of 36.0 hours. The corresponding numbers and ranges based on the self-reported data by the registered nurses working in the thirty emergency units during fieldwork, shown in Table 26, are: 8.8 (range 4-17), 242 (range 102-512), and 27.1 (range 17.1-37.3), respectively. As with most other measures, here too, inter-unit variability continues to be very high.

Both the average number of RN's and the total hours worked per RN are greater for emergency units having a high, compared to either medium or low, patient volume. They are also greater for emergency units operated by hospitals which have medical teaching affiliations than by hospitals which do not. The same holds true for institutions which have emergency personnel training programs compared to those which do not; and, to a lesser extent, also for institutions located in urban compared to non-urban areas. These findings are on the whole very similar to the corresponding findings about medical staffing discussed earlier, suggesting that some emergency units have richer nursing as well as medical staffing patterns than others.

Staff Capability for Different Levels of Patient Volume

In recent years, patient volume in the emergency units of hospitals has been increasing at a significant rate. It is likely to continue to increase, moreover, at least for the foreseeable future. In addition, of course, patient volume may change from one month to another, usually upwards but sometimes downwards as well. It would be of interest, therefore, to have some information about the staff capabilities of emergency units in this connection. One important issue concerns the relative ability of emergency units to handle a considerable increase in patient visits with current staffing levels, and without adverse effects on the quality of care. A second issue concerns the likely effect on the quality of care that a comparable decrease in patient visits might have, assuming again current staffing levels.

Data on both of these issues were obtained from the physicians (MDS) and registered nurses (RNS) working in the various emergency units, and also from the hospital administrators (HAS) of the various institutions. They are summarized in Tables 27 and 28. The question asked of the respondents concerning the first of the above issues was: "If, in the next two months, patient visits were to increase by 10%-15% but the quality of patient care were to remain at its current level, how well could the present staff of this emergency unit handle the increased patient volume?" The results are presented in Table 27.

On the average, the physicians working in the emergency units studied believe that their respective units could handle such an increase in patient volume fairly well, with "some minor difficulties" only. (The overall mean score for the 30 EU's is 2.07, on a six-point scale in which 1.00 corresponds to "without any difficulties".) It is also clear that the capabilities of individual units vary a great deal (the range of mean scores is 1.20-3.50, although not so greatly as might have been expected). The registered nurses are somewhat less optimistic than the physicians, but still believe that their units could (on the average) handle the increased volume with only "minor" to "moderate" difficulty. The corresponding estimates by hospital administrators show an intermediate level of optimism. Again, however, there is substantial inter-unit variability (see the ranges in Table 27) concerning the staff capabilities of the units studied. Regarding the various groupings of EU's, on the other hand, the results show no major differences in this

TABLE 27. THE CAPABILITY OF EMERGENCY UNITS FOR HANDLING A 10%-15% INCREASE IN PATIENT WORKLOAD WITH PRESENT STAFF AND AT CURRENT LEVELS OF CARE QUALITY[a]

Hospital Emergency Units (EU's) Involved		Capability Level as Assessed by		
		HAS	MDS	RNS
ALL EU'S IN THE STUDY SAMPLE (N=30 Hospital EU's)	Mean: Range:	2.36 (1.00-4.00)	2.07 (1.20-3.50)	2.48 (1.67-3.80)
YOUR HOSPITAL'S EU		--		
EU's with:				
Low Patient Volume (n=10)		2.15	1.87	2.72
Medium Pat. Volume (n=10)		2.48	1.96	2.40
High Patient Volume (n=10)		2.43	2.38	2.32
EU's in:				
Church Operated Hospitals (n=9)		2.17	2.17	2.63
Osteopathic Hospitals (n=3)		2.33	1.62	2.01
All Other Hospitals (n=18)		2.45	2.09	2.48
EU's Located in:				
SMSA (urban) Areas (n=21)		2.32	2.06	2.43
Non-SMSA Areas (n=9)		2.44	2.10	2.59
EU's in Hospitals Having:				
Medical Teaching Affiliations (n=17)		2.45	2.05	2.48
No Medical Teaching Affiliations (n=13)		2.23	2.09	2.48
EU's in Hospitals Having:				
Emergency Personnel Training Programs (n=15)		2.29	2.11	2.51
No Training Programs (n=15)		2.42	2.03	2.46

[a]The results are based on the responses of MDS, RNS, and HAS from each institution to the question: "If, in the next two months, patient visits were to increase by 10%-15% but the quality of patient care were to remain at its current level, how well could the present staff of this emergency unit handle the increase in patient volume?" The response alternatives were: (1) The present staff could handle the increased volume without any difficulties, (2) it could handle it with some minor difficulties, (3) it could handle it with moderate difficulties, (4) it could handle it, but with great difficulties, (5) it could handle it, but with very great difficulties, and (6) the present staff could not handle it at all. Thus, the lower the mean scores, the greater the capability of the EU's involved.

respect. The overall conclusion from the data is that, with present staffing levels, the emergency units in the sample apparently would be able to respond very well to a 10%-15% increase in patient visits.

As to the likely effects of a patient volume _decrease_ of the same magnitude on the quality of care, the results summarized in Table 28 provide some indication. These are based on the answers by the same three groups of respondents to the following question: "Considering the number of patients that the staff now sees on an average day, what effect would a _10%-15% decrease_ in patient visits have on the quality of care provided by this emergency unit?"

Overall, the registered nurses indicate that, on the average, the quality of care "would improve, but only a _little_" following the stipulated reduction in patient volume. The physicians, and also the administrators, indicate that the quality of care would improve "a little" to "very little." Apparently, the effect of 10%-15% decrease in patient visits would be very small, on the average, from the point of view of improvement in the current levels of the quality of care offered at the various emergency units. There is, nevertheless, considerable inter-unit variability in this respect, as the range of mean scores based on the data from each group of respondents shows (see Table 28). In some of the units, respondents estimate that the quality of care would improve "moderately" to "considerably" (depending upon the respondents involved) while in other units it would improve "very little" or even less than "very little."

Taken together, the results in Tables 27 and 28 suggest that Parkinson's law may apply also to health care institutions. On the average, the emergency units in the study sample could handle a substantial increase in patient volume with their present staff without adverse effects on the quality of care, with only minor to moderate difficulty. On the other hand, the quality

TABLE 28. THE LIKELY EFFECT ON THE QUALITY OF CARE OF A 10%-15% DECREASE IN THE PRESENT PATIENT WORKLOAD OF EMERGENCY UNITS[a]

Hospital Emergency Units (EU's) Involved		Likely Effect on Quality According to		
		HAS	MDS	RNS
ALL EU'S IN THE STUDY SAMPLE (N=30 Hospital EU's)	Mean: Range:	4.46 (2.00-5.50)	4.56 (2.67-5.67)	3.96 (2.75-5.50)
YOUR HOSPITAL'S EU		--		
EU's with:				
Low Patient Volume (n=10)		4.93	4.85	4.28
Medium Pat. Volume (n=10)		4.17	4.78	4.08
High Patient Volume (n=10)		4.27	4.03	3.51
EU's in:				
Church Operated Hospitals (n=9)		4.74	4.63	3.80
Osteopathic Hospitals (n=3)		4.67	4.96	4.49
All Other Hospitals (n=18)		4.28	4.45	3.95
EU's Located in:				
SMSA (urban) Areas (n=21)		4.41	4.54	3.99
Non-SMSA Areas (n=9)		4.56	4.60	3.88
EU's in Hospitals Having:				
Medical Teaching Affiliations (n=17)		4.22	4.69	3.94
No Medical Teaching Affiliations (n=13)		4.77	4.39	3.98
EU's in Hospitals Having:				
Emergency Personnel Training Programs (n=15)		4.43	4.60	3.94
No Training Programs (n=15)		4.48	4.51	3.97

[a] The results are based on the responses of MDS, RNS, and HAS from each institution to the question: "Considering the number of patients the staff now sees on an average day, what effect would a 10%-15% DECREASE in patient visits have on the quality of care provided by this emergency unit?" The response alternatives were: (1) The quality of care would improve very considerably, (2) quality would improve considerably, (3) quality would improve moderately, (4) quality would improve, but only a little, (5) quality would improve very little, and (6) the quality of care would not improve. Thus, the lower the mean scores, the more likely that the quality of patient care would improve.

of patient care would be unlikely to improve appreciably in the various units when patient volume decreased by as much as 10%-15%. The present staff of emergency units apparently would be able to respond to up or down fluctuations of this magnitude in the patient volume fairly well, but perhaps more effectively with respect to increases than decreases in patient volume.

Summary

In this chapter, based on data from hospital records and data provided by several groups of respondents, a great many findings about the staff resources of emergency units were presented and discussed. In addition to examining the staffing patterns (both medical and nursing) of the units, and differences in staffing patterns between selected groupings of units, staff size was considered in terms of both staff numbers and staff hours worked. Other findings dealt with the sufficiency and stability of staff resources, the relative success of emergency units in obtaining requested resources from their parent hospitals, and the access of units within the hospital to on-call medical specialists. Certain findings concerning the staff capability of emergency units for different levels of patient volume also were presented. In short, some of the most important aspects of the medical and nursing staff resources of the emergency units studied were examined in detail. (For some additional characteristics about the staff, mainly personal-demographic characteristics, see the Appendix at the end of the report.) The findings in this chapter, in addition to being important in their own right, therefore provide an excellent background for reviewing the results about the social, economic, and clinical efficiency of emergency units, which are presented in later chapters (Chapters 9, 10, and 11, respectively).

Chapter 3

CURRENT GOAL PRIORITIES, PROBLEMS, AND STRENGTHS

Among the most important organizational characteristics of emergency units are those involving overall goals, strengths, and weaknesses. The basic goal priorities, problems, and strengths of the units, as perceived by several key groups of resondents, are reviewed in this chapter. In the first section, findings regarding the goal priorities emphasized by the various EU's are presented, based on data from the physicians (MDS) and registered nurses (RNS) working in each unit, selected physicians from the rest of the hospital (HMDS), and the selected community respondents (CRS) who participated in the study. These findings are important not only because they summarize current goal priorities but also because they show the extent to which different key groups agree about the emphasis placed on particular unit goals.

In the second and third sections, respectively, the "most important" strengths and "major problems" of emergency units, again as perceived by several key groups, are summarized. The data regarding problems and strengths were obtained with open-ended interview questions. They are, therefore, likely to reflect those aspects or issues that the respondents themselves consider salient.

The Goal Priorities of Emergency Units

Emergency unit physicians (MDS) and registered nurses (RNS) were asked in their questionnaires to rank seven goal priorities <u>in order of their importance to the emergency unit</u> with which the respondents were associated. The specific goal priorities, in the sequence presented to the respondents, were: "maintaining a good reputation in the community"; "improving working conditions for the staff"; "minimizing patient waiting time"; "keeping the costs of the emergency service down"; "maintaining high standards of patient care"; "providing comprehensive emergency services"; and "maintaining a high level of patient satisfaction." The obtained data are summarized in Tables 29 and 30.

For the 30 EU's in the total sample, the different goal priorities are rank-ordered very similarly by physicians and nurses alike. Overall, both groups rank "maintaining high standards of patient care" as the most important priority of all, and "providing comprehensive emergency services" as second most important, followed by "maintaining a high level of patient satisfaction" in third place. At the other extreme, they both rank "improving working conditions for the staff" last (or in seventh place) in overall importance, and "keeping the costs of the emergency service down" next to last (or in sixth place). "Minimizing patient waiting time" is ranked fourth in overall importance by RNS and fifth by MDS (though the mean-rank score is identical, specifically 4.4, according to the data from both groups). And "maintaining a good reputation in the community" is ranked fourth by MDS, and fifth by RNS, among the seven goal priorities. Unlike the RNS, moreover, the MDS rank maintaining a good reputation and minimizing patient waiting time almost at exactly the same level (the RNS rank the latter as somewhat more important than the former), and do likewise for improving working conditions and keeping costs down (the RNS rank the latter as somewhat more important than the former).

Apart from the minor differences noted, the overall pattern of the relative importance of the seven goal priorities (viewed in relation to one another) is basically the same, according to both nurses and physicians. Furthermore, when considering the various subgroupings of emergency units instead of the

TABLE 29. BASIC GOAL PRIORITIES OF EMERGENCY UNITS AS RANK-ORDERED BY THE PHYSICIANS (MDS) WHO WORK THERE[a]

Hospital Emergency Units (EU's) Involved		"Maintaining a good reputation in the community"	"Improving working conditions for the staff"	"Minimizing patient waiting time"	"Keeping the costs of the emergency service down"	"Maintaining high standards of patient care"	"Providing comprehensive emergency services"	"Maintaining a high level of patient satisfaction"
ALL EU'S IN THE STUDY SAMPLE (N=30 Hospital EU's)	Mean:	4.3	5.4	4.4	5.3	1.6	2.9	3.4
	Range:	(3.2-5.5)	(4.2-6.7)	(2.6-5.3)	(3.7-6.7)	(1.0-2.6)	(1.5-5.0)	(2.3-5.0)
YOUR HOSPITAL'S EU								
EU's with:								
Low Patient Volume (n=10)		4.2	5.3	4.6	5.0	1.4	2.9	3.5
Medium Pat. Volume (n=10)		4.5	5.5	4.3	5.7	1.5	3.1	3.4
High Patient Volume (n=10)		4.3	5.5	4.3	5.3	1.8	2.9	3.3
EU's in:								
Small Hospitals (n=14)		4.4	5.3	4.7	5.3	1.4	2.8	3.5
Medium Hospitals (n=9)		4.3	5.5	4.3	5.2	1.6	3.1	3.1
Large Hospitals (n=7)		4.3	5.7	4.0	5.6	1.8	3.1	3.6
EU's in:								
Church Operated Hospitals (n=9)		4.3	5.5	4.6	5.3	1.4	2.8	3.6
Osteopathic Hospitals (n=3)		4.9	5.4	4.6	5.0	1.2	3.1	3.0
All Other Hospitals (n=18)		4.3	5.4	4.3	5.4	1.7	3.0	3.4
EU's Located in:								
SMSA (urban) Areas (n=21)		4.4	5.6	4.1	5.3	1.5	3.1	3.4
Non-SMSA Areas (n=9)		4.3	5.0	4.9	5.6	1.7	2.6	3.5
EU's in Hospitals Having:								
Medical Teaching Affiliations (n=17)		4.3	5.7	4.2	5.5	1.6	3.1	3.3
No Medical Teaching Affiliations (n=13)		4.4	5.1	4.7	5.1	1.6	2.7	3.6
EU's in Hospitals Having:								
Emergency Personnel Training Programs (n=15)		4.5	5.6	4.5	5.3	1.5	2.8	3.3
No Training Programs (n=15)		4.2	5.3	4.3	5.3	1.6	3.1	3.5

[a]The mean ranks shown for each goal priority are based on the responses of MDS from each EU to the following questionnaire item: "Hospital emergency units may emphasize different priorities and goals, some of which are listed below. Please rank these priorities in order of their importance to this emergency unit." Respondents were asked to: "Place 1 in front of the one which is the most important, 2 in front of the next most important, etc...., and 7 in front of the one that is least important." (The different goal priorities were presented in the questionnaire in exactly the same order as they appear in the columns of this table.) Thus, the lower the mean rank associated with a goal priority the greater the importance placed on that priority by the EU's involved, according to MDS.

TABLE 30. BASIC GOAL PRIORITIES OF EMERGENCY UNITS AS RANK-ORDERED BY
THE REGISTERED NURSES (RNS) WHO WORK THERE[a]

Hospital Emergency Units (EU's) Involved	"Maintaining a good reputation in the community"	"Improving working conditions for the staff"	"Minimizing patient waiting time"	"Keeping the costs of the emergency service down"	"Maintaining high standards of patient care"	"Providing comprehensive emergency services"	"Maintaining a high level of patient satisfaction"
ALL EU'S IN THE STUDY SAMPLE (N=30 Hospital EU's) Mean:	4.9	6.0	4.4	5.5	1.4	2.5	3.3
Range:	(3.8-6.2)	(5.1-7.0)	(3.4-5.4)	(3.8-6.4)	(1.0-2.0)	(1.7-3.5)	(2.7-4.4)
YOUR HOSPITAL'S EU							
EU's with:							
Low Patient Volume (n=10)	4.8	6.0	4.6	5.3	1.4	2.5	3.3
Medium Pat. Volume (n=10)	5.0	6.1	4.5	5.3	1.5	2.5	3.1
High Patient Volume (n=10)	4.8	6.0	4.0	5.9	1.5	2.5	3.4
EU's in:							
Small Hospitals (n=14)	4.9	6.0	4.5	5.3	1.4	2.5	3.3
Medium Hospitals (n=9)	4.8	6.1	4.5	5.5	1.6	2.4	3.2
Large Hospitals (n=7)	5.0	5.9	4.1	5.9	1.3	2.4	3.4
EU's in:							
Church Operated Hospitals (n=9)	5.0	6.0	4.4	5.5	1.4	2.3	3.3
Osteopathic Hospitals (n=3)	4.8	6.0	4.5	4.9	1.6	3.0	3.2
All Other Hospitals (n=18)	4.8	6.0	4.3	5.6	1.5	2.5	3.3
EU's Located in:							
SMSA (urban) Areas (n=21)	4.9	6.1	4.3	5.5	1.5	2.5	3.2
Non-SMSA Areas (n=9)	4.9	5.9	4.6	5.5	1.3	2.4	3.3
EU's in Hospitals Having:							
Medical Teaching Affiliations (n=17)	4.9	6.1	4.3	5.5	1.4	2.5	3.3
No Medical Teaching Affiliations (n=13)	4.8	6.0	4.5	5.5	1.5	2.4	3.3
EU's in Hospitals Having:							
Emergency Personnel Training Programs (n=15)	4.9	6.0	4.3	5.4	1.5	2.5	3.4
No Training Programs (n=15)	4.9	6.1	4.5	5.6	1.4	2.4	3.1

[a] The mean ranks shown for each goal priority are based on the responses of RNS from each EU to the following questionnaire item: "Hospital emergency units may emphasize different priorities and goals, some of which are listed below. Please rank these priorities in order of their importance to this emergency unit." Respondents were instructed to: "Place 1 in front of the one that is the most important, 2 in front of the next most important, etc...., and (7) in front of the one that is least important." (The different goal priorities were presented in the questionnaire in exactly the same order as they appear in the columns of this table.) Thus, the lower the mean rank associated with a goal priority the greater the importance placed on that priority by the EU's involved, according to RNS.

total sample, the rank-order of priorities based on the data from RNS (Table 30) remains the same for each particular grouping -- a remarkable consistency. In the case of the data from MDS (Table 29), there are some deviations from the overall pattern, but no great or numerous differences. For example, compared to the average situation characterizing the 30 EU's in the total sample, improving working conditions apparently is emphasized more than keeping costs down by emergency units in non-urban areas. For the total sample, on the other hand, the latter priority is emphasized just slightly more than the former.

Even when comparing the different subgroups of EU's on each specific goal priority, the mean-rank scores are very similar with only a few exceptions. In the case of the data from MDS (Table 29), the exceptions are: keeping costs down is emphasized more by EU's with a low compared to a medium patient volume; minimizing patient waiting time is emphasized more by EU's in urban compared to other areas, while the reverse is true with regard to improving working conditions; the latter is also emphasized less by the EU's of hospitals which have medical teaching affiliations than those which do not; and maintaining a good reputation is emphasized less by osteopathic than other institutions, while maintaining high standards is emphasized more by the former compared to church operated institutions. In the case of the data from RNS (Table 30) the exceptions are: minimizing patient waiting time is emphasized more by units with a high compared to a low (and possibly also medium) patient volume, while the reverse is true for keeping costs down; the latter goal priority is also less emphasized by non-osteopathic than by osteopathic institutions, and by EU's with a high compared to either a medium or a low patient volume.

Generally, then, those of the goal priorities which are most directly related to patient care are, on the average, more important to the emergency units than are other priorities, according to the nurses and physicians who work in the units. It is equally interesting that keeping costs down and improving working conditions are the least important of the seven priorities to the emergency units studied, again according to both RNS and MDS. Minimizing patient waiting time also is ranked relatively low, possibly reflecting the high incidence of non-emergency cases in most units.

It should be pointed out, however, that the situation of individual emergency units may differ from the above overall patterns -- and differ markedly for particular goal priorities. The range of mean-rank scores shown for each priority in Tables 29 and 30 is indicative of the variability which prevails across units. Examination of these scores reveals low inter-unit variability, according to the data from both MDS and RNS, for only one of the seven goal priorities -- maintaining high standards of care. According to the data from MDS, variability is especially high with respect to the relative importance of providing comprehensive emergency services (for some emergency units, in other words, this ranks very high while for others it ranks low compared to other goal priorities), and the importance of keeping costs down. According to the data from RNS, inter-unit variability is very high with respect to maintaining a good reputation and high with respect to keeping costs down. For the remaining goal priorities, the variability across EU's is moderately low based on the data from RNS but moderately high based on the data from MDS.

Goal priorities as seen by respondents other than the staff of the units. The selected physicians (HMDS) from the study hospitals also provided relevant data in this area. In their interviews, the HMDS were given the same list of seven goal priorities discussed above and asked to indicate which three of these priorities are emphasized the most by the emergency units of their respective hospitals. Because of their very high similarity to the results based on the data from MDS and RNS, discussed above, the results from the data provided by HMDS are not presented in table form. They need only be briefly discussed here.

With reference to all 30 EU's in the sample combined, these respondents too selected maintaining high standards of patient care as the top goal priority among the seven. This priority was mentioned as one of "the three most emphasized" by 30% of the HMDS (in the present case this also corresponds to 30% of all the mentions given by HMDS). The second most frequently chosen priority, mentioned by 25% of the same respondents, is providing comprehensive emergency services -- the same priority which was ranked second also by the MDS and by the RNS. And the third most emphasized priority according to the selected physicians (mentioned by 15% of the HMDS) is maintaining a high level of patient satisfaction -- the priority ranked third also by the MDS and by the RNS. The priority which places fourth according to the data from HMDS (based on the frequency with which it was mentioned) is maintaining a good reputation in the community (earlier ranked fourth by the MDS and fifth by the RNS). Finally, the pattern of findings for the total sample based on the data from HMDS is virtually the same also for each of the different groupings of EU's examined in the present report.

Thus, overall agreement as to the relative importance, or emphasis, placed by emergency units on particular goal priorities is very high among the three key groups of respondents -- the selected hospital physicians and the emergency unit physicians and registered nurses. The general pattern of findings is remarkably consistent regardless of the specific source of data, and consensus among the three groups involved is high, both when the total sample and when each of the different subgroupings of units are examined.

For individual emergency units, of course, the level of consensus among the three groups may differ.

Finally, the selected community respondents (CRS) who participated in the study also were asked their views about the goal priorities of the emergency units with which they are associated. The CRS, however, were asked only a general, open-ended question: "As far as you can tell, what are some of the priorities or goals that this emergency unit seems to emphasize at the present time?" Their responses were coded into seven different categories corresponding to the seven goal priorities specified above plus an additional residual category. The results based on the data from the selected community respondents are summarized in Table 31.

Very briefly, the three most frequently mentioned goal priorities by community respondents as those that are seemingly emphasized the most by the emergency units studied, are: maintaining high standards of patient care, which accounts for 41% of all the mentions given by CRS; minimizing patient waiting time, which accounts for 23% of all mentions; and providing comprehensive emergency services, which accounts for 21% of all mentions. (Maintaining a good reputation in the community places fourth in the present series.) The only major difference between this pattern and the patterns of findings based on the data from HMDS, MDS, and RNS concerns the appearance, for the first time, of patient waiting time as a high priority. The perception of community respondents in this respect is not supported by the other three groups of respondents.

Emergency Unit Strengths

The interviews completed by the various groups of respondents who participated in the study consisted of mostly open-ended questions about various

TABLE 31. BASIC GOAL PRIORITIES OF EMERGENCY UNITS AS PERCEIVED BY SELECTED RESPONDENTS FROM THE COMMUNITY (CRS)[a]

		Priorities Most Emphasized by the EU's, According to CRS		
Hospital Emergency Units (EU's) Involved	Total Mentions[b]	1st most frequently mentioned priority	2nd most frequently mentioned priority	3rd most frequently mentioned priority
ALL EU'S IN THE STUDY SAMPLE (N=30 Hospital EU's)	116	Maintaining high standards of patient care (41.4%)	Minimizing patient waiting time (23.3%)	Providing comprehensive emergency services (20.7%)
YOUR HOSPITAL'S EU				
EU's with:				
Low Patient Volume (n=10)	31	Maintaining high standards of patient care (38.7%)	Minimizing patient waiting time (29.0%)	Providing comprehensive emergency services (25.8%)
Medium Pat. Volume (n=10)	33	Maintaining high standards of patient care (42.4%)	Minimizing patient waiting time (27.3%)	Providing comprehensive emergency services (21.2%)
High Patient Volume (n=10)	52	Maintaining high standards of patient care (42.3%)	Maintaining a good reputation in the community (19.2%)	Providing comprehensive emergency services (17.3%); Minimizing patient waiting time (17.3%)
EU's in:				
Church Operated Hospitals (n=9)	37	Maintaining high standards of patient care (35.1%)	Providing comprehensive emergency services (27.0%)	Minimizing patient waiting time (24.3%)
Osteopathic Hospitals (n=3)	6	Maintaining high standards of patient care (50.0%)	Providing comprehensive emergency services (33.3%)	Minimizing patient waiting time (16.7%)
All Other Hospitals (n=18)	73	Maintaining high standards of patient care (43.8%)	Minimizing patient waiting time (23.3%)	Providing comprehensive emergency services (16.4%)
EU's Located in:				
SMSA (urban) Areas (n=21)	78	Maintaining high standards of patient care (41.0%)	Minimizing patient waiting time (24.4%)	Providing comprehensive emergency services (19.2%)
Non-SMSA Areas (n=9)	38	Maintaining high standards of patient care (42.1%)	Providing comprehensive emergency services (23.7%)	Minimizing patient waiting time (21.1%)
EU's in Hospitals Having:				
Medical Teaching Affiliations (n=17)	72	Maintaining high standards of patient care (45.8%)	Minimizing patient waiting time (22.2%)	Providing comprehensive emergency services (19.4%)
No Medical Teaching Affiliations (n=13)	44	Maintaining high standards of patient care (34.1%)	Minimizing patient waiting time (25.0%)	Providing comprehensive emergency services (22.7%)
EU's in Hospitals Having:				
Emergency Personnel Training Programs (n=15)	56	Maintaining high standards of patient care (35.7%)	Providing comprehensive emergency services (23.2%)	Maintaining a good reputation in the community (19.6%)
No Training Programs (n=15)	60	Maintaining high standards of patient care (46.7%)	Minimizing patient waiting time (26.7%)	Providing comprehensive emergency services (18.3%)

[a] These data are based on the responses of CRS associated with the various EU's to the question: "As far as you can tell, what are some of the priorities or goals that this Emergency Unit seems to emphasize at the present time?" Their responses were coded into the following general categories: (1) maintaining a good reputation in the community, (2) improving working conditions for the staff, (3) minimizing patient waiting time, (4) keeping the costs of the emergency service down, (5) maintaining high standards of patient care, (6) providing comprehensive emergency services, (7) maintaining a high level of patient satisfaction, and (8) general growth, expansion, or improvement of facilities.

[b] The mentions indicated for each grouping of EU's represent the sum of mentions for all hospital EU's in the grouping combined. The percentages enclosed in parentheses after each goal priority were computed using these summed mentions as a base.

aspects of the situation of emergency units. Included among such questions, at the beginning of each interview schedule, were two concerning "the most important strengths" of the emergency unit and the "major problems or key issues" faced by the unit. The strengths and problems mentioned in response to these open-ended questions were first coded into a large number of specific categories and then grouped into ten general categories for purposes of presentation in this report. These categories (also used to encompass the problems of emergency units discussed in a subsequent section of this chapter) are:

1. Organization and supervision: characteristics of the unit's organizational structure (e.g., roles, rules, influence, norms); adequacy of the medical, nursing, and administrative organization of the unit; and the effectiveness of the unit's medical, nursing, and administrative leadership or supervision.

2. Staff resources: the quantity, quality, and stability of the emergency unit's medical, nursing, and other staff resources (including the staff's potential to efficiently provide high quality patient care, but excluding responses referring explicitly to the staff's performance, which are included in #8, below).

3. Non-staff resources: the quantity and quality of the emergency unit's physical plant, equipment, and funds; and appropriate or inappropriate use of the unit's facilities by certain categories of patients (including non-emergency patients).

4. Work relations within the unit: the coordination of activities and work efforts within the unit, doctor-nurse relations, and the adequacy of relevant information available in the unit.

5. Staff identification (commitment) and satisfaction: staff identification with the emergency unit, and with the hospital; staff satisfaction with

the unit as a place to work; and staff satisfaction with financial and non-financial rewards.

6. <u>Costs, charges, and economic efficiency</u>: hospital charges for patient care, physician fees, costs, and efficient/inefficient use of resources.

7. <u>Strain and tension</u>: strain among emergency unit staff members; tension between some or all of the unit's staff and others outside the unit (including hospital staff, patients, and the community); and the presence or absence of conflicts.

8. <u>Staff performance or quality of care</u>: all aspects of good/poor staff performance; the quality of care provided to all kinds of patients from time of entry to time of exit from the unit; the job done by medical, nursing, and other staff; the comprehensiveness of services offered; and patient waiting time.

9. <u>Relations with the parent hospital</u>: characteristics of the hospital (e.g., its organizational structures and policies) that affect the autonomy, operation, or work of the emergency unit; and work relations between the emergency unit and other parts of the hospital (e.g., ancillary services, hospital administration, inpatient services).

10. <u>Relations with the community</u>: the emergency unit's relationships with various organizations in the community (e.g., hospitals, third-party payers, HSA's, police); how well community expectations are met by the emergency unit; and the ability of the unit to handle particular types of patients from the community or to function properly considering the stability, economic level, etc., of the population.

Tables 32, 33, and 34 summarize the data about the strengths of emergency units provided by emergency unit physicians (MDS), selected hospital physicians (HMDS), and hospital administrators (HAS), respectively. Relevant data were also obtained from the registered nurses (RNS) working in the various EU's. These are not presented in a separate table but will be discussed along with the data from MDS. The question answered by the respondents regarding strengths was: "What are the TWO or THREE most important areas, or respects, in which you consider this emergency unit to be particularly strong or especially outstanding?"

Overall, according to the physicians who work there (MDS), the emergency units in the study are strongest in the areas of staff performance or quality of care and staff resources. These two areas, taken together, account for about two-thirds of all strengths mentioned by the MDS (see Table 32). These particular strengths, moreover, are the same as the top two reported by the registered nurses (RNS) who work in the units. Furthermore, staff performance or quality of care is the strength most frequently mentioned by the MDS and RNS not only for the total sample but also for each of the various groupings of emergency units considered separately in this report. And staff resources is the area which is second most frequently mentioned as a strength by both MDS and RNS in all of the same groupings but one (the exception involves the data from MDS in the case of osteopathic hospital units, for which the second most often mentioned strength is non-staff resources).

Other areas in which the MDS and RNS see their units as being particularly strong, though less so than in the above two areas, include: relations with the parent hospital; relations with the community; and the emergency unit's non-staff resources. Together with staff performance or quality of care and staff resources, these areas account for 96% of all the strengths mentioned by the physicians and 90% of those mentioned by the registered nurses of the emergency units studied.

For the sample as a whole, relations with the parent hospital is the area cited third most often by the MDS as one of the greatest strengths of

TABLE 32. THE MOST IMPORTANT STRENGTHS OF EMERGENCY UNITS, AS ASSESSED
BY THE PHYSICIANS (MDS) WHO WORK THERE[a]

		The Three Strengths Most Frequently Mentioned by MDS		
Hospital Emergency Units (EU's) Involved	Total Mentions[b]	First	Second	Third
ALL EU'S IN THE STUDY SAMPLE (N=30 Hospital EU's)	509	Staff performance or quality of care (36.5%)	Staff resources (29.1%)	Relations with parent hospital (12.8%)
YOUR HOSPITAL'S EU				
EU's with:				
Low Patient Volume (n=10)	182	Staff performance or quality of care (36.8%)	Staff resources (25.3%)	Relations with parent hospital (12.1%); Non-staff resources (12.1%)
Medium Pat. Volume (n=10)	138	Staff performance or quality of care (33.3%)	Staff resources (28.3%)	Relations with parent hospital (21.7%)
High Patient Volume (n=10)	189	Staff performance or quality of care (38.6%)	Staff resources (33.3%)	Relations with the community (12.2%)
EU's in:				
Church Operated Hospitals (n=9)	175	Staff performance or quality of care (38.3%)	Staff resources (32.6%)	Relations with parent hospital (9.7%); Non-staff resources (9.7%)
Osteopathic Hospitals (n=3)	39	Staff performance or quality of care (46.2%)	Non-staff resources (12.8%)	Relations with parent hospital (12.8%); Relations with the community (12.8%)
All Other Hospitals (n=18)	295	Staff performance or quality of care (34.2%)	Staff resources (29.5%)	Relations with parent hospital (14.6%)
EU's Located in:				
SMSA (urban) Areas (n=21)	352	Staff performance or quality of care (39.2%)	Staff resources (29.5%)	Relations with parent hospital (12.2%)
Non-SMSA Areas (n=9)	157	Staff performance or quality of care (30.6%)	Staff resources (28.0%)	Relations with parent hospital (14.0%)
EU's in Hospitals Having:				
Medical Teaching Affiliations (n=17)	293	Staff performance or quality of care (38.6%)	Staff resources (32.1%)	Relations with parent hospital (12.3%)
No Medical Teaching Affiliations (n=13)	216	Staff performance or quality of care (33.8%)	Staff resources (25.0%)	Relations with parent hospital (13.4%)
EU's in Hospitals Having:				
Emergency Personnel Training Programs (n=15)	277	Staff performance or quality of care (37.2%)	Staff resources (32.9%)	Relations with parent hospital (11.2%)
No Training Programs (n=15)	232	Staff performance or quality of care (35.8%)	Staff resources (24.6%)	Relations with parent hospital (14.7%)

[a]The results are based on the responses of MDS from the various EU's to the following open-ended question: "What are the TWO or THREE most important areas, or respects, in which you consider this Emergency Unit to be <u>particularly strong or especially outstanding</u>?" Their responses were first coded into a large number of specific categories and then collapsed into the following ten general categories: (1) Organization or supervision, (2) staff resources, (3) non-staff resources, (4) work relations in the unit, (5) staff identification and satisfaction, (6) costs and charges, (7) strain and tension, (8) staff performance or quality of care, (9) relations with parent hospital, and (10) relations with the community.

[b]The mentions indicated for each grouping of EU's represent the sum of mentions for all hospital EU's in the grouping combined. The percentages enclosed in parentheses after each strength were computed using the summed mentions as a base. Of all the MDS in the study, 88% mentioned at least one strength, 74% mentioned at least two, and 43% mentioned three.

emergency units. Concerning some of the various groupings of EU's, however, certain other areas are mentioned just as frequently, or even more frequently. For example, physicians in units with a high patient volume refer to <u>relations with the community</u> as a major strength almost twice as often as they refer to <u>relations with the parent hospital</u> (12% vs. 7%). Other such deviations from the general pattern are shown in Table 32.

Again for the sample as a whole, unlike the physicians, the registered nurses mention <u>non-staff resources</u> third most often as one of the greatest strengths of their emergency units. In the case of certain EU groupings, however, the nurses cite <u>relations with the community</u> more often than <u>non-staff resources</u>. The groupings in question include: units with a high patient volume, the units of not church operated hospitals, the units of hospitals with medical teaching affiliations, also emergency personnel training programs, and the units of hospitals in urban areas. Finally, it is rather interesting that the RNS, unlike the MDS, do not include relations with the parent hospital among the top three strengths of their units.

<u>The strengths of EU's as seen by respondents not working in the units</u>. The selected physicians (HMDS) and administrators (HAS) from the participating hospitals also provided data about the major strengths of emergency units. The results based on these data are presented in Table 33 and Table 34, respectively. In general, these are consistent with the results obtained in the case of emergency unit nurses and physicians discussed above.

Considering first the total sample, nearly two-thirds of all the strengths mentioned by the HMDS, and also by the HAS, concern <u>staff performance or quality of care</u> and <u>staff resources</u>. These respondents, however, cite <u>staff resources</u> somewhat more frequently than do those working within the emergency

TABLE 33. THE MOST IMPORTANT STRENGTHS OF EMERGENCY UNITS, AS ASSESSED BY SELECTED PHYSICIANS (HMDS) IN THEIR RESPECTIVE PARENT HOSPITALS[a]

Hospital Emergency Units (EU's) Involved	Total Mentions[b]	The Three Strengths Most Frequently Mentioned by HMDS		
		First	Second	Third
ALL EU'S IN THE STUDY SAMPLE (N=30 Hospital EU's)	470	Staff performance or quality of care (35.1%)	Staff resources (30.9%)	Relations with parent hospital (10.4%); Relations with the community (10.4%)
YOUR HOSPITAL'S EU				
EU's with:				
Low Patient Volume (n=10)	91	Staff resources (33.0%)	Staff performance or quality of care (28.6%)	Non-staff resources (16.5%)
Medium Pat. Volume (n=10)	180	Staff performance or quality of care (34.4%)	Staff resources (31.1%)	Relations with parent hospital (13.3%)
High Patient Volume (n=10)	199	Staff performance or quality of care (38.7%)	Staff resources (29.6%)	Relations with the community (13.6%)
EU's in:				
Church Operated Hospitals (n=9)	97	Staff resources (34.0%)	Staff performance or quality of care (26.8%)	Relations with parent hospital (12.4%)
Osteopathic Hospitals (n=3)	59	Staff resources (40.7%)	Staff performance or quality of care (37.3%)	Relations with parent hospital (6.8%)
All Other Hospitals (n=18)	314	Staff performance or quality of care (37.3%)	Staff resources (28.0%)	Relations with the community (11.5%)
EU's Located in:				
SMSA (urban) Areas (n=21)	355	Staff performance or quality of care (37.5%)	Staff resources (30.1%)	Relations with parent hospital (10.1%)
Non-SMSA Areas (n=9)	115	Staff resources (33.0%)	Staff performance or quality of care (27.8%)	Non-staff resources (13.0%)
EU's in Hospitals Having:				
Medical Teaching Affiliations (n=17)	325	Staff performance or quality of care (38.8%)	Staff resources (29.2%)	Relations with the community (10.8%)
No Medical Teaching Affiliations (n=13)	145	Staff resources (34.5%)	Staff performance or quality of care (26.9%)	Non-staff resources (13.8%)
EU's in Hospitals Having:				
Emergency Personnel Training Programs (n=15)	254	Staff performance or quality of care (39.4%)	Staff resources (32.3%)	Relations with the community (10.2%)
No Training Programs (n=15)	216	Staff performance or quality of care (30.1%)	Staff resources (29.2%)	Relations with parent hospital (13.4%)

[a] The results are based on the responses of HMDS from the various hospitals to the following open-ended question: "What are the TWO or THREE most important areas, or respects, in which you consider this Emergency Unit to be particularly strong or especially outstanding?" Their responses were first coded into a large number of specific categories and then collapsed into the following ten general categories: (1) Organization or supervision, (2) staff resources, (3) non-staff resources, (4) work relations in the unit, (5) staff identification and satisfaction, (6) costs and charges, (7) strain and tension, (8) staff performance or quality of care, (9) relations with the parent hospital, and (10) relations with the community.

[b] The mentions indicated for each grouping of EU's represent the sum of mentions for all hospital EU's in the grouping combined. The percentages enclosed in parentheses after each strength were computed using the summed mentions as a base. Of all HMDS in the sample 90% mentioned at least one strength, 76% mentioned at least two, and 53% mentioned three.

TABLE 34. THE MOST IMPORTANT STRENGTHS OF EMERGENCY UNITS, AS ASSESSED BY HOSPITAL ADMINISTRATOR RESPONDENTS (HAS)[a]

Hospital Emergency Units (EU's) Involved	Total Mentions[b]	The Three Strengths Most Frequently Mentioned by HAS		
		First	Second	Third
ALL EU'S IN THE STUDY SAMPLE (N=30 Hospital EU's)	184	Staff resources (29.9%)	Staff performance or quality of care (29.3%)	Relations with the community (19.0%)
YOUR HOSPITAL'S EU		--	--	--
EU's with:				
Low Patient Volume (n=10)	59	Relations with the community (27.1%)	Staff resources (25.4%)	Staff performance or quality of care (23.7%)
Medium Pat. Volume (n=10)	56	Staff performance or quality of care (37.5%)	Staff resources (30.4%)	Non-staff resources (14.3%)
High Patient Volume (n=10)	69	Staff resources (33.3%)	Staff performance or quality of care (27.5%)	Relations with the community (21.7%)
EU's in:				
Church Operated Hospitals (n=9)	58	Relations with the community (25.9%)	Staff performance or quality of care (24.1%)	Staff resources (20.7%)
Osteopathic Hospitals (n=3)	17	Staff resources (41.2%)	Staff performance or quality of care (29.4%)	Non-staff resources (11.8%)
All Other Hospitals (n=18)	109	Staff resources (33.0%)	Staff performance or quality of care (32.1%)	Relations with the community (17.4%)
EU's Located in:				
SMSA (urban) Areas (n=21)	138	Staff resources (32.6%)	Staff performance or quality of care (29.7%)	Relations with the community (15.9%)
Non-SMSA Areas (n=9)	46	Staff performance or quality of care (28.3%)	Relations with the community (28.3%)	Staff resources (21.7%)
EU's in Hospitals Having:				
Medical Teaching Affiliations (n=17)	113	Staff performance or quality of care (35.4%)	Staff resources (29.2%)	Relations with the community (15.0%)
No Medical Teaching Affiliations (n=13)	71	Staff resources (31.0%)	Relations with the community (25.4%)	Staff performance or quality of care (19.7%)
EU's in Hospitals Having:				
Emergency Personnel Training Programs (n=15)	100	Staff resources (33.0%)	Staff performance or quality of care (23.0%)	Relations with the community (21.0%)
No Training Programs (n=15)	84	Staff performance or quality of care (36.9%)	Staff resources (26.2%)	Relations with the community (16.7%)

[a] The results are based on the responses of HAS from the various hospitals to the following open-ended question: "What are the TWO or THREE most important areas, or respects, in which you consider this Emergency Unit to be <u>particularly strong or especially outstanding</u>?" Their responses were first coded into a large number of specific categories and then collapsed into the following ten general categories: (1) Organization or supervision, (2) staff resources, (3) non-staff resources, (4) work relations in the unit, (5) staff identification and satisfaction, (6) costs and charges, (7) strain and tension, (8) staff performance or quality of care, (9) relations with the parent hospital, and (10) relations with the community.

[b] The mentions indicated for each grouping of EU's represent the sum of mentions for all hospital EU's in the grouping combined. The percentages enclosed in parentheses after each strength were computed using the summed mentions as a base. Of all HAS in the sample 98% mentioned at least one strength, 97% mentioned at least two, and 75% mentioned three.

units. Other areas in which the selected hospital physicians and administrators consider the emergency units to be particularly strong include: <u>relations with the community</u>, <u>non-staff resources</u>, and <u>relations with the parent hospital</u>. These three areas are mentioned with about equal frequency by the HMDS, while the HAS mention <u>relations with the community</u> more than twice as often as the other two areas. These five areas together account for 93% of all the strengths cited by the hospital administrators and 95% of those cited by the selected hospital physicians in the study.

The data also show some differences across emergency unit groupings in the pattern of strengths identified by HMDS and HAS respondents. For example, HAS from hospitals with emergency personnel training programs mention <u>staff resources</u> as one of the top strengths of emergency units more often than <u>staff performance or quality of care</u>. The reverse pattern characterizes the EU's of hospitals without such training programs. The HAS also mention <u>relations with the community</u> as a strength more often in the case of hospitals in non-urban areas, hospitals whose emergency units have a low patient volume, and church operated hospitals than in the case of other institutions. Other findings show that the HMDS associated with institutions having medical teaching affiliations most often mention <u>staff performance or quality of care</u> as a strength, while those associated with institutions not having such affiliations mention <u>staff resources</u> most often. Another interesting difference is that the HMDS from hospitals whose emergency units have a low patient volume consider <u>non-staff resources</u> as a strength more than do their counterparts in hospitals whose emergency units have a high or medium patient volume.

Before concluding this section, it might be noted that the selected community respondents (CRS) also were asked about the major strengths of the emergency units with which they are associated (data now shown). For the total sample, the top three areas of strength indicated by these respondents are: <u>staff performance or quality of care</u> (accounting for 38% of all responses); <u>relations with the community</u> (accounting for 27%); and unit <u>staff resources</u> (accounting for 19%). The relatively high frequency with which CRS mention <u>relations with the community</u> probably can be attributed to their direct familiarity with, and/or sensitivity about, the performance of emergency units in this area.

Finally, some readers may wish to examine some of the specific findings about emergency unit strengths shown in the above four-table series -- Tables 31, 32, 33, and 34 -- in greater detail. And most readers in the participating institutions will want to compare their own emergency unit's situation to the more general patterns discussed above. The strengths of a particular unit may or may not conform to the general pattern, regardless of the specific source(s) of data considered, and this would be important to know. Moreover, a complete picture of a unit's strengths, and weaknesses, can be developed only after reviewing all of the findings in all of the chapters included in the present report.

The Current Major Problems of Emergency Units

Although some of the greatest strengths of emergency units are in the areas of <u>staff resources</u> and <u>relations with the community</u>, some of the most important problems faced by these units are apparently in the same areas. The data concerning the "major problems or key issues" facing the emergency units in the study sample are discussed in this section. The problems mentioned by the physicians (MDS) working in the emergency units, by the registered nurses (RNS) of the units, and by the hospital administrator (HAS) respondents are summarized in Tables 35, 36, and 37, respectively.

The data in Tables 35 and 36 show that, according to the doctors and nurses working in the emergency units, the majority of the problems faced by EU's are concentrated in the area of resources. More specifically, for the sample as a whole, staff resources and non-staff resources together account for 58% of all the problems mentioned by the MDS and 63% of all those mentioned by the RNS. (Staff resources were mentioned by certain respondents both as a strength, e.g., "good medical staff," and as a problem, e.g., "not enough nurses.") However, staff resources are more problematic than non-staff resources according to the RNS, while the reverse is the case according to the MDS.

Emergency unit physicians, particularly those in units with a medium patient volume and in hospitals with medical teaching affiliations, cite more problems with non-staff than with staff resources. In osteopathic hospital units, the MDS cite non-staff resources somewhat less, and relations with the parent hospital somewhat more, often as a problem than do their counterparts in other hospitals. In contrast, the RNS cite staff resources more often than non-staff resources as problem areas. This is particularly true in the case of hospitals whose emergency units have a low patient volume, and in the case of osteopathic and church operated institutions.

Other areas in which both the physicians and registered nurses working in the various EU's see problems include: relations with the community (mentioned by 17% of the MDS, and 9% of the RNS); relations with the parent hospital (8% of MDS, 9% of RNS); and staff performance or quality of care (8% of MDS, 6% of RNS). Additionally a few of the problems cited by nurses concern the emergency unit's organization and supervision (8% of RNS). In general, problems in these latter areas are mentioned much less frequently by both groups of respondents than are problems in the resource areas.

TABLE 35. THE CURRENT MAJOR PROBLEMS OF EMERGENCY UNITS, AS ASSESSED BY
THE PHYSICIANS (MDS) WHO WORK THERE[a]

Hospital Emergency Units (EU's) Involved	Total Mentions[b]	The Three Problems Most Frequently Mentioned by MDS		
		First	Second	Third
ALL EU'S IN THE STUDY SAMPLE (N=30 Hospital EU's)	402	Non-staff resources (32.1%)	Staff resources (26.1%)	Relations with the community (16.7%)
YOUR HOSPITAL'S EU				
EU's with:				
Low Patient Volume (n=10)	152	Non-staff resources (28.3%)	Staff resources (25.7%)	Relations with the community (21.7%)
Medium Pat. Volume (n=10)	120	Non-staff resources (40.0%)	Staff resources (29.2%)	Relations with the community (14.2%)
High Patient Volume (n=10)	130	Non-staff resources (29.2%)	Staff resources (23.8%)	Relations with the community (13.1%)
EU's in:				
Church Operated Hospitals (n=9)	148	Non-staff resources (35.1%)	Staff resources (27.7%)	Relations with the community (16.9%)
Osteopathic Hospitals (n=3)	32	Staff resources (28.1%)	Relations with parent hospital (21.9%)	Relations with the community (18.8%)
All Other Hospitals (n=18)	222	Non-staff resources (32.4%)	Staff resources (24.8%)	Relations with the community (16.2%)
EU's Located in:				
SMSA (urban) Areas (n=21)	293	Non-staff resources (34.1%)	Staff resources (25.9%)	Relations with the community (16.0%)
Non-SMSA Areas (n=9)	109	Non-staff resources (26.6%)	Staff resources (26.6%)	Relations with the community (18.3%)
EU's in Hospitals Having:				
Medical Teaching Affiliations (n=17)	223	Non-staff resources (35.4%)	Staff resources (25.6%)	Relations with the community (16.1%)
No Medical Teaching Affiliations (n=13)	179	Non-staff resources (27.9%)	Staff resources (26.8%)	Relations with the community (17.3%)
EU's in Hospitals Having:				
Emergency Personnel Training Programs (n=15)	202	Non-staff resources (30.2%)	Staff resources (21.8%)	Relations with the community (18.8%)
No Training Programs (n=15)	200	Non-staff resources (34.0%)	Staff resources (30.5%)	Relations with the community (14.5%)

[a] The results are based on the responses of MDS from the various EU's to the following open-ended question: "At the present time, what sorts of problems does the Emergency Unit of this hospital face? What would you say are the major problems or key issues?" Their responses were first coded into a large number of specific categories and then collapsed into the following ten general categories: (1) Organization or supervision, (2) staff resources, (3) non-staff resources, (4) work relations in the unit, (5) staff identification and satisfaction, (6) costs and charges, (7) strain and tension, (8) staff performance or quality of care, (9) relations with the parent hospital, and (10) relations with the community.

[b] The mentions indicated for each grouping of EU's represent the sum of mentions for all hospital EU's in the grouping combined. The percentages enclosed in parentheses after each problem were computed using the summed mentions as a base. Of all MDS in the sample 85% mentioned at least one major problem, 52% mentioned at least two, and 26% mentioned three.

TABLE 36. THE CURRENT MAJOR PROBLEMS OF EMERGENCY UNITS, AS ASSESSED BY THE REGISTERED NURSES (RNS) WHO WORK THERE[a]

Hospital Emergency Units (EU's) Involved	Total Mentions[b]	The Three Problems Most Frequently Mentioned by RNS		
		First	Second	Third
ALL EU'S IN THE STUDY SAMPLE (N=30 Hospital EU's)	551	Staff resources (34.1%)	Non-staff resources (28.7%)	Relations with parent hospital (8.5%); relations with the community (8.5%)
YOUR HOSPITAL'S EU				
EU's with:				
Low Patient Volume (n=10)	155	Staff resources (39.4%)	Non-staff resources (25.2%)	Relations with parent hospital (11.6%)
Medium Pat. Volume (n=10)	163	Staff resources (37.4%)	Non-staff resources (30.7%)	Organization or supervision (10.4%)
High Patient Volume (n=10)	233	Non-staff resources (29.6%)	Staff resources (28.3%)	Relations with the community (11.2%)
EU's in:				
Church Operated Hospitals (n=9)	154	Staff resources (40.3%)	Non-staff resources (26.0%)	Relations with parent hospital (10.4%)
Osteopathic Hospitals (n=3)	61	Staff resources (36.1%)	Non-staff resources (19.7%)	Relations with parent hospital (14.8%)
All Other Hospitals (n=18)	336	Non-staff resources (31.5%)	Staff resources (31.0%)	Relations with the community (8.9%)
EU's Located in:				
SMSA (urban) Areas (n=21)	401	Staff resources (31.7%)	Non-staff resources (27.9%)	Relations with parent hospital (9.7%); relations with the community (9.7%)
Non-SMSA Areas (n=9)	150	Staff resources (40.7%)	Non-staff resources (30.7%)	Organization or supervision (8.7%)
EU's in Hospitals Having:				
Medical Teaching Affiliations (n=17)	327	Staff resources (33.0%)	Non-staff resources (27.5%)	Relations with the community (10.1%)
No Medical Teaching Affiliations (n=13)	224	Staff resources (35.7%)	Non-staff resources (30.4%)	Organization or supervision (9.4%)
EU's in Hospitals Having:				
Emergency Personnel Training Programs (n=15)	313	Staff resources (33.5%)	Non-staff resources (26.5%)	Relations with the community (9.9%)
No Training Programs (n=15)	238	Staff resources (34.9%)	Non-staff resources (31.5%)	Organization or supervision (8.8%)

[a]The results are based on the responses of RNS from the various EU's to the following open-ended question: "At the present time, what sorts of problems does the Emergency Unit of this hospital face? What would you say are the major problems or key issues?" Their responses were first coded into a large number of specific categories and then collapsed into the following ten general categories: (1) Organization or supervision, (2) staff resources, (3) non-staff resources, (4) work relations in the unit, (5) staff identification and satisfaction, (6) costs and charges, (7) strain and tension, (8) staff performance or quality of care, (9) relations with the parent hospital, and (10) relations with the community.

[b]The mentions indicated for each grouping of EU's represent the sum of mentions for all hospital EU's in the grouping combined. The percentages enclosed in parentheses after each problem were computed using the summed mentions as a base. Of all RNS in the sample 96% mentioned at least one major problem, 69% mentioned at least two, and 33% mentioned three.

Two key groups of respondents not working in the emergency units -- hospital administrators (HAS) and the selected physicians (HMDS) -- also were asked about the current major problems of the units. The data from hospital administrators are summarized in Table 37; those from the selected physicians are not presented in tabular form. These outside respondents (both HAS and HMDS), like the doctors and nurses who work in the units, cite staff resources and non-staff resources as the top two major problem areas. The third most frequently mentioned problem area, again by both HAS and HMDS, is that of relations with the community -- the same area which placed third also according to the data from the physicians who work in the emergency units.

Overall, when the total sample is considered, staff resources, non-staff resources, and relations with the community together account for two-thirds of all the problems mentioned by either hospital administrators or the selected hospital physicians. However, the relative frequency with which these three problem areas are mentioned by the HAS differs considerably across emergency unit groupings. For units with a low patient volume, for example, staff resources are mentioned as problems by these respondents more often than non-staff resources or relations with the community. For units with a medium patient volume, problems with non-staff resources are mentioned by the same respondents as often as are problems with staff resources. For the same units, moreover, relations with the community are mentioned much less frequently by the HAS as a problem than they are for units having either a low or a high patient volume. Comparable differences across emergency unit groupings with respect to the frequency with which particular problems are mentioned occur significantly less in the data provided by HMDS (not shown in table form). As with most other findings, however, the reader is once again reminded that the situation of individual emergency units may well differ greatly from the more general patterns discussed.

TABLE 37. THE CURRENT MAJOR PROBLEMS OF EMERGENCY UNITS, AS ASSESSED BY THE HOSPITAL ADMINISTRATOR RESPONDENTS (HAS)[a]

		The Three Problems Most Frequently Mentioned by HAS		
Hospital Emergency Units (EU's) Involved	Total Mentions[b]	First	Second	Third
ALL EU'S IN THE STUDY SAMPLE (N=30 Hospital EU's)	151	Staff resources (26.5%)	Non-staff resources (20.5%)	Relations with the community (20.5%)
YOUR HOSPITAL'S EU		--	--	--
EU's with:				
Low Patient Volume (n=10)	45	Staff resources (31.1%)	Non-staff resources (17.8%)	Relations with the community (17.8%)
Medium Pat. Volume (n=10)	51	Staff resources (29.4%)	Non-staff resources (29.4%)	Relations with the community (9.8%); Costs and charges (9.8%)
High Patient Volume (n=10)	55	Relations with the community (32.7%)	Staff resources (20.0%)	Non-staff resources (14.5%)
EU's in:				
Church Operated Hospitals (n=9)	45	Staff resources (28.9%)	Relations with the community (24.4%)	Non-staff resources (15.6%)
Osteopathic Hospitals (n=3)	16	Staff resources (31.3%)	Non-staff resources (18.8%)	Costs and charges (18.8%); Relations with parent hospital (18.8%)
All Other Hospitals (n=18)	90	Staff resources (24.4%)	Non-staff resources (23.3%)	Relations with the community (22.2%)
EU's Located in:				
SMSA (urban) Areas (n=21)	117	Staff resources (27.4%)	Non-staff resources (22.2%)	Relations with the community (19.7%)
Non-SMSA Areas (n=9)	34	Staff resources (23.5%)	Relations with the community (23.5%)	Non-staff resources (14.7%)
EU's in Hospitals Having:				
Medical Teaching Affiliations (n=17)	96	Staff resources (25.0%)	Relations with the community (24.0%)	Non-staff resources (19.8%)
No Medical Teaching Affiliations (n=13)	55	Staff resources (29.1%)	Non-staff resources (21.8%)	Relations with the community (14.5%)
EU's in Hospitals Having:				
Emergency Personnel Training Programs (n=15)	84	Relations with the community (25.0%)	Staff resources (22.6%)	Non-staff resources (19.0%)
No Training Programs (n=15)	67	Staff resources (31.3%)	Non-staff resources (22.4%)	Relations with the community (14.9%)

[a] The results are based on the responses of HAS from the various hospitals to the following open-ended question: "At the present time, what sorts of problems does the Emergency Unit of this hospital face? What would you say are the major problems or key issues?" Their responses were first coded into a large number of specific categories and then collapsed into the following ten general categories: (1) Organization or supervision, (2) staff resources, (3) non-staff resources, (4) work relations in the unit, (5) staff identification and satisfaction, (6) costs and charges, (7) strain and tension, (8) staff performance or quality of care, (9) relations with the parent hospital, and (10) relations with the community.

[b] The mentions indicated for each grouping of EU's represent the sum of mentions for all hospital EU's in the grouping combined. The percentages enclosed in parentheses after each problem were computed using the summed mentions as a base. Of all HAS in the sample 94% mentioned at least one major problem, 81% mentioned at least two, and 47% mentioned three.

Summary

The results presented in this chapter indicate considerable agreement among the various groups of respondents regarding the top goal priorities, most important strengths, and current major problems of the emergency units studied. The physicians (MDS) and registered nurses (RNS) working in the units, for example, as well as the selected hospital physicians (HMDS), all rank the goal priorities of their respective units very similarly. In general, they indicate that the priorities most directly related to the patient care provided (maintaining high standards of care, providing comprehensive services, and maintaining a high level of patient satisfaction -- in that order) are the most important ones or the ones that are emphasized the most by the emergency units.

Minimizing patient waiting time and maintaining a good reputation in the community are generally emphasized less, according to the same respondents. However, the selected community respondents (CRS) indicate that minimizing patient waiting time is one of the top priorities of emergency units. (This disparity may reflect the different kinds of patients with whom various respondents come in contact, or it may reflect a difference in perspectives or even perhaps misperception by the CRS.) Finally, the data show that keeping the costs of the emergency service down and improving working conditions for the staff are the least emphasized among the seven goal priorities considered.

Other findings in this chapter show that <u>staff performance or quality of care</u> places in either first or second place among the most important strengths of emergency units mentioned by each of the several groups of respondents. This appears to be consistent with the high emphasis placed on the quality of patient care by the emergency units. Another aspect, <u>staff resources</u>, also is generally considered as a top strength, occupying second or first place among the strengths most mentioned (when staff performance places first, staff resources places second, and vice versa). This same area, however, also occupies a prominent place among the current major problems of emergency units cited by the respondents. Other frequently mentioned strengths include relations with the parent hospital and relations with the community -- areas that are also frequently seen as problems.

Concerning problems, the non-staff resources of emergency units are mentioned first or second most often by all responding groups (the same resources are seen as one of the top three strengths of emergency units by one of the groups -- the RNS). The same is true, as pointed out above, regarding staff resources. Other problems among the three most often mentioned by at least one of the several groups of respondents include relations with the community and relations with the parent hospital. These same areas, however, also are seen as strengths by at least one group of respondents.

Apart from these general patterns, the findings show a number of interesting differences for emergency units in the various groupings studied, i.e., the groupings based on hospital size and location, medical teaching affiliation, emergency unit patient volume, etc. They also show certain differences among the several groups of respondents who provided the data. Differences of both of these kinds occur with respect to all of the topics considered in this chapter -- the goal priorities, the most important strengths, and the current major problems of emergency units. Generally, however, they are neither great nor numerous. The most important of these differences have been discussed. Finally, inter-unit variability on each of the measures examined also exists and must be kept in mind when considering the situation of individual emergency units. We next turn to the areas of leadership and influence over the operations of emergency units.

Chapter 4

PERCEIVED LEADERSHIP EFFECTIVENESS AND THE INFLUENCE OF VARIOUS GROUPS

Reviewed in this chapter are findings regarding the leadership of emergency units and the influence that various key groups have on how these units operate. The effectiveness of medical, nursing, and administrative leadership, as assessed by certain respondents in each case, is discussed in the first section. The second section focuses on the amount of influence that particular groups have, and also the influence that they should have, on how the emergency units operate. These influence patterns are based on data from the physicians (MDS) working in the various EU's and from the hospital administrators (HAS) who participated in the study as respondents.

Potentially, the leadership of an emergency unit is related to organizational effectiveness in a number of important ways. Where the leadership is strong, for example, work problems are likely to be resolved more adequately than in units where the leadership is ineffective or weak. The adequacy of problem solving, in turn, can increase both the quality of the services offered by the unit and the efficiency with which services are provided. Effective leadership, moreover, is likely to correlate positively with the availability and stability of resources. Further, leadership may be related to the influence that different groups exercise on how a unit operates.

In emergency units having effective medical, nursing, and administrative leadership, the amount of influence that all relevant groups have on how the unit functions -- or the "total amount of influence" exercised by all relevant groups together -- is likely to be substantial. The total amount of influence has been found, in different types of organizations, to correlate with various criteria of organizational effectiveness, including staff satisfaction. Thus, emergency units with strong leadership are likely to be more effective than others not only with respect to solving work problems and obtaining resources, and with respect to the quality of services provided, but also with respect to the satisfaction of those who do the work.

Medical, Nursing, and Administrative Leadership

Concerning the leadership of emergency units, data were obtained from key hospital administrators (HAS), the selected hospital physicians (HMDS) not working in the units, and the supervising nurses (SRNS) of the units. In all cases, the respondents were asked to assess the relative effectiveness of leadership. The results presented in Table 38 pertain to medical leadership. Overall, considering all of the 30 EU's in the study sample, the data show that the medical leadership of the emergency units is regarded as better than "fairly effective," on the average, but less than "very effective." This is true regardless of the specific source of data (the overall mean scores based on the data from HMDS, SRNS, and HAS, respectively, are 2.32, 2.44, and 2.63). The data also indicate that medical leadership is evaluated as somewhat more effective by the selected hospital physicians than by the administrators, with the supervising nurses of emergency units occupying an intermediate position in this respect.

There also appear to be some differences in the perceived effectiveness of medical leadership between certain groupings of emergency units, at least based on the data from hospital administrators. For example, medical leadership is seen by HAS as relatively more effective in the units of urban compared to non-urban area hospitals, and the units of hospitals with medical

TABLE 38. RELATIVE EFFECTIVENESS OF THE MEDICAL LEADERSHIP OF EMERGENCY UNITS, AS ASSESSED BY CERTAIN GROUPS OF RESPONDENTS[a]

Hospital Emergency Units (EU's) Involved		Leadership Effectiveness According to		
		SRNS	HAS	HMDS
ALL EU'S IN THE STUDY SAMPLE (N=30 Hospital EU's)	Mean: Range:	2.44 (1.00-4.00)	2.63 (1.00-4.50)	2.32 (1.67-3.14)
YOUR HOSPITAL'S EU		--	--	
EU's with:				
Low Patient Volume (n=10)		2.35	2.75	2.25
Medium Pat. Volume (n=10)		2.50	2.57	2.35
High Patient Volume (n=10)		2.47	2.58	2.37
EU's in:				
Church Operated Hospitals (n=9)		2.67	3.04	2.29
Osteopathic Hospitals (n=3)		2.83	2.17	2.29
All Other Hospitals (n=18)		2.26	2.51	2.34
EU's Located in:				
SMSA (urban) Areas (n=21)		2.53	2.45	2.30
Non-SMSA Areas (n=9)		2.22	3.06	2.37
EU's in Hospitals Having:				
Medical Teaching Affiliations (n=17)		2.50	2.47	2.26
No Medical Teaching Affiliations (n=13)		2.36	2.85	2.40
EU's in Hospitals Having:				
Emergency Personnel Training Programs (n=15)		2.41	2.59	2.31
No Training Programs (n=15)		2.47	2.68	2.33

[a] The results, presented here in the form of mean scores, are based on the responses of SRNS, HAS, and HMDS associated with the various institutions, to the following question: "Based on your knowledge and observation, how would you characterize the medical leadership of this emergency unit?" (The wording differed slightly in the interview completed by HMDS.) The response alternatives were: (1) Extremely effective, (2) very effective, (3) fairly effective, (4) not so effective, and (5) not effective at all. Using the data from each group of respondents, mean scores were first computed separately for each EU and then averaged for the EU's in the different categories. The lower the mean score, the more effective the leadership in all cases.

teaching affiliations compared to those without such affiliations. It is also seen by HAS as more effective in osteopathic than in church operated hospitals, but the SRNS disagree in this case. According to the SRNS, medical leadership is least effective in the units of osteopathic hospitals. The data from HMDS show no differences between one grouping of emergency units and another, when the various groupings are properly compared.

More important, the effectiveness of medical leadership varies greatly across individual emergency units, according to the data from both hospital administrators and the supervising nurses (see the ranges of unit mean scores in Table 38). In some of the units, medical leadership is regarded "extremely effective" while in others it is regarded "not so effective" by both HAS and SRNS respondents. Inter-unit variability is more modest according to the data from selected hospital physicians (HMDS).

The results concerning administrative and nursing leadership are all summarized in Table 39. First, they show that, on the average, both hospital administrators and the selected physicians consider the nursing leadership of emergency units as "very effective." But, according to both respondent groups, especially the HAS, nursing leadership is less effective in emergency units with a medium than a low or high patient volume. In addition, it is somewhat less effective in the units of osteopathic hospitals compared to other not church operated hospitals and to church operated institutions. (Between the latter two groupings there is no difference.)

Finally, as the range of unit mean scores indicates, the effectiveness of nursing leadership as perceived by HAS, varies greatly across individual emergency units. As perceived by HMDS, on the other hand, it varies only moderately.

Table 39 also summarizes the evaluations by selected hospital physicians (HMDS) of the administrative leadership of the emergency units in their

TABLE 39. RELATIVE EFFECTIVENESS OF THE ADMINISTRATIVE AND NURSING LEADERSHIP OF EMERGENCY UNITS, AS ASSESSED BY CERTAIN GROUPS OF RESPONDENTS[a]

Hospital Emergency Units (EU's) Involved		Administrative Leadership Effectiveness According to	Nursing Leadership Effectiveness According to	
		HMDS	HMDS	HAS
ALL EU'S IN THE STUDY SAMPLE (N=30 Hospital EU's)	Mean: Range:	2.33 (1.14-3.33)	2.04 (1.00-2.71)	2.13 (1.00-3.50)
YOUR HOSPITAL'S EU				--
EU's with:				
Low Patient Volume (n=10)		2.29	1.93	2.05
Medium Pat. Volume (n=10)		2.37	2.22	2.40
High Patient Volume (n=10)		2.32	1.99	1.95
EU's in:				
Church Operated Hospitals (n=9)		2.32	1.90	2.20
Osteopathic Hospitals (n=3)		2.62	2.23	2.50
All Other Hospitals (n=18)		2.28	2.08	2.04
EU's Located in:				
SMSA (urban) Areas (n=21)		2.36	2.01	2.14
Non-SMSA Areas (n=9)		2.24	2.13	2.11
EU's in Hospitals Having:				
Medical Teaching Affiliations (n=17)		2.31	2.10	2.18
No Medical Teaching Affiliations (n=13)		2.35	1.97	2.08
EU's in Hospitals Having:				
Emergency Personnel Training Programs (n=15)		2.35	2.03	2.13
No Training Programs (n=15)		2.30	2.06	2.13

[a] The results are based on data provided by HMDS and HAS associated with the various institutions in response to the following item: "Based on your knowledge and observation, how would you characterize the.... leadership of this emergency unit?" One question dealing with <u>administrative leadership</u> was asked of HMDS, and a similar question about <u>nursing leadership</u> was asked of HMDS and of HAS. The response alternatives were: (1) Extremely effective, (2) very effective, (3) fairly effective, (4) not so effective, and (5) not effective at all. Using the data from each respondent group to each question, mean scores were first computed separately for each EU and then averaged for the EU's in the different categories. The <u>lower</u> the mean score, the more effective the leadership in all cases.

respective institutions. According to these respondents, the effectiveness of administrative leadership (i.e., the leadership provided by hospital administration for the emergency units) varies for individual EU's from "extremely effective" to less than "fairly effective." Concerning the various groupings of EU's, however, the data show no appreciable differences, with the exception that administrative leadership is seen as more effective for the units of non-osteopathic compared to osteopathic institutions. For all other groupings, administrative leadership is seen almost as "very effective," on the average, as it is for the study sample as a whole.

The Influence of Key Groups

Emergency unit physicians (MDS) and the hospital administrators (HAS) who completed questionnaires for the study were both asked to indicate the amount of influence that each of six groups currently has on how the emergency unit operates. In addition, they were asked to indicate how much influence the same groups should have. The relevant groups are: the Board of Trustees, or governing authority, of the hospital; Hospital Administration; the doctors who work in the emergency unit; the nurses who work in the emergency unit; the patients of the unit; and the "community outside." The results about the current, or actual, influence of these groups based on the data from MDS and HAS are presented in Tables 40 and 41, respectively, followed by the findings about the preferred, or desired, influence by the same respondents for the same groups.

Considering first all 30 EU's in the sample, the overall mean scores in Table 40 show that, on the average, the doctors who work in the units (i.e., the MDS) themselves have the greatest amount of influence, among the six groups, on how their respective units operate. The doctors are followed,

TABLE 40. THE INFLUENCE OF VARIOUS GROUPS ON HOW THE EMERGENCY UNITS OPERATE, ACCORDING TO THE DOCTORS (MDS) WHO WORK THERE[a]

Hospital Emergency Units (EU's) Involved		The Doctors Working in the EU	The Nurses Working in the EU	Hospital Administration	The Hospital's Board of Trustees	The EU Patients	The Community Outside
ALL EU'S IN THE STUDY SAMPLE (N=30 Hospital EU's)	Mean:	2.05	2.26	2.07	2.85	3.02	3.33
	Range:	(1.33-3.00)	(1.50-3.17)	(1.25-3.67)	(2.00-4.00)	(2.11-4.50)	(2.60-4.50)
YOUR HOSPITAL'S EU							
EU's with:							
Low Patient Volume (n=10)		2.05	2.14	1.85	2.90	3.15	3.40
Medium Pat. Volume (n=10)		2.06	2.39	2.17	2.85	3.10	3.51
High Patient Volume (n=10)		2.03	2.25	2.18	2.78	2.80	3.07
EU's in:							
Church Operated Hospitals (n=9)		2.13	2.19	1.84	2.84	3.14	3.43
Osteopathic Hospitals (n=3)		2.13	2.74	2.56	3.16	3.07	3.56
All Other Hospitals (n=18)		1.99	2.21	2.10	2.80	2.95	3.24
EU's Located in:							
SMSA (urban) Areas (n=21)		2.03	2.31	2.03	2.85	2.99	3.36
Non-SMSA Areas (n=9)		2.08	2.14	2.16	2.84	3.10	3.26
EU's in Hospitals Having:							
Medical Teaching Affiliations (n=17)		1.96	2.27	2.14	2.96	2.98	3.38
No Medical Teaching Affiliations (n=13)		2.15	2.24	1.97	2.70	3.07	3.26
EU's in Hospitals Having:							
Emergency Personnel Training Programs (n=15)		2.06	2.28	2.05	2.78	2.92	3.23
No Training Programs (n=15)		2.03	2.23	2.08	2.92	3.12	3.42

[a] The results, presented here in the form of mean scores, are based on the responses of MDS to the following multiple-part question: "Generally, how much influence does each of the following have on how this emergency unit operates?" (The order in which the referent groups appeared in the question was: Board of Trustees, Hospital Administration, Doctors, Nurses, Patients, the Community.) The response alternatives were: (1) Very considerable influence, (2) considerable influence, (3) moderate influence, (4) little influence, and (5) very little or no influence. Mean scores regarding the influence of each group were first computed separately for each EU and then averaged for the EU's in each category. The lower the mean scores, the higher the level of influence attributed by MDS to the particular groups.

very closely, by Hospital Administration in second place, and by the nurses who are working in the various emergency units in third place. In fact, the level of influence attributed to these three groups by MDS respondents is almost the same and corresponds to "considerable influence." (The relevant mean influence scores for the identified groups are 2.05, 2.07, and 2.26, respectively.) The remaining groups apparently have much less influence, on the average, on how the emergency units operate. Next most influential after the nurses, but at a good distance, are the trustees who, according to the MDS, have slightly more than "moderate influence" (the relevant mean score is 2.85). The patients (who are said to have "moderate" influence) are next, followed by the community (which is said to have somewhat less than "moderate" influence) in last place.

Thus, as seen by the physicians (MDS) who work in the emergency units studied, three of the six groups -- the doctors themselves, Hospital Administration, and the nurses -- are very influential while the other three are not. (The same conclusion emerges from the data provided by hospital administrator respondents.)

It is also interesting to note that the influence of each of the six groups involved, according to the data from MDS, on the average is about the same for emergency units in urban and non-urban areas, in hospitals with and without medical teaching affiliations, and in hospitals with and without emergency personnel training programs. On the other hand, the influence of nurses, trustees, and Hospital Administration is generally lower in the units of osteopathic compared to non-osteopathic hospitals. And, the influence of patients and of the community is generally greater in emergency units with a high, compared to a medium or low, patient volume, while the reverse is true regarding the influence of Hospital Administration.

Finally, the data in Table 40 show that the amount of influence attributed to each of the six groups by MDS respondents varies widely across individual emergency units (see the ranges of mean scores). Inter-unit variability is especially high concerning the influence of Hospital Administration and of patients. The patients of some of the units, for example, are seen as having "considerable" influence while those of other units are seen as having "little" to "very little" influence. The influence of the other groups, including the doctors and nurses who work in the units, also varies substantially across individual EU's, but less.

The data from hospital administrators (HAS) about the influence that the same six groups have are summarized in Table 41. On the average, these respondents too indicate that the doctors, the nurses, and Hospital Administration have significantly more influence on how the emergency units operate than do the patients, the community, or the trustees. The doctors who work in the units have the greatest influence ("considerable" to "very considerable" influence, on the average), and the nurses are next (with "considerable" influence), followed by Hospital Administration (with almost "considerable" influence). The patients are next, at some distance, followed (almost exactly at the same level) by the community and the trustees. The last two groups are seen by administrators as having somewhat less than "moderate" influence.

Thus, administrators (HAS) agree with the physicians (MDS) that the three most influential groups are the doctors, the nurses, and Hospital Administration. However, comparison of the overall mean scores in Table 41 and Table 40 also shows that the physicians attribute more influence to the trustees than do the administrators (2.85 vs. 3.22). They also attribute somewhat more influence to Hospital Administration than do the administrators. In contrast, the HAS attribute more influence to the doctors who work in the

TABLE 41. THE INFLUENCE OF VARIOUS GROUPS ON HOW THE EMERGENCY UNITS OPERATE,
ACCORDING TO HOSPITAL ADMINISTRATOR RESPONDENTS (HAS)[a]

Hospital Emergency Units (EU's) Involved		Level of Influence Attributed to					
		The Doctors Working in the EU	The Nurses Working in the EU	Hospital Administration	The Hospital's Board of Trustees	The EU Patients	The Community Outside
ALL EU'S IN THE STUDY SAMPLE (N=30 Hospital EU's)	Mean: Range:	1.77 (1.00-3.00)	2.01 (1.00-3.00)	2.29 (1.00-3.50)	3.22 (1.00-4.33)	2.86 (1.00-4.00)	3.21 (1.00-4.50)
YOUR HOSPITAL'S EU		--	--	--	--	--	--
EU's with:							
Low Patient Volume (n=10)		1.72	1.97	2.45	3.42	2.88	3.20
Medium Pat. Volume (n=10)		1.88	2.07	2.23	3.07	3.07	3.50
High Patient Volume (n=10)		1.72	1.98	2.18	3.18	2.62	2.93
EU's in:							
Church Operated Hospitals (n=9)		1.81	1.96	2.19	3.56	3.07	3.07
Osteopathic Hospitals (n=3)		1.50	2.17	2.83	3.67	3.33	3.67
All Other Hospitals (n=18)		1.80	2.00	2.25	2.98	2.67	3.20
EU's Located in:							
SMSA (urban) Areas (n=21)		1.75	2.06	2.46	3.46	2.79	3.25
Non-SMSA Areas (n=9)		1.83	1.89	1.89	2.67	3.00	3.11
EU's in Hospitals Having:							
Medical Teaching Affiliations (n=17)		1.69	1.98	2.30	3.30	2.95	3.34
No Medical Teaching Affiliations (n=13)		1.88	2.04	2.27	3.12	2.73	3.04
EU's in Hospitals Having:							
Emergency Personnel Training Programs (n=15)		1.72	1.97	2.29	3.43	2.87	3.22
No Training Programs (n=15)		1.82	2.04	2.29	3.01	2.84	3.20

[a] The results, presented here in the form of mean scores, are based on the responses of HAS to the following multiple-part question: "Generally, how much influence does each of the following have on how this emergency unit operates?" (The order is which the referent groups appeared in the question was: Board of Trustees, Hospital Administration, Doctors, Nurses, Patients, the Community.) The response alternatives were: (1) Very considerable influence, (2) considerable influence, (3) moderate influence, (4) little influence, and (5) very little or no influence. Mean scores regarding the influence of each group were first computed separately for each EU and then averaged for the EU's in each category. The lower the mean scores, the higher the level of influence attributed by HAS to the particular groups.

units than do the MDS (1.77 vs. 2.05). The HAS also attribute somewhat more influence to each of the remaining groups -- the nurses, patients, and community -- than do the MDS.

When considering the various groupings of emergency units instead of the total sample, the data from administrators (Table 41) show a great many differences. First, the trustees have less influence on how the emergency units operate in hospitals with than without emergency personnel training programs. (For institutions with and without medical teaching affiliation there is no difference.) They also have less influence in the case of urban compared to non-urban EU's, in the case of church operated and osteopathic institutions compared to other institutions, and in the case of EU's with a low (compared to other than low) patient volume. Hospital Administration also has less influence on how EU's with a low, compared to other than low, patient volume operate, and also in the case of urban compared to non-urban area EU's, and osteopathic compared to non-osteopathic EU's.

The patients of emergency units have more influence, on the average, in hospitals which are not church operated (excluding osteopathic) than in those which are church operated, and in EU's with a high compared to a medium patient volume. The community also has more influence in EU's with a high compared to a medium patient volume. It similarly has more influence in the EU's of non-osteopathic (whether or not church operated) compared to osteopathic institutions. In contrast, the doctors have more influence in the latter than in the former institutions. Apart from this single difference, however, the doctors have about the same amount of influence in all of the different groupings of EU's, and the same applies in the case of the nurses without exception.

Finally, as was the case with the data from physician respondents, the data from administrators show great differences across individual emergency units in the amount of influence that each of the six groups has. The greatest variability across individual EU's concerns the influence exercised by the community and by trustees (for both of these groups, influence ranges from "very considerable" to less than "little"). And the smallest variability, which is still very substantial, concerns the influence exercised by the doctors and by the nurses of the unit (again for both of these groups, influence ranges from "very considerable" to "moderate").

Preferred, or desired, influence patterns. The above findings on the current influence of the various groups can be also compared to the influence that the same groups should have on how the emergency units operate, again according to the administrators (HAS) and physicians (MDS). The findings on these preferred patterns of influence are summarized in Table 42 based on the data from HAS and Table 43 based on the data from MDS.

In brief, Table 42 shows that hospital administrators believe that, on the average, the doctors and nurses who work in the emergency unit should have (as they now do) the greatest amount of influence on how the unit operates (incidentally, an identical amount of influence). Hospital Administration should be next, close behind, followed by the patients, the community, and the trustees -- in that order.

Moreover, a comparison of Tables 41 and 42 shows that, from the perspective of administrators (HAS), the doctors working in the emergency units studied have the right amount of influence on how the units operate. The nurses have almost the right amount, but not quite; their influence should be somewhat higher than at present. The other four groups, however, have less influence than is seen as appropriate by HAS respondents. They each "should have" appreciably more influence on the average than is now the case.

TABLE 42. THE AMOUNT OF INFLUENCE THAT VARIOUS GROUPS SHOULD HAVE ON HOW THE EMERGENCY UNITS OPERATE, ACCORDING TO HOSPITAL ADMINISTRATOR RESPONDENTS (HAS)[a]

Hospital Emergency Units (EU's) Involved		The Doctors Working in the EU	The Nurses Working in the EU	Hospital Administration	The Hospital's Board of Trustees	The EU Patients	The Community Outside
ALL EU'S IN THE STUDY SAMPLE (N=30 Hospital EU's)	Mean:	1.73	1.73	1.89	2.64	2.27	2.50
	Range:	(1.00-2.50)	(1.00-3.00)	(1.00-3.00)	(1.00-4.00)	(1.00-4.50)	(1.00-4.50)
YOUR HOSPITAL'S EU		--	--	--	--	--	--
EU's with:							
Low Patient Volume (n=10)		1.87	1.77	2.02	2.78	2.30	2.68
Medium Pat. Volume (n=10)		1.68	1.78	1.73	2.28	2.38	2.38
High Patient Volume (n=10)		1.65	1.63	1.92	2.85	2.12	2.43
EU's in:							
Church Operated Hospitals (n=9)		1.96	1.80	1.87	2.76	2.37	2.54
Osteopathic Hospitals (n=3)		1.17	1.67	2.33	3.33	2.33	2.67
All Other Hospitals (n=18)		1.71	1.70	1.82	2.46	2.20	2.45
EU's Located in:							
SMSA (urban) Areas (n=21)		1.64	1.80	2.08	2.87	2.29	2.55
Non-SMSA Areas (n=9)		1.94	1.56	1.44	2.11	2.22	2.39
EU's in Hospitals Having:							
Medical Teaching Affiliations (n=17)		1.65	1.73	1.89	2.80	2.26	2.50
No Medical Teaching Affiliations (n=13)		1.85	1.73	1.88	2.42	2.27	2.50
EU's in Hospitals Having:							
Emergency Personnel Training Programs (n=15)		1.74	1.73	1.96	2.99	2.44	2.78
No Training Programs (n=15)		1.72	1.72	1.82	2.29	2.09	2.22

[a] The results, presented here in the form of mean scores, are based on the responses of HAS to the following multiple-part question: "Generally, how much influence should each of the following have on how this emergency unit operates?" (The order in which the referent groups appeared in the question was: Board of Trustees, Hospital Administration, Doctors, Nurses, Patients, the Community.) The response alternatives were: (1) Very considerable influence, (2) considerable influence, (3) moderate influence, (4) little influence, and (5) very little or no influence. Mean scores representing the influence that each group should have according to HAS were first computed separately for each EU and then averaged for the EU's in each category. The lower the mean scores, the higher the preferred level of influence for the particular groups.

Similar comparisons, based on the corresponding findings in Tables 41 and 42, can be made with respect to each of the various groupings of EU's for which data are shown.

Results about the preferred influence patterns for the various groups based on the data from physicians (MDS) are summarized in Table 43. The physicians too believe that they should have the greatest amount of influence (even more than they now have) on how their respective emergency units operate, and that the nurses should be next, though at some distance, followed by Hospital Administration, but at a considerably greater distance, in third place. In fourth, fifth, and sixth place, respectively, should be the patients of the unit, the trustees, and the community.

As might be expected, however, the preferred level of influence for each particular group differs considerably across individual emergency units (see the ranges of unit mean scores in Table 43). Generally, based on the inter-unit variability in each case, the physicians agree more across EU's about the influence that they and the nurses should have than about the influence that each of the other four groups should have; they agree least about the influence that the patients and the community should have. (The administrators, Table 42, similarly agree more about the influence that the doctors and nurses, and also Hospital Administration, should have, and less about the influence that the other three groups should have.)

It is also clear from the findings (Tables 43 and 42) that the stated preferences of physicians (MDS) differ from those of the administrators (HAS) in a number of ways. Overall, the physicians would prefer somewhat more influence for the doctors who work in the emergency unit, and somewhat less influence for the nurses, than would the administrators. In varying degrees, they would also prefer less influence for each of the other groups than would

TABLE 43. THE AMOUNT OF INFLUENCE THAT VARIOUS GROUPS SHOULD HAVE ON HOW THE EMERGENCY UNITS OPERATE, ACCORDING TO THE DOCTORS (MDS) WHO WORK THERE[a]

		Level of Influence Preferred for					
Hospital Emergency Units (EU's) Involved		The Doctors Working in the EU	The Nurses Working in the EU	Hospital Administration	The Hospital's Board of Trustees	The EU Patients	The Community Outside
ALL EU'S IN THE STUDY SAMPLE (N=30 Hospital EU's)	Mean:	1.51	1.91	2.53	2.99	2.70	3.01
	Range:	(1.00-2.33)	(1.33-2.33)	(1.50-3.80)	(2.00-4.00)	(1.80-4.50)	(2.20-4.50)
YOUR HOSPITAL'S EU							
EU's with:							
Low Patient Volume (n=10)		1.51	1.91	2.40	2.91	2.72	3.06
Medium Pat. Volume (n=10)		1.58	1.94	2.63	3.00	2.84	3.20
High Patient Volume (n=10)		1.42	1.89	2.56	3.05	2.55	2.78
EU's in:							
Church Operated Hospitals (n=9)		1.52	1.97	2.23	2.76	2.69	3.03
Osteopathic Hospitals (n=3)		1.32	1.87	3.03	3.45	2.54	2.81
All Other Hospitals (n=18)		1.53	1.89	2.60	3.02	2.74	3.04
EU's Located in:							
SMSA (urban) Areas (n=21)		1.51	1.92	2.59	3.03	2.70	3.06
Non-SMSA Areas (n=9)		1.50	1.91	2.41	2.89	2.71	2.90
EU's in Hospitals Having:							
Medical Teaching Affiliations (n=17)		1.46	1.87	2.67	3.11	2.66	3.07
No Medical Teaching Affiliations (n=13)		1.56	1.97	2.35	2.82	2.75	2.94
EU's in Hospitals Having:							
Emergency Personnel Training Programs (n=15)		1.49	1.97	2.56	3.08	2.66	3.02
No Training Programs (n=15)		1.52	1.86	2.50	2.89	2.74	3.01

[a] The results, presented here in the form of mean scores, are based on the responses of MDS to the following multiple-part question: "Generally, how much influence should each of the following have on how this emergency unit operates?" (The order in which the referent groups appeared in the question was: Board of Trustees, Hospital Administration, Doctors, Nurses, Patients, the Community.) The response alternatives were: (1) Very considerable influence, (2) considerable influence, (3) moderate influence, (4) little influence, and (5) very little or no influence. Mean scores representing the influence that each group should have according to MDS were first computed separately for each EU and then averaged for the EU's in each category. The lower the mean scores, the higher the preferred level of influence for the particular groups.

the administrators. The discrepancy is largest (2.53 vs. 1.89) concerning the influence that Hospital Administration should have (it is next largest concerning the community's influence).

The data from MDS in Table 43 about preferred influence can be also compared to the data in Table 40, from the same respondents, about current influence patterns. The two tables together show a number of interesting findings. Considering the total sample, for example, the MDS believe that the doctors who work in the emergency units, and also the nurses (more so than the doctors, however) should have more influence, on the average, than they presently have on how the unit operates. The patients and the community also should have somewhat more influence than at present, according to the MDS. (The administrators agree with the physicians in this connection, but they would like to increase the influence of patients, community, and nurses, even more than would the physicians.) Hospital Administration, on the other hand, should have less influence than currently, according to the MDS. And, the trustees should have about the same amount of influence as they presently do.

Total influence. Finally, certain additional comparisons can be made on the basis of the results in the preceding four tables -- Tables 40, 41, 42, and 43 -- after adding together the influence scores for the six groups in each case. The resulting sum of scores represents the total amount of influence that the six groups together have, or should have, on how an emergency unit operates. The total amount of current influence attributed to these groups by physicians (MDS) is, on the average, about the same as the total amount attributed to them by hospital administrators (HAS). However, the total amount of influence that these groups should have is greater based on the stated preferences of HAS than the preferences of MDS. This finding may indicate that administrators, more than physicians, tend to believe (perhaps only implicitly) that any one group's influence could be increased without the other groups necessarily losing influence.*

Summary

The results presented in this chapter suggest a number of interesting conclusions regarding leadership and influence in the emergency units studied. For example, nursing leadership is evaluated more favorably than is either medical or administrative leadership. Further, the respondent groups involved are in greater agreement about the effectiveness of nursing leadership than about the effectiveness of medical leadership. The results also show that there are large differences across individual emergency units in the perceived effectiveness of medical, nursing, and administrative leadership.

Concerning influence, hospital administrators and the physicians who work in the various emergency units are in agreement that the influence of the latter group on how the units operate is, on the average, greater (and should be greater) than that of any of the other key groups specified. They are also in agreement that the groups working in the hospital (emergency unit doctors, the nurses, and Hospital Administration) should, and do, have more influence than the other groups (the trustees, patients, and the community). However, they are only in partial agreement as to which group's influence should be increased, or decreased, and by how much, over current levels.

---

*According to the administrators, it will be recalled, all six groups, especially those which are seen as having the least influence, should have more influence on how an emergency unit operates than they currently have; according to the physicians, on the other hand, several of the groups should have more while some (e.g., Hospital Administration) should have less than they now do.

Differences across individual emergency units in the amount of influence that the hospital administrators believe each of the six groups actually has, also should have, are very great; and the corresponding differences based on the data from physicians are only slightly smaller. There are also a number of differences, according to the data from both of these groups of respondents, in the current and preferred influence patterns for the six groups when the emergency units are grouped according to such things as patient volume, location, and affiliation.

Finally, though not discussed in the preceding pages, the results tend to suggest some relationships between leadership effectiveness and influence patterns when the various groupings of emergency units are examined in greater detail. Although the differences tend to be small, the groupings in which hospital administrators see medical leadership to be the most effective tend to be those in which the administrators also indicate that the doctors who work in the emergency unit do, and should, have the greatest influence on how the unit operates. Similarly, differences in the effectiveness of administrative leadership, as perceived by the selected hospital physician respondents, tend to be congruent with differences in the influence (both current and preferred) that administrators and emergency unit physicians attribute to Hospital Administration. However, no comparable relationships are suggested by the findings concerning nursing leadership effectiveness and the influence of nurses on how the emergency units operate. There appears to be some limited evidence, in short, of possible relationships between leadership effectiveness and the influence of certain groups on how emergency units operate. Such relationships, as well as the relationship (if any) between leadership effectiveness and the "total amount of influence" attributed to all six groups together, will be the subject of more thorough investigation in the forthcoming analyses of the research.

Chapter 5

WORK RELATIONS AND PROBLEM SOLVING WITHIN THE EMERGENCY UNIT

This chapter assesses the nature of work relations among the staff working in the various emergency units. (Relations with the parent hospital and with the outside community are considered in the two chapters which follow next.) First, it examines the adequacy of coordination of work efforts -- how well staff activities fit together, the extent to which the staff take into account each other's work problems and needs, and the extent to which they can rely on others to do their job right. Second, it examines the use and effectiveness of different types of, or approaches to, problem solving within the units. Third, it considers certain important aspects of doctor-nurse relations, including task-centered communication, joint planning, and mutual understanding. Finally, it examines the level of tension between emergency unit nurses and physicians, and also the level of tension among the doctors who work in the unit.

The staff of emergency units are constantly faced with, and must resolve, a variety of work problems, including not only clinical but also coordination and communication problems, task allocation problems, role autonomy and discretion problems, and many other problems that they encounter because of their close interdependence at work. The clinical, economic, and social efficiency of an emergency unit depend on the relative success of the staff in dealing with these problems. Inadequate problem solving can generate tensions, affect staff satisfaction and commitment adversely, and impair staff performance and organizational effectiveness.

Overall Coordination of Staff Efforts and Activities

Adequate coordination in emergency units can not be achieved in a programmed fashion, or through advanced planning and scheduling or standardization of activities, because the work tends to be highly variable and unpredictable and because the staff must be always able to respond quickly to the needs of a great variety of patients (some of whom arrive in a serious or life-threatening condition). Under these circumstances, most of the necessary coordination can be achieved only through a great deal of informal cooperation, good communication, and spontaneous adjustments by all involved. Staff members must be able to anticipate and take into account each other's work problems and needs; to avoid creating problems or interferences with each other's duties and responsibilities; and to rely on one another to a high degree. Only then will their activities fit together properly and their efforts converge toward the accomplishment of the unit's objectives.

Data on these and other important aspects of work relations within the emergency units studied were obtained from the physicians and nurses working in the units and from other respondents. The coordination data are discussed in the present section. The first table, Table 44, shows the results on (a) how well the jobs and activities of the staff fit together -- an indicator of the adequacy of overall coordination, and (b) the extent to which the staff make an effort to avoid creating problems in their mutual work activities -- an indicator of "preventive" coordination.

On the whole, the findings show that staff efforts in the emergency units are, on the average, well coordinated. According to the data from both physicians (MDS) and registered nurses (RNS), the different jobs and activities around the patient fit together "very well" (the overall mean scores describing the average situation in the 30 EU's are 2.08 and 2.00, respectively, based on

TABLE 44. ADEQUACY OF THE OVERALL COORDINATION OF STAFF EFFORTS IN THE EMERGENCY UNITS, ACCORDING TO THE DOCTORS (MDS) AND NURSES (RNS) WHO WORK THERE[a]

Hospital Emergency Units (EU's) Involved		How Well Jobs and Activities Fit Together[b]		Staff Effort to Avoid Creating Problems[c]	
		MDS	RNS	MDS	RNS
ALL EU'S IN THE STUDY SAMPLE (N=30 Hospital EU's)	*Mean:*	2.08	2.00	2.27	2.25
	Range:	(1.57-2.71)	(1.40-2.43)	(1.60-3.00)	(1.60-3.00)
YOUR HOSPITAL'S EU					
EU's with:					
Low Patient Volume (n=10)		2.20	1.97	2.28	2.18
Medium Pat. Volume (n=10)		2.00	1.98	2.22	2.30
High Patient Volume (n=10)		2.04	2.04	2.32	2.28
EU's in:					
Church Operated Hospitals (n=9)		2.34	2.01	2.44	2.26
Osteopathic Hospitals (n=3)		1.86	1.91	2.43	2.36
All Other Hospitals (n=18)		1.99	2.01	2.16	2.23
EU's Located in:					
SMSA (urban) Areas (n=21)		2.03	1.96	2.23	2.29
Non-SMSA Areas (n=9)		2.19	2.09	2.37	2.18
EU's in Hospitals Having:					
Medical Teaching Affiliations (n=17)		2.01	1.98	2.22	2.20
No Medical Teaching Affiliations (n=13)		2.18	2.02	2.34	2.32
EU's in Hospitals Having:					
Emergency Personnel Training Programs (n=15)		2.10	1.98	2.20	2.20
No Training Programs (n=15)		2.06	2.01	2.35	2.31

Table 44 Continues

TABLE 44
(Continued)

---

[a] The results, presented here in the form of mean scores, are based on the responses of MDS and RNS to a pair of interview questions about the coordination of work efforts in their respective EU's. Using the data from each question and each group of respondents, mean scores were first computed separately for each EU and then averaged for the EU's in the different categories.

[b] The question was: "Overall, how well do the different jobs and activities around the patient fit together in this emergency unit?" The response alternatives were: (1) Extremely well, (2) very well, (3) fairly well, (4) not so well, and (5) not well at all. Thus, the lower the score, the better the fit of jobs and activities.

[c] The question was: "To what extent do the people in this emergency unit make an effort to avoid creating problems or interferences with each other's duties and responsibilities?" The response alternatives were: (1) To a very great extent, (2) a great extent, (3) a fair extent, (4) a small extent, and (5) to a very small extent or not at all. Thus, the lower the score the greater the effort to avoid creating problems.

the data from MDS and RNS). Moreover, individual emergency units do not deviate greatly from this general pattern (unlike the case with most measures in most chapters of the present report). Inter-unit variability on this measure is small to moderate (see the ranges of unit mean scores in Table 44). Further, the different groupings of emergency units score very similarly on the present measure, with one exception -- according to the data from MDS activities fit together better, on the average, in the units of hospitals which are not church operated than in the units of those which are. The data from RNS, however, do not show such a difference.

The adequacy of preventive coordination in the units, as indicated by the extent to which the different staff "make an effort to avoid creating problems or interferences with each other's duties and responsibilities" is also high on the average, again according to the data from both MDS and RNS. Inter-unit variability is greater on this measure compared to the first one, whether the data from MDS or RNS are considered, but still only moderate. Again, moreover, the different groupings of emergency units score similarly, with one exception -- according to the MDS, but not the RNS, the staff in the units of hospitals which are not church operated (excluding osteopathic institutions) make a greater effort to avoid creating problems than do the staff in the units of osteopathic and church operated hospitals.

While there is still some room for improvement with respect to both of the above measures, overall coordination in the emergency units in the sample apparently is quite good. In part, this is probably due to the consideration that the staff accord to one another -- something that is confirmed by the results in Table 45. These results indicate the extent to which the emergency unit staff "take into account each other's work problems and needs," according to the hospital administrators (HAS), and the physicians (MDS), registered

TABLE 45. EXTENT TO WHICH THE VARIOUS PEOPLE WHO WORK IN THE EMERGENCY UNITS TAKE INTO ACCOUNT EACH OTHER'S WORK PROBLEMS AND NEEDS[a]

Hospital Emergency Units (EU's) Involved		Extent Staff Take Into Account Each Other's Work Needs, According to			
		HAS	MDS	RNS	LPNS
ALL EU'S IN THE STUDY SAMPLE (N=30 Hospital EU's)	Mean:	2.33	2.32	2.22	1.98
	Range:	(1.50-3.50)	(1.89-3.00)	(1.40-3.00)	(1.00-3.00)
YOUR HOSPITAL'S EU		--			
EU's with:					
Low Patient Volume (n=10)		2.28	2.33	2.32	2.20
Medium Pat. Volume (n=10)		2.32	2.37	2.20	1.83
High Patient Volume (n=10		2.40	2.26	2.15	1.96
EU's in:					
Church Operated Hospitals (n=9)		2.37	2.48	2.37	2.04
Osteopathic Hospitals (n=3)		2.17	2.41	2.17	1.83
All Other Hospitals (n=18)		2.34	2.22	2.16	1.99
EU's Located in:					
SMSA (urban) Areas (n=21)		2.31	2.34	2.24	1.81
Non-SMSA Areas (n=9)		2.39	2.27	2.19	2.67
EU's in Hospitals Having:					
Medical Teaching Affiliations (n=17)		2.44	2.30	2.13	1.90
No Medical Teaching Affiliations (n=13)		2.19	2.35	2.35	2.12
EU's in Hospitals Having:					
Emergency Personnel Training Programs (n=15)		2.36	2.31	2.23	1.94
No Training Programs (n=15)		2.31	2.33	2.22	2.02

[a] The results, presented here in the form of mean scores, are based on the answers of respondents to the following question: "Here in the emergency unit, to what extent do the different people who have to work together take into account each other's work problems and needs as they go about doing their own work activities?" The response alternatives ranged from "(1) To a very great extent,"... to "(5) To a very small extent or not at all." Using the data from each group of respondents, mean scores were first computed separately for each EU and then averaged for the EU's in the different categories. The lower the mean score, the greater the extent to which EU staff members take into account each other's work problems and needs.

nurses (RNS), and practical nurses (LPNS) working in the various emergency units.

All four of these respondent groups agree that, on the average, the staff of the 30 EU's involved generally take into account each other's work problems and needs to a "great extent," or nearly so. For the total sample, the overall mean scores, based on the data from the four groups, are between 1.98 and 2.33, with 2.00 corresponding exactly to "to a great extent." Across individual emergency units, however, the relevant mean scores range from 1.00 (signifying "to a very great extent") to 3.50 (signifying a level exactly midway between "to a fair extent" and "to a small extent"), depending on the particular source of data examined. Thus, there is sufficient inter-unit variability to suggest that the situation of the units in the present area is not uniformly favorable, although on the average it may be quite good -- as it apparently is. Among the various EU groupings, on the other hand, the relevant mean scores differ little, except in the case of the data provided by LPNS. From the perspective of these respondents, the staff of medium patient volume units take into account each other's problems and needs better than do the staff of low patient volume units, and the same applies to the staff of urban compared to non-urban area units.

The last table in the present series, Table 46, shows the extent to which emergency unit nurses and physicians feel that they can rely on others, whose work is related to their own, to do their jobs properly. On the average, the practical nurses (LPNS) who work in the emergency units full-time report that they can rely on others almost to "a very great extent." For individual EU's the range is from "to a very great extent" to slightly better than "to a fair extent." The registered nurses (RNS) and also the physicians (MDS) who work in the units both report that, on the average, they can rely on others to

TABLE 46. EXTENT TO WHICH THE VARIOUS PEOPLE WHO WORK IN THE EMERGENCY UNITS CAN RELY ON THE PERFORMANCE OF CO-WORKERS[a]

		Reliability as Reported by		
Hospital Emergency Units (EU's) Involved		MDS	RNS	LPNS
ALL EU'S IN THE STUDY SAMPLE (N=30 Hospital EU's)	*Mean:* *Range:*	2.06 (1.60-2.67)	1.95 (1.33-2.50)	1.36 (1.00-2.67)
YOUR HOSPITAL'S EU				
EU's with:				
Low Patient Volume (n=10)		2.17	1.97	1.53
Medium Pat. Volume (n=10)		2.04	1.95	1.23
High Patient Volume (n=10)		1.98	1.92	1.36
EU's in:				
Church Operated Hospitals (n=9)		2.22	2.05	1.58
Osteopathic Hospitals (n=3)		2.33	1.69	1.25
All Other Hospitals (n=18)		1.94	1.94	1.31
EU's Located in:				
SMSA (urban) Areas (n=21)		2.07	1.96	1.32
Non-SMSA Areas (n=9)		2.05	1.93	1.50
EU's in Hospitals Having:				
Medical Teaching Affiliations (n=17)		2.04	1.86	1.30
No Medical Teaching Affiliations (n=13)		2.10	2.06	1.48
EU's in Hospitals Having:				
Emergency Personnel Training Programs (n=15)		1.98	1.93	1.28
No Training Programs (n=15)		2.15	1.97	1.44

[a] The results, presented here in the form of mean scores, are based on the responses of MDS, RNS, and LPNS to the following question: "In this emergency unit, to what extent do you feel that you can rely on others whose work is related to yours (or affects your work) to do their jobs right?" The response alternatives ranged from "(1) To a very great extent,"... to "(5) To a very small extent or not at all." Using the data from each group of respondents, mean scores were first computed separately for each EU and then averaged for the EU's in the different categories. The lower the mean score, the more the staff can rely on others.

"a great extent." For individual EU's, the range in each case is from midway between "a very great" and "a great" extent to midway between "a great extent" and "a fair extent." In other words, inter-unit variability on the present measure is small according to the data from both MDS and RNS.

In view of these findings, it is not surprising that the various groupings of EU's differ little from one another on the level of reported reliance on others by the staff -- a generally high level. The only differences are: (a) in osteopathic hospital units the physicians feel that they can rely on others somewhat less than they do in the units of other not church operated hospitals; and (b) in osteopathic hospital units the nurses, both RNS and LPNS, feel that they can rely on others somewhat more than they do in the units of church operated hospitals. Generally, then, based on all of the measures examined in the present section, it appears that the coordination of activities in the emergency units studied is on the whole adequate.

Problem Solving Within the Emergency Units

The various problems facing the emergency units, including that of coordination, can be dealt with in a number of different ways, some of which may be used more, or prove more effective, than others. These often reflect differences in strategies or approaches to problem solving. In the present study, relevant data were obtained concerning the following five approaches or types of problem solving:

(a) careful and precise timing and scheduling of tasks and work activities;

(b) correcting immediately any departures from the proper way of doing things;

(c) improving the staff's understanding of work requirements;

(d) making sure that existing rules and regulations are followed by all concerned; and

(e) trying to find better ways of doing things.

Data about the relative use of each of these approaches/types were obtained from the supervising nurses (SRNS) of the emergency units, and data about the relative effectiveness of each were obtained from the physicians (MDS) working in the units. In both respects, the respondents were asked to rank-order the five approaches (in relation to one another), from most to least used in the case of SRNS and from most to least effective in the case of MDS. Table 47 summarizes the data concerning use.

Considering first the "average" situation of the 30 EU's in the sample, the results in Table 47 show that by far the most used approach of all is "improving the staff's understanding of work requirements," and the least used is "careful and precise timing and scheduling of activities." The second, third, and fourth most used approaches -- all being used almost equally as much but substantially less than the most used approach -- are: "making sure that rules and regulations are followed," "trying to find better ways of doing things," and "correcting departures from the proper way of doing things." This last, or fourth most used, approach is apparently used substantially more than is "careful and precise timing," which is the least used of the five approaches.

Furthermore, the results show only moderate variability across individual emergency units with respect to the most used approach (improving the staff's understanding), in sharp contrast to each of the other four approaches with respect to which inter-unit variability is extremely high (see the ranges of mean rank scores in Table 47). In fact, there are emergency units in which any one of the five approaches is used the most (of all five), and there are

TABLE 47. COMPARATIVE USE OF DIFFERENT TYPES OF PROBLEM SOLVING IN THE EMERGENCY UNITS, ACCORDING TO THE SUPERVISING NURSES (SRNS)[a]

Hospital Emergency Units (EU's) Involved		Improving staff's understanding of work requirements	Making sure that existing rules/regulations are followed	Trying to find better ways of doing things	Correcting departures from proper way of doing things	Careful and precise timing and scheduling of activities
ALL EU'S IN THE STUDY SAMPLE (N=30 Hospital EU's)	Mean: Range:	1.6 (1.0-3.0)	2.9 (1.0-5.0)	3.0 (1.0-5.0)	3.1 (1.0-5.0)	4.0 (1.0-5.0)
YOUR HOSPITAL'S EU		--	--	--	--	--
EU's in:						
Small Hospitals (n=14)		1.5	3.1	2.6	3.3	4.3
Medium Hospitals (n=9)		1.6	2.4	3.2	3.6	4.2
Large Hospitals (n=7)		1.9	3.1	3.6	2.1	3.0
EU's in:						
Church Operated Hospitals (n=9)		1.6	3.1	2.8	3.4	4.1
Osteopathic Hospitals (n=3)		1.2	2.5	2.7	3.2	4.2
All Other Hospitals (n=18)		1.6	2.9	3.2	2.9	3.9
EU's Located in:						
SMSA (urban) Areas (n=21)		1.6	2.8	3.1	3.0	3.8
Non-SMSA Areas (n=9)		1.6	3.0	2.9	3.3	4.3
EU's in Hospitals Having:						
Medical Teaching Affiliations (n=17)		1.7	2.8	3.3	2.7	3.7
No Medical Teaching Affiliations (n=13)		1.5	3.0	2.6	3.6	4.8
EU's in Hospitals Having:						
Emergency Personnel Training Programs (n=15)		1.5	2.5	3.6	3.1	3.7
No Training Progrmas (n=15)		1.7	3.3	2.4	3.1	4.3

Table 47 Continues

TABLE 47
(Continued)

---

[a]The results, presented here in the form of mean rank scores, are based on the responses of SRNS to the following questionnaire item: "In emergency units like this, work problems may be handled in a number of different ways, some of which may be used more than others. Listed below are some ways that are perhaps being used here. Please rank them from the one that is generally used the most to the one that is used the least in this emergency unit. (Place 1 in front of the way that is most used, 2 in front of the next most used way, etc...., and 5 in front of the least used way.)" The sequence in which the five types of problem solving appeared in the questionnaire was: Timing and scheduling, correcting, improving staff's understanding, finding better ways of doing things, and following rules and regulations. Based on the rankings provided by SRNS, mean rank scores were first computed separately for each EU and then averaged for the EU's in the different categories. The lower the mean rank, the greater the use of the particular type of problem solving.

other units in which the same approach is used the least (except for "improving the staff's understanding" which in none of the 30 units is used the least). Apparently, problem solving patterns vary widely from one emergency unit to another.

Patterns of use also differ among groupings of emergency units. First, on the average, the emergency units of large hospitals apparently rely relatively more on "careful and precise timing and scheduling," and also on "correcting departures from the proper way of doing things," than do the units of small and medium-size hospitals; the units of medium-size hospitals rely more on compliance with "existing rules and regulations" than do those of either small or large hospitals; and the units of small hospitals rely more on "trying to find better ways of doing things" than do their counterparts in other hospitals. Second, the emergency units of osteopathic hospitals (like medium-size hospitals) rely relatively more on existing rules and regulations than do the units of other hospitals. Third, the units of hospitals which have medical teaching affiliations, compared to those which do not, rely relatively more on "correcting departures from the proper way of doing things" and also on "careful and precise timing and scheduling." Finally, the units of hospitals which have emergency personnel training programs, compared to those which do not, on the average rely relatively more on existing rules and regulations and on "careful and precise timing and scheduling" and less on "trying to find better ways of doing things."

Problem solving effectiveness. The data from emergency unit physicians (MDS) on the relative effectiveness of the same five approaches or types of problem solving are summarized in Table 48. Considering first the total sample, the results show the following order of overall effectiveness for the different

TABLE 48. THE RELATIVE EFFECTIVENESS OF DIFFERENT TYPES OF PROBLEM SOLVING IN THE EMERGENCY UNITS, ACCORDING TO THE DOCTORS (MDS) WHO WORK THERE[a]

Hospital Emergency Units (EU's) Involved		Improving staff's understanding of work requirements	Making sure that existing rules/ regulations are followed	Trying to find better ways of doing things	Correcting departures from proper way of doing things	Careful and precise timing and scheduling of activities
ALL EU'S IN THE STUDY SAMPLE (N=30 Hospital EU's)	Mean:	2.1	3.3	2.8	2.9	3.7
	Range:	(1.0-3.4)	(2.0-5.0)	(1.0-3.9)	(1.8-4.0)	(2.6-4.7)
YOUR HOSPITAL'S EU						
EU's in:						
Small Hospitals (n=14)		2.0	3.5	2.8	2.9	3.6
Medium Hospitals (n=9)		2.3	3.1	2.8	2.8	3.6
Large Hospitals (n=7)		2.2	3.7	2.7	3.1	3.8
EU's in:						
Church Operated Hospitals (n=9)		2.1	3.1	3.0	3.0	3.7
Osteopathic Hospitals (n=3)		1.3	3.3	2.8	3.1	3.8
All Other Hospitals (n=18)		2.3	3.4	2.7	2.9	3.7
EU's Located in:						
SMSA (urban) Areas (n=21)		2.1	3.1	2.8	2.9	3.7
Non-SMSA Areas (n=9)		2.1	3.6	2.8	2.8	3.6
EU's in Hospitals Having:						
Medical Teaching Affiliations (n=17)		2.2	3.3	2.7	2.9	3.8
No Medical Teaching Affiliations (n=13)		2.0	3.2	2.9	2.9	3.5
EU's in Hospitals Having:						
Emergency Personnel Training Programs (n=15)		2.0	3.2	2.8	3.0	3.8
No Training Programs (n=15)		2.2	3.3	2.8	2.8	3.5

Table 48 Continues

TABLE 48
(Continued)

---

[a] The results, presented here in the form of mean rank scores, are based on the responses of MDS to the following questionnaire item: "In emergency units like this, work problems may be handled in a number of different ways, some of which may be more effective than others. Listed below are some ways that are perhaps used here. Please rank them from the one that is generally most effective to the one that is least effective in this emergency unit. (Place 1 in front of the way that is most effective, 2 in front of the next most effective way, etc...., and 5 in front of the least effective way.)" Of all the MDS questioned, only 12% did not provide complete data. The obtained data were treated in exactly the same way as the parallel data in Table 47.

approaches: "improving the staff's understanding" (most effective); "trying to find better ways of doing things"; "correcting departures from the proper way of doing things"; "making sure that existing rules and regulations are followed"; and "careful and precise timing and scheduling of activities" (least effective).

The results also show, however, that inter-unit variability concerning the effectiveness of each of the five approaches is high to very high in every case, but not as high as the variability found (in Table 47) concerning the relative use of the same approaches. Differences among emergency unit groupings on the effectiveness measure are very few (in contrast to the use measure). Specifically, "making sure that existing rules and regulations are followed" is on the average relatively more effective in the emergency units of medium-size hospitals than the units of large hospitals; and "improving the staff's understanding" is relatively more effective in the units of osteopathic than the units of non-osteopathic hospitals (although even in the latter institutions this is the most effective approach of all).

Finally, a comparison of the results in Table 47 and Table 48, reveals an interesting picture. First, the approach which is most used in the various emergency units (considering the total sample) -- "improving the staff's understanding of work requirements" -- is also the most effective of the five approaches to problem solving on the average. And, conversely, the approach which is used the least among the five -- "careful and precise timing and scheduling of activities" -- is also the least effective on the average. The other three approaches occupy intermediate positions. One of them, however, namely "making sure that existing rules and regulations are followed" is apparently used more than its relative effectiveness would warrant, according to the data. And the remaining two approaches are perhaps used somewhat less than their relative effectiveness might suggest.

Reliance on bureaucratic vs. professional means. Still another way to look at problem solving patterns within the emergency units is to examine the degree to which the staff relies on formal arrangements vs. professional norms as a means for ensuring that "everyone contributes properly to the work and operation of the unit." The two measures in Table 49, based on data from the physicians (MDS) working in the various units, provide appropriate material for such an examination. One measure indicates the degree to which the units rely on "regularly scheduled meetings or conferences, written reports, and the like," and the second indicates the degree to which they rely on "the autonomy and discretion of the professional staff."

First, as might be expected from the findings already presented in this chapter, it is clear that the emergency units studied on the average rely on the autonomy and discretion of the professional staff to a significantly higher degree than they do on such things as scheduled meetings and written reports. The overall mean score for the 30 EU's is 2.29 on the former measure vs. 2.85 on the latter (the former score signifies almost "a high degree" of reliance, while the latter signifies "a fair degree").

Second, the variability across individual emergency units with respect to relying on the autonomy and discretion of the staff is only moderate (the range of unit mean scores is from 1.50 to 3.20), while with respect to the other measure it is high (from 1.80 to 4.00). The results also show that, on the average, the emergency units of hospitals which are not church operated (both osteopathic and non-osteopathic) rely more on the autonomy and discretion of the staff than do the units of church operated hospitals, and that the units of medium size hospitals rely less on formal meetings and reports than do the units of large hospitals. More important, for each and every one of the various groupings of units examined (see Table 49), the findings show

TABLE 49. RELIANCE BY EMERGENCY UNIT PERSONNEL ON CERTAIN MEANS FOR INSURING PROPER PERFORMANCE CONTRIBUTIONS TO THE WORK OF THE UNIT ACCORDING TO PHYSICIANS (MDS)[a]

Hospital Emergency Units (EU's) Involved		Degree of Reliance on	
		Regular meetings or conferences, written reports, and the like	The autonomy and discretion of the professional staff
ALL EU'S IN THE STUDY SAMPLE (N=30 Hospital EU's)	Mean: Range:	2.85 (1.80-4.00)	2.29 (1.50-3.20)
YOUR HOSPITAL'S EU			
EU's with:			
Low Patient Volume (n=10)		2.89	2.30
Medium Pat. Volume (n=10)		3.02	2.20
High Patient Volume (n=10		2.65	2.35
EU's in:			
Church Operated Hospitals (n=9)		2.80	2.54
Osteopathic Hospitals (n=3)		3.05	2.06
All Other Hospitals (n=18)		2.84	2.20
EU's Located in:			
SMSA (urban) Areas (n=21)		2.88	2.24
Non-SMSA Areas (n=9)		2.79	2.40
EU's in Hospitals Having:			
Medical Teaching Affiliations (n=17)		2.72	2.25
No Medical Teaching Affiliations (n=13)		3.02	2.34
EU's in Hospitals Having:			
Emergency Personnel Training Programs (n=15)		2.76	2.29
No Training Programs (n=15)		2.95	2.29

[a] The results, presented here in the form of mean scores, are based on the responses of MDS to the following multiple-part question: "Emergency unit personnel often <u>rely</u> on different arrangements or bases to ensure that everyone contributes properly to the work and operation of the unit. Generally, to what degree do the personnel of this unit <u>rely on</u>... for this particular purpose?" The response alternatives ranged from "(1) To a very high degree,"... to "(5) To a very small degree." Thus, the <u>lower</u> the score the <u>higher</u> the reliance. Of all the MDS questioned, 87% provided complete data.

(in varying degrees) greater reliance on staff autonomy and discretion than on scheduled meetings and written reports for ensuring that every one contributes properly to the work and operation of the unit. In summary, the findings in the present section concerning problem solving within the emergency units are very consistent with those in the preceding section concerning coordination in the units.

Work Relations Between Nurses and Physicians in the Units

The next three tables present findings concerning certain specific aspects of doctor-nurse relations within the emergency units. Two such aspects are: (a) the degree of discretion or judgment that doctors allow the registered nurses to exercise (considering the latter's training and professional experience), as reported by the registered nurses (RNS) themselves; and (b) the degree of "help or advice" regarding patient care that nurses "can get" from the doctors when they need it, or how helpful the doctors are in this area, as perceived by the nurses -- both RNS and LPNS. The results on both of these measures are presented in Table 50.

Considering all the emergency units in the sample, the RNS on the average report that the doctors allow them to use almost exactly "the right amount of discretion" (the overall mean score on this measure for the 30 EU's is 1.91). Across individual emergency units, the situation in this respect differs only moderately (from midway between "more than enough" and "about the right amount" of discretion to "somewhat less discretion than they should"). Furthermore all of the various groupings of EU's score very similarly on the present measure, there being no significant difference from one grouping to another. Obviously, from the perspective of the registered nurses this is a favorable situation.

TABLE 50. DISCRETION ALLOWED AND HELP PROVIDED BY PHYSICIANS TO THE NURSES WORKING IN EMERGENCY UNITS, AS REPORTED BY THE NURSES (RNS, LPNS)[a]

Hospital Emergency Units (EU's) Involved		Degree of Allowed Discretion[b]	Degree of Physician Helpfulness[c]	
		RNS	RNS	LPNS
ALL EU'S IN THE STUDY SAMPLE (N=30 Hospital EU's)	*Mean:* *Range:*	1.91 (1.43-3.00)	2.28 (1.67-3.00)	2.17 (1.00-3.00)
YOUR HOSPITAL'S EU				
EU's with:				
Low Patient Volume (n=10)		1.81	2.48	2.60
Medium Pat. Volume (n=10)		2.01	2.25	2.21
High Patient Volume (n=10)		1.91	2.11	1.90
EU's in:				
Church Operated Hospitals (n=9)		1.85	2.33	2.37
Osteopathic Hospitals (n=3)		2.11	2.30	2.17
All Other Hospitals (n=18)		1.91	2.26	2.11
EU's Located in:				
SMSA (urban) Areas (n=21)		1.95	2.25	2.03
Non-SMSA Areas (n=9)		1.83	2.37	2.75
EU's in Hospitals Having:				
Medical Teaching Affiliations (n=17)		1.98	2.19	2.11
No Medical Teaching Affiliations (n=13)		1.82	2.41	2.29
EU's in Hospitals Having:				
Emergency Personnel Training Programs (n=15)		1.88	2.23	2.05
No Training Programs (n=15)		1.95	2.33	2.30

Table 50 Continues

TABLE 50
(Continued)

---

^aThe results, presented here in the form of mean scores, are based on data from the RNS and LPNS in the various emergency units.

^bThe question was: "Considering the training and professional experience that you have had, how do you feel about the amount of <u>discretion or judgment</u> that the doctors in the Emergency Unit allow you to use at work?" The response alternatives were: "(1) More than enough discretion, (2) about the right amount of discretion, (3) somewhat less discretion than they should, and (4) much less discretion than they should." Thus, the lower the mean score, the greater the amount of discretion allowed.

^cThe question was: "When you need <u>help or advice from the doctors here</u> in deciding what to do for emergency patients, how do you feel about the help or advice that you <u>can get</u> from them?" Responses to this open-ended question were coded into five categories as follows: (1) The doctors are extremely helpful or extremely willing to offer advice, (2) they are very helpful, (3) they are fairly helpful, (4) they are not so helpful, and (5) the doctors are not at all helpful. Thus, the <u>lower</u> the score, the <u>greater</u> the helpfulness.

Concerning the helpfulness of physicians, the results are nearly as favorable from the point of view of the nurses. Both the RNS and the LPNS who work in the various units report that, on the average, the physicians of the unit are generally "very helpful" (or almost "very helpful"). The range across individual EU's again is moderate (though somewhat higher based on the data from LPNS than from RNS), from "extremely"/"very" helpful to exactly "fairly helpful." As for differences among the various groupings of EU's, the results show only a few. First, the physicians working in units with a high patient volume are seen, by both RNS and LPNS, as more helpful on the average than are the physicians working in units with a low patient volume. And, second, the physicians working in urban area units are seen by the LPNS, but not the RNS, as more helpful on the average than are the physicians working in non-urban area units.

Another two aspects of doctor-nurse relations which are important to consider are: (a) the adequacy with which the doctors in the unit "explain things to nursing personnel about the condition and needs of patients"; and (b) the sufficiency of "joint planning" between doctors and nurses, from the standpoint of "being able to provide patients with care of the highest quality possible." Data for measuring both of these aspects were obtained from the registered nurses (RNS) working in the emergency units. They are summarized in Table 51.

On the whole, these results are not as favorable as for the preceding aspects of doctor-nurse relations. The overall mean scores for the 30 EU's in the study sample indicate that, on the average, the physicians explain the condition and needs of patients to the nurses considerably less than "very adequately" (and close to only "fairly adequately"). Further, the amount of "joint planning" is perceived by RNS to be, on the average, somewhat

TABLE 51. ADEQUACY WITH WHICH EMERGENCY UNIT PHYSICIANS EXPLAIN PATIENT NEEDS TO THE NURSES, AND THE ADEQUACY OF JOINT PLANNING BY NURSES AND PHYSICIANS, AS REPORTED BY THE NURSES (RNS)[a]

Hospital Emergency Units (EU's) Involved		Adequacy of Physician Explanations[b]	Adequacy of Joint Planning[c]
ALL EU'S IN THE STUDY SAMPLE (N=30 Hospital EU's)	Mean: Range:	2.70 (1.80-3.57)	2.65 (2.00-3.44)
YOUR HOSPITAL'S EU			
EU's in:			
Small Hospitals (n=14)		2.77	2.65
Medium Hospitals (n=9)		2.75	2.84
Large Hospitals (n=7)		2.47	2.41
EU's in:			
Church Operated Hospitals (n=9)		2.82	2.83
Osteopathic Hospitals (n=3)		2.45	2.44
All Other Hospitals (n=18)		2.67	2.60
EU's Located in:			
SMSA (urban) Areas (n=21)		2.62	2.60
Non-SMSA Areas (n=9)		2.88	2.78
EU's in Hospitals Having:			
Medical Teaching Affiliations (n=17)		2.66	2.57
No Medical Teaching Affiliations (n=13)		2.75	2.76
EU's in Hospitals Having:			
Emergency Personnel Training Programs (n=15)		2.66	2.71
No Training Programs (n=15)		2.73	2.60

Table 51 Continues

TABLE 51
(Continued)

---

[a]The results, presented here in the form of mean scores, are based on the responses of RNS from the various emergency units.

[b]The question was: "In general, how adequately do the doctors here explain things to nursing personnel about the condition and needs of patients?" The response alternatives ranged from "(1) Extremely adequately,"... to "(5) Not adequately at all." Thus, the lower the score, the higher the adequacy of physician explanations.

[c]The question was: "From the standpoint of being able to provide patients with care of the highest quality possible, how much joint planning, would you say, is there between the doctors and nurses in this emergency unit?" The response alternatives were: "(1) There is probably more than sufficient joint planning, (2) about the right amount of joint planning, (3) somewhat less joint planning than is needed, (4) much less than is needed, and (5) there is no joint planning at all that I know of." Thus, the lower the score, the more adequate the amount of joint planning.

less than sufficient (less than "the right amount"). Inter-unit variability on both measures is moderate (from "very adequately" to midway between "fairly adequately" and "not so adequately" for the first measure, and from "about the right amount" to midway between "somewhat less joint planning than is needed" to "much less... than is needed" for the second). The results also show that physician explanations are more adequate, on the average, in the units of large than either medium-size or small hospitals, and that joint planning between doctors and nurses is also more adequate in the units of large (and possibly also medium-size) than the units of small hospitals. Among the other emergency unit groupings there are no significant differences on either measure.

The final aspect of work relations between doctors and nurses in the emergency units to be examined in this section concerns the mutual understanding between the two groups -- the degree to which each group "understands and appreciates the work problems and needs" of the other. In any organizational setting where the work of two key groups is highly interdependent, mutual understanding is critical for coordination and successful performance. Both the physicians (MDS) and the registered nurses (RNS) in the various units, therefore, were asked about their own understanding of the problems and needs of the other group, as well as about the other group's understanding of their own problems and needs. The findings from these data are all summarized in Table 52.

First, it is clear, MDS and RNS are in agreement that the nursing staff has a significantly better understanding of the work problems and needs of the medical staff than the medical staff has of the problems and needs of the nursing staff. On the average, for all the EU's in the sample, the nursing staff's understanding is "very good" according to MDS and midway

TABLE 52. LEVEL OF MUTUAL UNDERSTANDING OF THEIR WORK PROBLEMS AND NEEDS ON THE PART OF THE DOCTORS AND NURSES WORKING IN THE EMERGENCY UNITS[a]

		Degree to Which the			
		Nursing Staff Understand the Work Problems of the Medical Staff, According to[b]		Medical Staff Understand the Work Problems of the Nursing Staff, According to[c]	
Hospital Emergency Units (EU's) Involved		MDS	RNS	MDS	RNS
ALL EU'S IN THE STUDY SAMPLE (N=30 Hospital EU's)	Mean: Range:	2.11 (1.56-3.00)	2.51 (1.73-3.29)	2.46 (1.62-3.33)	3.08 (2.27-4.10)
YOUR HOSPITAL'S EU					
EU's in:					
Small Hospitals (n=14)		2.18	2.55	2.59	3.12
Medium Hospitals (n=9)		1.93	2.49	2.28	3.20
Large Hospitals (n=7)		2.19	2.46	2.42	2.85
EU's in:					
Church Operated Hospitals (n=9)		2.30	2.50	2.57	3.16
Osteopathic Hospitals (n=3)		2.44	2.55	2.90	2.96
All Other Hospitals (n=18)		1.96	2.51	2.32	3.06
EU's Located in:					
SMSA (urban) Areas (n=21)		2.12	2.46	2.46	3.02
Non-SMSA Areas (n=9)		2.08	2.63	2.45	3.23
EU's in Hospitals Having:					
Medical Teaching Affiliations (n=17)		2.11	2.52	2.43	3.07
No Medical Teaching Affiliations (n=13)		2.11	2.49	2.49	3.09
EU's in Hospitals Having:					
Emergency Personnel Training Programs (n=15)		2.07	2.43	2.39	3.04
No Training Programs (n=15)		2.15	2.59	2.52	3.13

Table 52 Continues

TABLE 52
(Continued)

---

^aThe results, presented here in the form of mean scores, are based on the responses of MDS and RNS from the various emergency units to a pair of complementary questions.

^bThe question was: "On the whole, to what extent does the nursing staff understand and appreciate the work problems and needs of the medical staff in this emergency unit?" The response alternatives were: "(1) They have an excellent understanding, (2) a very good understanding, (3) a good understanding, (4) a fair understanding, and (5) they have a rather poor understanding." Thus, the lower the score, the better the understanding.

^cThe question was: "On the whole, to what extent does the medical staff understand and appreciate the work problems and needs of the nursing staff of this emergency unit?" The response alternatives were identical to those in the preceding question. Thus, the lower the score, the better the understanding.

between "very good" and "good" according to RNS. The nurses themselves, therefore, are more critical than the physicians on this matter. The medical staff's understanding, on the average, is midway between "very good" and "good" according to the physicians themselves, and just "good" according to the nurses. Again, the RNS are more critical than the MDS.

Second, when the EU's are grouped on the basis of such things as hospital size, location, affiliations, etc., the above patterns again emerge from the data. For each and every grouping of EU's, in other words, the findings are virtually the same as for the total sample. Furthermore, the different groupings of units score very similarly on the two measures, based on the data from both MDS and RNS, with only a very few exceptions.

The exceptions are as follows. According to MDS, the nursing staff's understanding of the work problems and needs of the medical staff is higher in the units of hospitals which are not church operated (excluding osteopathic hospitals) than in the units of either the osteopathic or the church operated institutions. Further, the same trend holds regarding the medical staff's understanding of the problems of the nursing staff. Also according to MDS, the medical staff in the units of medium-size hospitals has a better understanding of the problems of nurses than it does in the units of small hospitals. This is not supported by the data from RNS. According to the RNS, the medical staff in the units of medium-size hospitals has the least understanding -- an understanding that is lower than that of the medical staff working in the units of large hospitals.

Lastly, the results in Table 52 show moderate variability across individual emergency units with respect to each staff's understanding of the problems and needs of the other. The variability is greater for the levels of understanding as assessed by the nurses than as assessed by the doctors.

It is greatest (ranging from "very good" to "fair") for the understanding that the medical staff has of the problems and needs of the nursing staff according to the RNS. Finally, readers may notice, the above findings concerning mutual understanding between medical and nursing staff are similar to those discussed earlier in this chapter (see Table 45) concerning the extent to which the different people who are working in the emergency units take into account each other's work problems and needs.

Tension Among Key Staff

Inadequate communication between doctors and nurses, insufficient joint planning, lack of sufficient mutual understanding, and deficient problem solving in an emergency unit often can lead to tensions and conflicts which, in turn, can lead to further deterioration of work relations. In a work situation such as that of emergency units, some tension among the staff is unavoidable. When the level of tension is relatively low, serious problems are unlikely. But, if considerable tension persists for any length of time, it will probably undermine work relations, successful problem solving, and effective performance. For these reasons, data about the level of prevailing tension between doctors and nurses in the emergency units also were collected. These were obtained from the hospital administrators (HAS) who participated in the study as respondents and from the physicians (MDS) and registered nurses (RNS) of the units. They are summarized in Table 53.

The three groups of respondents are in agreement that, on the average, tension between doctors and nurses in the emergency units studied is "low" to "very low" -- a finding which is consistent with most other data concerning the nature of work relations in the units. Of the respondents, the HAS perceive relatively more tension than that reported by MDS, with the RNS occupying

TABLE 53. TENSION BETWEEN DOCTORS AND NURSES IN THE EMERGENCY UNITS, AS REPORTED BY CERTAIN GROUPS OF RESPONDENTS[a]

		Level of Tension, According to[b]		
Hospital Emergency Units (EU's) Involved		HAS	MDS	RNS
ALL EU'S IN THE STUDY SAMPLE (N=30 Hospital EU's)	*Mean:* *Range:*	3.27 (1.50–4.00)	3.79 (2.50–4.60)	3.54 (2.33–4.29)
YOUR HOSPITAL'S EU		--		
EU's in:				
Small Hospitals (n=14)		3.39	3.68	3.67
Medium Hospitals (n=9)		3.15	4.03	3.56
Large Hospitals (n=7)		3.19	3.71	3.28
EU's in:				
Church Operated Hospitals (n=9)		3.04	3.60	3.46
Osteopathic Hospitals (n=3)		3.33	3.80	3.79
All Other Hospitals (n=18)		3.38	3.89	3.54
EU's Located in:				
SMSA (urban) Areas (n=21)		3.34	3.85	3.52
Non-SMSA Areas (n=9)		3.11	3.66	3.59
EU's in Hospitals Having:				
Medical Teaching Affiliations (n=17)		3.25	3.80	3.38
No Medical Teaching Affiliations (n=13)		3.31	3.79	3.76
EU's in Hospitals Having:				
Emergency Personnel Training Programs (n=15)		3.20	3.84	3.57
No Training Programs (n=15)		3.34	3.74	3.52

[a] The results, reported here in the form of mean scores, are based on data from the HAS, MDS, and RNS in the various institutions.

[b] The question was: "All things considered, how much tension (friction, strain, or conflict) would you say is there between... doctors in the emergency unit and nurses in the emergency unit?" The response alternatives were: "(1) A high level of tension, (2) a moderate level of tension, (3) a low level of tension, (4) a very low level of tension, and (5) no tension at all." Thus, the lower the score, the higher the level of tension; and, conversely, the higher the score, the lower the level of tension.

an intermediate position. Even in their case, however, the reported level of tension is low on the average. Across individual emergency units, however, the level of tension between doctors and nurses varies considerably -- from midway between "high" and "moderate" to "very low" as perceived by HAS, from midway between "moderate" and "low" to almost "no tension at all" as perceived by the MDS, and from "moderate" to "very low" as perceived by the RNS. Apparently, in some of the units the level of tension is undesirably high for good work relations.

The general pattern of low tension that characterizes the total sample is also prevalent in the various groupings of emergency units considered separately. Moreover, with only a few exceptions, the different groupings score very similarly on the tension measure according to the data from all three of the respondent groups -- HAS, MDS, and RNS. The exceptions are as follows: (a) on the average, tension between doctors and nurses is somewhat higher in the units of the church operated hospitals than the units of the other hospitals, according to all of the respondent groups; (b) based on the data from MDS only, the level of tension is somewhat lower in the units of medium-size hospitals than the units of either large or small hospitals; and (c) based on the data from RNS only, the level of tension is somewhat higher in the units of large compared to other hospitals, and also in the units of hospitals which have medical teaching affiliations compared to those which do not. Overall, of course, the important finding is that the prevailing tension between doctors and nurses in the 30 EU's studied is quite low on the average.

Finally, the same groups of respondents were also asked a question about tension between "some doctors in the emergency unit *and* other doctors in the emergency unit." The results from this measure are presented in Table 54.

TABLE 54. TENSION AMONG DOCTORS WITHIN THE EMERGENCY UNIT, AS REPORTED BY DOCTORS AND OTHER RESPONDENTS[a]

Hospital Emergency Units (EU's) Involved		Level of Tension Among Doctors, According to		
		MDS	RNS	HAS
ALL EU'S IN THE STUDY SAMPLE (N=30 Hospital EU's)	Mean: Range:	3.88 (2.75-5.00)	3.58 (2.55-4.67)	3.19 (1.50-4.70)
YOUR HOSPITAL'S EU				--
EU's in:				
Small Hospitals (n=14)		3.70	3.51	3.18
Medium Hospitals (n=9)		4.11	3.72	3.30
Large Hospitals (n=7)		3.94	3.55	3.10
EU's in:				
Church Operated Hospitals (n=9)		3.70	3.45	2.96
Osteopathic Hospitals (n=3)		4.06	3.86	3.33
All Other Hospitals (n=18)		3.94	3.60	3.29
EU's Located in:				
SMSA (urban) Areas (n=21)		3.98	3.64	3.28
Non-SMSA Areas (n=9)		3.64	3.44	3.00
EU's in Hospitals Having:				
Medical Teaching Affiliations (n=17)		4.00	3.60	3.20
No Medical Teaching Affiliations (n=13)		3.73	3.56	3.19
EU's in Hospitals Having:				
Emergency Personnel Training Programs (n=15)		3.89	3.72	3.23
No Training Programs (n=15)		3.87	3.44	3.16

[a]The results, presented here in the form of mean scores, are based on data from MDS, RNS, and HAS in the various institutions. The question was: "All things considered, how much tension (friction, strain, or conflict) would you say is there between... some doctors in the emergency unit and other doctors in the emergency unit?" The response alternatives ranged from: "(1) A high level of tension,"... to "(5) No tension at all." Thus, the lower the score, the higher the level of tension; and, conversely, the higher the score, the lower the level of tension.

Overall, they are very similar to the above results concerning tension between doctors and nurses. The HAS again report somewhat more tension among the doctors working in the emergency units than do the MDS (who report the least tension) or the RNS. According to all three groups of respondents, nevertheless, the average level of tension in the 30 EU's is "low" to "very low."

The results also show, however, substantial inter-unit variability on this measure, regardless of the specific source of data (HAS, MDS, or RNS) examined. In some of the individual emergency units, apparently, tension between doctors and nurses is almost non-existent while in other units it may be "very low," "low," or even higher (but in no case "high"). For each of the various groupings of EU's, the average level of tension does not deviate significantly from the overall pattern that characterizes the total sample. There are a few differences, however, between some of the groupings. First, all of the respondents see somewhat more tension among the doctors of church operated units than among the doctors of other units. Second, MDS report somewhat more tension among the doctors in the units of small hospitals than among the doctors in other units. And third, according to all of the respondents, there is a slight trend for tension to be slightly lower in urban than non-urban area units and in the units of hospitals which have medical teaching affiliations, also emergency personnel training programs, than of hospitals which do not.

Summary

This chapter focused on the nature of work relations and problem solving within the emergency units studied. Findings were presented about the coordination of staff efforts and mutual facilitation of work, the use and effectiveness of different approaches to problem solving, certain important aspects of doctor-nurse relations (including the exercise of professional discretion, communication and joint planning, and mutual understanding of work problems and needs), and tension between the staff in the unit. On the whole, the findings show that work relations in the emergency units are generally quite good on the average. They also show, as might be expected, that there is still room for improvement for most aspects examined, and that the situation of individual emergency units is not uniformly positive (although, in general, inter-unit variability on the measures in the present chapter is not as great as for most of the measures in most of the other chapters). The nature of work relations between the emergency units and their present hospitals will be considered next.

Chapter 6

WORK RELATIONS WITH THE PARENT HOSPITAL

The effectiveness of an emergency unit depends not only upon the nature of work relations and problem solving within the unit, but also upon the unit's work relations with others in the hospital who may be providing relevant services or support. Effectiveness is determined in part by what occurs internally within the subsystem itself, in other words, and in part by the subsystem's transactions with its relevant organizational environment. Work relations with the parent hospital are especially important in this connection, but relations with the outside community are also relevant.

Chapter 5 focused exclusively on work relations among the staff with the emergency unit, and Chapter 7 will discuss relations with the community. The present chapter, on the other hand, is concerned with the relations between emergency units and their parent hospitals. Some of the findings previously discussed in the areas of resources (Chapter 2), goal priorities and current problems (Chapter 3), and leadership and influence (Chapter 4) also are indicative, at least by inference, of the nature of work relations between emergency units and the hospital. The present chapter, however, deals much more directly with this latter area. Specifically, it examines the following: (a) institutional mechanisms for monitoring the work or performance of the emergency unit; (b) hospital administration's relations with the emergency unit; and (c) the nature of work interaction between emergency unit staff and other staff or groups in the hospital.

Institutional Monitoring

One important aspect of EU-hospital relations involves the issue of institutional "control" by the hospital over the emergency units. The influence patterns discussed in Chapter 4 are indicative of the amount of control exercised by various key groups over the emergency unit. They do not, however, address the question of whether any special organizational structures, or mechanisms, are being used by the various institutions for reviewing the work and performance of emergency units. The data in Table 55 do.

First, at each of the institutions participating in the research, the chief executive officer was asked whether the institution has an emergency department committee or an emergency room committee. The data show that 23 of the hospitals have such a committee (data are missing for one of the thirty institutions). Those which do not include three large, three small, and one medium-size hospitals. Next, those who responded affirmatively to the question were asked to indicate "how active" the emergency department committee is. The results (not included in Table 55) show that this committee is "very active," or meets at least once a month, in almost half of the hospitals involved (11 of the 23). In the remaining institutions it is only "fairly active," or meets several times a year, and even less active than that in two cases. The results also indicate that, on the average, emergency room committees are somewhat less active in osteopathic and medium-size hospitals than in other institutions.

Additional data about institutional control mechanisms were obtained from both hospital administrators (HAS) and the physicians (MDS) working in the various emergency units in response to the following item: "Some hospitals have _formal_ mechanisms for _monitoring the performance or the quality of work_ of their emergency unit. At the present time, does this institution have any such mechanisms?" The results are presented in Table 55. Hospitals are

TABLE 55. NUMBER OF INSTITUTIONS HAVING EMERGENCY DEPARTMENT COMMITTEES AND FORMAL MECHANISMS FOR MONITORING THE WORK OF THE EMERGENCY UNIT[a]

Hospital Emergency Units (EU's) Involved		An Emergency Department (Room) Committee[b] HAS	Formal Mechanisms for Monitoring EU Performance or the Quality of Work[c] HAS	MDS
ALL EU'S IN THE STUDY SAMPLE	n:	23	23	20
	%:	(79.3%)	(82.1%)	(69.0%)
EU's in:				
Small Hospitals		11	9	10
Medium Hospitals		8	7	4
Large Hospitals		4	7	6
EU's in:				
Church Operated Hospitals		7	8	7
Osteopathic Hospitals		3	1	2
All Other Hospitals		13	14	11
EU's Located in:				
SMSA (urban) Areas		17	17	14
Non-SMSA Areas		6	6	6
EU's in Hospitals Having:				
Medical Teaching Affiliations		13	15	11
No Medical Teaching Affiliations		10	8	9
EU's in Hospitals Having:				
Emergency Personnel Training Programs		10	12	8
No Training Programs		13	11	12

Table 55 Continues

TABLE 55
(Continued)

---

[a] According to data from hospital administrator respondents (HAS) and the physicians (MDS) working in the emergency units.

[b] Data provided by the chief executive officer of each hospital, in response to the question: "At the present time, does this hospital have an Emergency Room Committee or an Emergency Department Committee?" (Data are missing for one of the thirty institutions.)

[c] Data based on the answers of HAS and MDS respondents to the item: "Some hospitals have formal mechanisms for monitoring the performance or the quality of work of their emergency unit. At the present time, does this institution have any such mechanisms?" An institution is counted as having such formal mechanisms if at least two-thirds of the respondents from the group involved answered affirmatively. (It is interesting to note that 17% of all the MDS in the study responded "I don't know" to this question; and sufficient data were not provided by MDS for one institution. In the case of HAS, sufficient data were not provided for two of the thirty institutions in the sample.)

counted as having such formal mechanisms if at least two-thirds of the HAS and MDS respondents in each case answered affirmatively. It is interesting to note that 17% of all the physicians who were asked the question responded "I don't know." (In the case of HAS, relevant data are available for 28, and in the case of MDS for 29, of the 30 institutions in the sample.)

According to the data from administrators, 23 of the hospitals have formal mechanisms for monitoring the performance of their emergency unit; according to the data from physicians, 20 of them do. Practically all of the large hospitals, but only about two-thirds of the remaining institutions, apparently have such mechanisms. These findings, along with those about emergency department committees, suggest that formal institutional controls over the work of the emergency units are either lacking or weak in about half of the hospitals. Considering also the fact that the physicians working in the various units are the most influential group of all with respect to how the unit operates (see Chapter 4), it would appear that emergency units enjoy a rather high degree of autonomy from their parent hospital in most cases.

Relations with Hospital Administration

How positive or strained the work relations between hospital administration and the emergency unit are may have important consequences for the operation and effectiveness of emergency units. There are, of course, numerous different aspects to this relationship, which may manifest themselves in all of the major areas investigated by the study (and especially in the areas of resources discussed in Chapter 2, goals and strengths, discussed in Chapter 3, and leadership and influence, discussed in Chapter 4). Here, two overall aspects of the relations between the administration and the unit are examined -- the kind of understanding that hospital administration has of the work problems and needs of the emergency unit, and the level of prevailing tension between emergency unit staff and hospital administration. Data on each aspect were obtained from the principals involved -- the hospital administrators (HAS) from the different institutions and the physicians (MDS) and supervising nurses (SRNS) of each emergency unit.

The level of understanding attributed to hospital administration by the three groups is shown in Table 56. According to the physicians, hospital administration on the average has a "good" (but not a "very good" or "excellent") understanding of the work problems and needs of the emergency unit (the overall mean score for the 30 EU's is 3.05). For individual emergency units, the level of understanding varies greatly, from clearly "very good" to midway between "fair" and "rather poor" (the relevant mean scores ranging from 1.87 to 4.67). Interestingly, moreover, while the understanding which hospital administration has varies impressively across institutions, it averages at about the same level for emergency units in each of the various groupings examined (i.e., the groupings according to hospital size, location, teaching affiliations, etc.). There is only one exception to this -- the administration in osteopathic institutions is seen by MDS to have a lower level of understanding than the administration in other institutions. According to the supervising nurses, however, exactly the opposite is the case.

On the whole, the supervising nurses evaluate the hospital administration's understanding more favorably than do the physicians, regarding it better than just "good" on the average (the overall mean score is 2.63 in their case, compared to 3.05 in the case of MDS). Their evaluations too, however, show the prevalence of extreme differences across individual EU's in the administration's level of understanding. (Unit mean scores range from 1.00, signifying "excellent" understanding to 4.50, signifying a level midway between "fair"

TABLE 56. HOSPITAL ADMINISTRATION'S UNDERSTANDING OF THE WORK PROBLEMS AND NEEDS OF THE EMERGENCY UNIT STAFF[a]

Hospital Emergency Units (EU's) Involved		Administration's Understanding, According to		
		HAS	MDS	SRNS
ALL EU'S IN THE STUDY SAMPLE (N=30 Hospital EU's)	Mean:	2.49	3.05	2.63
	Range:	(1.50-4.00)	(1.87-4.67)	(1.00-4.50)
YOUR HOSPITAL'S EU		--		--
EU's in:				
Small Hospitals (n=14)		2.32	3.13	2.54
Medium Hospitals (n=9)		2.72	2.93	2.94
Large Hospitals (n=7)		2.55	3.05	2.43
EU's in:				
Church Operated Hospitals (n=9)		2.54	3.05	2.93
Osteopathic Hospitals (n=3)		2.33	3.80	2.33
All Other Hospitals (n=18)		2.50	2.93	2.54
EU's Located in:				
SMSA (urban) Areas (n=21)		2.52	3.07	2.67
Non-SMSA Areas (n=9)		2.44	3.00	2.54
EU's in Hospitals Having:				
Medical Teaching Affiliations (n=17)		2.61	3.13	2.59
No Medical Teaching Affiliations (n=13)		2.35	2.95	2.69
EU's in Hospitals Having:				
Emergency Personnel Training Programs (n=15)		2.51	3.02	2.27
No Training Programs (n=15)		2.48	3.08	3.00

[a]The results, presented here in the form of mean scores, are based on the responses of HAS, MDS, and SRNS from each institution to the following question: "On the whole, to what extent does Hospital Administration understand and appreciate the work problems and needs of the emergency unit staff?" The response alternatives were: "(1) Hospital Administration has an excellent understanding, (2) a very good understanding, (3) a good understanding, (4) a fair understanding, and (5) a rather poor understanding." Thus, the lower the score, the better the understanding. Mean scores were first computed separately for each EU and then averaged for the EU's in the different categories.

and "rather poor.") With reference to the various groupings of EU's, the data from SRNS indicate that, on the average, the administration in osteopathic hospitals and hospitals having emergency personnel training programs has a better understanding of the work problems and needs of the emergency unit, while the administration in medium-size hospitals has a poorer understanding, as compared to the administration in the other relevant groupings.

Finally, as might be expected, the administrators themselves give the most favorable evaluation. On the average, according to the data from HAS, hospital administration has a level of understanding exactly midway between "very good" and "good." Even in their case, however, inter-unit variability on this measure is very great (unit mean scores range from 1.50 to 4.00, the latter indicating only "fair" understanding). Overall, the evaluations provided by HAS are more similar to those provided by SRNS than by MDS, both when considering the results for the total sample and when examining the various groupings of EU's.

Concerning the level of prevailing tension between emergency unit staff and hospital administration (as assessed by HAS, MDS, and RNS), the results are presented in Table 57. On this measure, the assessment provided by hospital administrators is on the whole more similar to that provided by physicians than by the registered nurses working in the emergency units, although the three groups are close to each other. The registered nurses are slightly more critical on the average than are the other two groups.

For the EU's in the total sample, the level of tension between emergency unit staff and hospital administration is somewhere between "low" and "very low," on the average, according to all three groups. In each case, however, as the range of mean scores indicates, there is considerable inter-unit variability (across EU's, the level of tension ranges from less than "very

TABLE 57. TENSION BETWEEN EMERGENCY UNIT STAFF AND HOSPITAL ADMINISTRATION[a]

Hospital Emergency Units (EU's) Involved		Level of Tension, According to		
		HAS	MDS	RNS
ALL EU'S IN THE STUDY SAMPLE (N=30 Hospital EU's)	Mean: Range:	3.48 (2.33-4.50)	3.45 (2.33-4.40)	3.20 (2.08-4.00)
YOUR HOSPITAL'S EU		--		
EU's in:				
Small Hospitals (n=14)		3.54	3.28	3.27
Medium Hospitals (n=9)		3.50	3.57	2.97
Large Hospitals (n=7)		3.33	3.64	3.33
EU's in:				
Church Operated Hospitals (n=9)		3.61	3.37	3.16
Osteopathic Hospitals (n=3)		3.17	2.89	2.59
All Other Hospitals (n=18)		3.46	3.58	3.31
EU's Located in:				
SMSA (urban) Areas (n=21)		3.42	3.53	3.15
Non-SMSA Areas (n=9)		3.61	3.28	3.30
EU's in Hospitals Having:				
Medical Teaching Affiliations (n=17)		3.46	3.58	3.27
No Medical Teaching Affiliations (n=13)		3.50	3.29	3.10
EU's in Hospitals Having:				
Emergency Personnel Training Programs (n=15)		3.51	3.58	3.39
No Training Programs (n=15)		3.44	3.32	3.00

[a]The results, reported here in the form of mean scores, are based on the responses of HAS, MDS, and RNS from each institution to the question: "All things considered, how much _tension_ (friction, strain, or conflict) would you say is there between... Emergency Unit staff _and_ Hospital Administration?" The response alternatives were: (1) A high level of tension, (2) a moderate level of tension, (3) a low level of tension, (4) a very low level of tension, and (5) no tension at all. Thus, the _lower_ the score, the _higher_ the level of tension; and, conversely, the higher the score the lower the level of tension.

low" to "moderate"). All three groups report more tension in osteopathic compared to other hospitals. In addition, physicians report more tension in the case of small compared to other hospitals, and also in the case of hospitals without as contrasted to those with medical teaching affiliations. The registered nurses, on the other hand, report somewhat more tension in the case of medium size hospitals and in the case of hospitals which do not have emergency personnel training programs. Overall, the results concerning tension, like those concerning level of understanding, suggest generally positive but not unproblematic relations with hospital administration.

Relations with Other Hospital Staff or Units

The above three groups of respondents were also asked a question about tension "between doctors in the emergency unit and hospital staff outside the unit." The results are presented in Table 58. In this case, it is the emergency unit physicians (MDS) who report the least tension, while the administrators (HAS) report the most (still, however, a relatively low level); the registered nurses (RNS) occupy an intermediate position in this respect.

On the average, for all the EU's in the study, the level of tension is somewhere between "low" and "very low," according to all three groups of respondents. Again, however, in each case the data show a good deal of interunit variability regarding the level of prevailing tension. With reference to the various groupings of EU's, the results once again show very few significant differences specifically. On the average, both the hospital administrators and the physicians working in the emergency units of osteopathic hospitals report more tension than their counterparts in other hospitals, either church operated or not (the data from registered nurses also are consistent with this finding). Thus, overall, the level of tension between emergency

TABLE 58. TENSION BETWEEN DOCTORS IN THE EMERGENCY UNIT AND HOSPITAL STAFF OUTSIDE THE UNIT[a]

		Level of Tension, According to		
Hospital Emergency Units (EU's) Involved		HAS	MDS	RNS
ALL EU'S IN THE STUDY SAMPLE (N=30 Hospital EU's)	Mean: Range:	3.17 (2.00-4.50)	3.61 (2.00-4.40)	3.35 (2.67-4.33)
YOUR HOSPITAL'S EU		--		
EU's in:				
Small Hospitals (n=14)		3.25	3.52	3.46
Medium Hospitals (n=9)		3.06	3.81	3.26
Large Hospitals (n=7)		3.14	3.54	3.24
EU's in:				
Church Operated Hospitals (n=9)		3.28	3.58	3.36
Osteopathic Hospitals (n=3)		2.50	3.22	3.17
All Other Hospitals (n=18)		3.22	3.69	3.37
EU's Located in:				
SMSA (urban) Areas (n=21)		3.17	3.63	3.30
Non-SMSA Areas (n=9)		3.17	3.56	3.45
EU's in Hospitals Having:				
Medical Teaching Affiliations (n=17)		3.12	3.56	3.24
No Medical Teaching Affiliations (n=13)		3.23	3.67	3.49
EU's in Hospitals Having:				
Emergency Personnel Training Programs (n=15)		3.12	3.68	3.46
No Training Programs (n=15)		3.21	3.54	3.24

[a]The results, reported here in the form of mean scores, are based on the responses of HAS, MDS, and RNS from the various institutions to the question: "All things considered, how much tension (friction, strain, or conflict) would you say is there between... Doctors in the Emergency Unit and Hospital Staff outside the emergency unit?" The response alternatives ranged from "(1) A high level of tension,"... to "(5) No tension at all." Thus, the lower the score the higher the level of tension; and, conversely, the higher the score the lower the level of tension.

unit doctors and other hospital staff outside the unit, like the level of tension between emergency unit staff and hospital administration, appears to be generally low in the emergency units studied.

A different way to assess work relations is to ascertain how satisfactory such relations are to the other party. Accordingly, the selected physicians (HMDS) from each hospital were also asked to provide certain information about their work relations with the emergency unit. These physicians, it will be recalled, are key physicians within the hospital but outside the emergency unit who have important contacts (either of a clinical or of an organizational nature) with the staff of the unit. The specific question was: "From your point of view, how satisfactory are your work contacts with the emergency unit?" The data which they provided are summarized in Table 59.

The results are even more positive than those above concerning tension. On the average, for the 30 EU's in the study sample, the data show that the selected physicians consider their work contacts with their respective emergency units to be "very satisfactory." Moreover, inter-unit variability in this connection is only moderate (unit mean scores range from 1.00, which corresponds to "completely satisfactory," to 2.71, which corresponds to better than "moderately satisfactory," while the overall mean score is 2.12). Once again, however, work relations are somewhat less satisfactory in the case of osteopathic compared to non-osteopathic institutions. Apart from this exception, the different groupings of EU's show no differences whatsoever on this measure.

Finally, since an emergency unit depends (or relies) on other hospital units -- with some of which it interacts a great deal -- for a variety of important services or support, the study also inquired about the responsiveness of these other units (or "services"). The data were obtained from the

TABLE 59. THE QUALITY OF THE WORK CONTACTS OF SELECTED HOSPITAL PHYSICIANS (HMDS) WITH THE EMERGENCY UNIT[a]

Hospital Emergency Units (EU's) Involved	Quality of Work Contacts
ALL EU'S IN THE STUDY SAMPLE (N=30 Hospital EU's)	Mean: 2.12 Range: (1.00-2.71)
YOUR HOSPITAL'S EU	
EU's in:	
Small Hospitals (n=14)	2.15
Medium Hospitals (n=9)	2.19
Large Hospitals (n=7)	1.95
EU's in:	
Church Operated Hospitals (n=9)	2.18
Osteopathic Hospitals (n=3)	2.42
All Other Hospitals (n=18)	2.03
EU's Located in:	
SMSA (urban) Areas (n=21)	2.07
Non-SMSA Areas (n=9)	2.23
EU's in Hospitals Having:	
Medical Teaching Affiliations (n=17)	2.12
No Medical Teaching Affiliations (n=13)	2.11
EU's in Hospitals Having:	
Emergency Personnel Training Programs (n=15)	2.01
No Training Programs (n=15)	2.22

[a] The results, reported here in the form of mean scores, are based on the answers of HMDS from each hospital to the following open-ended question: "From your point of view, how satisfactory are your work contacts with the Emergency Unit?" Their answers were coded on a five-point scale, ranging from "(1) Completely satisfactory,"... to "(5) not satisfactory at all." Thus, the lower the mean scores the higher the quality of work contacts.

registered nurses (RNS) working in the various emergency units, because of their direct knowledge and experience concerning this matter, in response to the following question: "When you request the services, assistance, or support of others in the hospital (outside the emergency unit), on the whole, how satisfactory are your requests met by...(each of certain parties)?" The referent parties included: (a) "the inpatient medical services or departments in the hospital"; (b) "ancillary services from various units in the hospital (outside the emergency unit)"; (c) "the services of medical specialists from the hospital who are 'on call' to the emergency unit"; and (d) "administrative services or support from the hospital." The findings are presented in Table 60.

The overall mean scores based on the data about each of the four kinds of requests, or units, involved all fall on the positive side of the scale, indicating that the emergency units' requests, on the average, are being met satisfactorily by these other hospital units. For inpatient services, ancillary services, on-call specialists, and administrative support, the specific scores are 2.16, 2.20, 2.29, and 2.45, respectively. The first three indicate a level of responsiveness which is close to "very satisfactory," and the fourth indicates a level midway between "very" and "fairly" satisfactory. Moreover, inter-unit variability in each case is only moderately high (see the relevant range of unit mean scores shown under each overall mean score in Table 60).

Equally important, when examining the various groupings of EU's, the results show few differences from the overall pattern concerning each of the hospital units or services involved. There are no significant differences whatsoever between the average scores of emergency units in urban vs. nonurban areas, in hospitals having vs. not having teaching affiliations, or in hospitals having vs. not having emergency personnel training programs. Concerning the remaining groupings, there are only two exceptions that should be noted.

TABLE 60. ADEQUACY WITH WHICH OTHERS IN THE HOSPITAL MEET EMERGENCY UNIT NURSES' REQUESTS FOR SERVICES OR SUPPORT, AS REPORTED BY THE NURSES (RNS)[a]

		Requests for Service/Support from			
Hospital Emergency Units (EU's) Involved		Inpatient Medical Units	Ancillary Services	On-call Medical Specialists	Hospital Administration
ALL EU'S IN THE STUDY SAMPLE (N=30 Hospital EU's)	Mean: Range:	2.16 (1.50-2.87)	2.20 (1.50-3.12)	2.29 (1.30-3.10)	2.45 (1.60-3.23)
YOUR HOSPITAL'S EU					
EU's in:					
Small Hospitals (n=14)		2.10	2.21	2.30	2.52
Medium Hospitals (n=9)		2.37	2.31	2.39	2.60
Large Hospitals (n=7)		1.99	2.05	2.13	2.13
EU's in:					
Church Operated Hospitals (n=9)		2.28	2.34	2.37	2.51
Osteopathic Hospitals (n=3)		2.16	2.28	2.51	2.68
All Other Hospitals (n=18)		2.10	2.13	2.21	2.39
EU's Located in:					
SMSA (urban) Areas (n=21)		2.16	2.21	2.27	2.42
Non-SMSA Areas (n=9)		2.15	2.19	2.32	2.54
EU's in Hospitals Having:					
Medical Teaching Affiliations (n=17)		2.16	2.24	2.24	2.42
No Medical Teaching Affiliations (n=13)		2.15	2.16	2.35	2.49
EU's in Hospitals Having:					
Emergency Personnel Training Programs (n=15)		2.10	2.18	2.28	2.38
No Training Programs (n=15)		2.21	2.22	2.29	2.53

[a] The results, reported here in the form of mean scores, are based on the responses of RNS from the various emergency units to the question: "When you request the services, assistance, or support of others in the hospital (outside the emergency unit), on the whole, how satisfactorily are your requests met by... ?" The response alternatives were: (1) Completely satisfactorily, (2) very satisfactorily, (3) fairly satisfactorily, (4) not so satisfactorily, and (5) not satisfactorily at all. Thus, the lower the score, the more satisfactorily requests are met.

First, there is a trend for the emergency units of osteopathic and, to a lesser extent, church operated hospitals to score somewhat less favorably, on the average, than their counterparts in other hospitals. Second, there is a similar trend for the emergency units of large hospitals to score more favorably on the average then their counterparts in medium- and small-size hospitals. This latter trend is sufficiently pronounced to indicate significant difference between large and other hospitals with regard to administrative support, and between large and medium-size hospitals with regard to the responsiveness of inpatient medical services.

Apparently, work relations between emergency units and these other important hospital units, or services, are quite good on the whole, although the situation of individual emergency units in this respect varies from better than "very satisfactory" to only "fairly satisfactory." The reader, incidentially, may wish to compare these findings with some of those discussed in previous chapters, particularly those in Chapter 2 about the sufficiency of emergency unit resources (Tables 15 and 16), the success of emergency units in obtaining requested staff resources from the hospital (Table 17), and the access of emergency units to medical specialists on call (Table 20).

Summary

In this chapter, certain findings concerning the emergency units' relations with their parent hospitals were presented and discussed. Institutional mechanisms for monitoring the performance of emergency units are either lacking or weak in about half of the hospitals. This may be a problem worthy of further study. Hospital administration's understanding of the work problems and needs of the emergency units varies a great deal from one unit to another, but for the total sample it is quite good (though not "very good" or "excellent").

Tension between emergency unit staff and hospital administration or other hospital staff, appears to be generally low. And the responsiveness of other hospital units, or services to the requests of the emergency unit is generally considered satisfactory. Inter-unit variability on these measures is moderately high to high, depending upon the specific measure examined. Overall, work relations with the parent hospital are favorable for the emergency units.

Chapter 7

RELATIONS WITH THE COMMUNITY

Emergency units interact, on a frequent basis, not only with other units of the hospital but also with a variety of organizations in the community outside -- other health care institutions, city health department, police and fire departments, ambulance companies, and other health or community agencies. The kind of work relations that the staff of an emergency unit have with personnel from these outside organizations can either aid or hinder the work of the unit. Good work relations within the unit and with the parent hospital are essential to effective performance but not sufficient. Relations with the external environment also must be satisfactory for an emergency unit to operate efficiently. Favorable relations with police and ambulance personnel, for example, may facilitate the patient entry process. Moreover, good external relations can foster inter-institutional collaboration, patient transfer arrangements, and joint activities for improving emergency services on a community-wide basis. The adequacy of an emergency unit's relations with the external organizational environment, therefore, is not only relevant but also important to examine. This is the task of the present chapter.

First, the chapter reviews certain findings concerning the staff's information about relevant outside health agencies and regulatory bodies, and the extent of each institution's collaboration with other health care institutions regarding emergency service matters. Second, it examines the adequacy of inter-institutional arrangements for patient transfers, and the staff's contacts with people from various outside organizations. Third, it examines the level of prevailing tension between emergency unit staff and the community. Fourth, it considers the quality of work relations between the selected community respondents (CRS) who participated in the study and the various emergency units with which these individuals are associated. Finally, the chapter reviews certain data concerning particular aspects of the community which, according to various groups of respondents, may be causing special problems or difficulties for each emergency unit.

Information About Health Agencies and Extent of Inter-Institutional Collaboration

Relations between hospitals and various federal, state, and professional health agencies and regulatory bodies have become increasingly more complex and more important to hospital functioning and to the work of emergency units. Consequently, the study specifically inquired about the information that hospital administrators (HAS) and the physicians (MDS) and supervising nurses (SRNS) who work in the various EU's have about such agencies. The question asked of each group was: "From the point of view of being able to do your work properly, on the whole, how adequate is the information that you have about the requirements and workings of... [e.g., HSA's, PSRO's, EMS,...] these outside health agencies and regulatory bodies?" The data are summarized in Table 61.

On the average, hospital administrators report that the information which they have is almost midway between "very adequate" and "fairly adequate," ranging across individual institutions from "completely adequate" to less than "fairly adequate." The physicians and supervising nurses of emergency units, on the other hand, report that their information is only "fairly adequate" on the average, ranging across EU's from "very adequate" to midway between "not so adequate" and "not adequate at all." Of the three groups, the physicians

TABLE 61. ADEQUACY OF INFORMATION WITHIN THE INSTITUTION ABOUT
OUTSIDE HEALTH AGENCIES AND REGULATORY BODIES[a]

Hospital Emergency Units (EU's) Involved		Adequacy of Information on the Part of		
		HAS	MDS	SRNS
ALL EU'S IN THE STUDY SAMPLE (N=30 Hospital EU's)	Mean: Range:	2.39 (1.00-3.50)	3.20 (2.20-4.20)	2.91 (2.00-4.50)
YOUR HOSPITAL'S EU		--		--
EU's with:				
Low Patient Volume (n=10)		2.50	3.11	3.17
Medium Pat. Volume (n=10)		2.50	3.43	2.90
High Patient Volume (n=10)		2.17	3.05	2.65
EU's in:				
Church Operated Hospitals (n=9)		2.46	3.22	3.07
Osteopathic Hospitals (n=3)		2.67	2.72	2.67
All Other Hospitals (n=18)		2.31	3.10	2.86
EU's Located in:				
SMSA (urban) Areas (n=21)		2.51	3.22	2.91
Non-SMSA Areas (n=9)		2.11	3.14	2.91
EU's in Hospitals Having:				
Medical Teaching Affiliations (n=17)		2.51	3.26	2.88
No Medical Teaching Affiliations (n=13)		2.23	3.11	2.94
EU's in Hospitals Having:				
Emergency Personnel Training Programs (n=15)		2.54	3.12	2.91
No Training Programs (n=15)		2.23	3.28	2.90

[a] The results, reported here in the form of mean scores, are based on the responses of HAS, MDS, and SRNS from the various institutions to the following question: "From the point of view of being able to do your work properly, on the whole, how adequate is the information that you have about the requirements and workings of... outside health agencies and regulatory bodies?" The response alternatives ranged from "(1) Completely adequate,"... to "(5) Not adequate at all." Thus, the lower the score the more adequate the information. Mean scores were first computed separately for each EU and then averaged for the EU's in the different categories.

are apparently the least well informed in this area. Obviously there is considerable room for improvement according to the data.

It is also interesting that the adequacy of information reported by the three groups does not differ between institutions having and not having medical teaching affiliations. The same applies with respect to emergency personnel training programs. The administrators of hospitals in urban areas, however, have less adequate information compared to their colleagues in non-urban areas. Administrators in hospitals whose emergency units have a high patient volume, on the other hand, report more adequate information than do those in institutions whose EU's have either a medium or a low patient volume. The most adequately informed physicians, and supervising nurses, also are those working in the high-volume units. Finally, with reference to institutional control, HAS from osteopathic hospitals and MDS and SRNS from church operated hospitals feel the least adequately informed, while HAS from not church operated hospitals (excluding osteopathic) and MDS and SRNS from osteopathic hospitals feel the most adequately informed about outside health agencies and regulatory bodies.

Inter-institutional collaboration. Hospital administrators and the supervising nurses of emergency units also were asked about the extent to which their institutions are collaborating with others, for the purpose of providing "better or less costly emergency medical services" or for the purpose of establishing or maintaining "special emergency care facilities or a regional system" The data from the two groups have been combined for each hospital in the study, and the results are presented in Table 62. Clearly, the extent of inter-institutional collaboration for either purpose is extremely variable, ranging across indi-

TABLE 62. EXTENT OF INSTITUTIONAL COLLABORATION WITH OTHER HOSPITALS OR EMERGENCY UNITS, AS REPORTED BY HOSPITAL ADMINISTRATOR (HAS) AND SUPERVISING NURSE (SRNS) RESPONDENTS FROM EACH INSTITUTION[a]

Hospital Emergency Units (EU's) Involved		Extent of Collaboration to	
		Provide Better or Less Costly Emergency Medical Services	Establish or Maintain Special Emergency Care Facilities or a Regional System
ALL EU'S IN THE STUDY SAMPLE (N=30 Hospital EU's)	Mean:	3.05	2.65
	Range:	(1.00-4.50)	(1.00-4.33)
YOUR HOSPITAL'S EU			
EU's with:			
Low Patient Volume (n=10)		3.39	2.82
Medium Pat. Volume (n=10)		3.07	2.86
High Patient Volume (n=10)		2.68	2.29
EU's in:			
Church Operated Hospitals (n=9)		3.47	2.91
Osteopathic Hospitals (n=3)		3.36	3.06
All Other Hospitals (n=18)		2.79	2.46
EU's Located in:			
SMSA (urban) Areas (n=21)		3.08	2.66
Non-SMSA Areas (n=9)		2.97	2.64
EU's in Hospitals Having:			
Medical Teaching Affiliations (n=17)		2.95	2.60
No Medical Teaching Affiliations (n=13)		3.18	2.73
EU's in Hospitals Having:			
Emergency Personnel Training Programs (n=15)		2.96	2.68
No Training Programs (n=15)		3.14	2.62

[a] The results, reported here in the form of mean scores, are based on the combined responses of HAS and SRNS from each institution to the following multiple-part question: "At the present time, to what extent is this hospital or emergency unit collaborating with other hospitals, emergency units, or other relevant service agencies (in order) to...?" The response alternatives ranged from "(1) To a very great extent,"... to "(5) To a very small extent or not at all." Thus, the lower the mean score the greater the extent of collaboration.

vidual hospitals from "very great" to less than "small" (midway between "small" and "very small or none at all").

For all 30 hospitals in the sample, the average level of inter-institutional collaboration is higher with respect to establishing or maintaining special emergency care facilities than with respect to providing better or less costly emergency medical services. But even with respect to the former it is rather low. The overall mean scores are 2.65 (which signifies collaboration midway between "to a great extent" and "to a fair extent" but closer to the latter) and 3.05 (which corresponds almost exactly to "to a fair extent"), respectively. In this area too, therefore, there seems to be considerable room for improvement in relations with the relevant environment.

Considering next the various groupings of hospitals/emergency units, the results show no differences in the average level of collaboration for hospitals in urban vs. nonurban areas, hospitals with vs. without medical teaching affiliations, or hospitals with vs. without emergency personnel training programs. In contrast, inter-institutional collaboration, for both of the above purposes, is greater in the case of hospitals whose emergency units have a high than a low or medium patient volume. It is similarly greater for not church operated hospitals (excluding osteopathic) than for either church operated or osteopathic hospitals (these latter two kinds of institutions do not differ on the collaboration measure). Even more important to remember, however, is the fact that the variability across individual hospitals (shown by the range of mean scores) is extremely great regarding the extent of reported collaboration for either of the two purposes specified. Some of the hospitals are doing a great deal and some are doing very little, with the remaining occupying the intermediate positions which themselves cover a rather broad range.

Work Contacts with Other Organizations and Patient Transfer Arrangements

The same key respondents, i.e., hospital administrators (HAS) and supervising nurses (SRNS), also provided an assessment of the work contacts between emergency unit staff and personnel from: (a) police departments; (b) private ambulance companies; (c) local health departments; and (d) health systems agencies. The combined data from HAS and RNS respondents associated with each institution studied are summarized in Table 63, separately with reference to each kind of personnel involved. Overall, these work contacts are apparently more adequate than the extent of inter-institutional collaboration discussed above.

Comparatively, the work contacts of emergency units are on the average most satisfactory with the personnel of police departments, least satisfactory with the personnel of health systems agencies, and at an intermediate level with ambulance personnel and personnel from local health departments. Even with health systems agencies, however, the work contacts of emergency units on the whole are better than "fairly satisfactory" (actually midway between "very" and "fairly" satisfactory) according to the respondents. Contacts with police departments are "very satisfactory" (the overall mean score for the 30 EU's being 2.01 in this case). The variability on the measure in question across individual EU's is moderately high to high, depending upon the work contacts considered. It is lowest in the case of contacts with police departments and highest in the case of contacts with health systems agencies. Generally, of course, the work contacts of emergency units with the personnel of the several organizations specified are quite good, on the average, according to the data.

With reference to the various groupings of emergency units, the results show a number of interesting trends. First, for some reason, the EU's of hospitals with teaching affiliations, and also training programs, tend to

TABLE 63. ADEQUACY OF THE WORK-RELATED CONTACTS OF THE EMERGENCY UNIT STAFF WITH RELEVANT ORGANIZATIONS IN THE COMMUNITY, ACCORDING TO HOSPITAL ADMINISTRATOR (HAS) AND SUPERVISING NURSE (SRNS) RESPONDENTS[a]

Hospital Emergency Units (EU's) Involved		Adequacy of Contacts With			
		Police Department Personnel	Private Ambulance Services Personnel	Local Health Department Personnel	Health Systems Agency (HSA) Personnel
ALL EU'S IN THE STUDY SAMPLE (N=30 Hospital EU's)	*Mean:*	2.01	2.21	2.26	2.43
	Range:	(1.20-3.00)	(1.40-3.67)	(1.50-3.50)	(1.00-3.50)
YOUR HOSPITAL'S EU					
EU's in:					
Small Hospitals (n=14)		1.92	2.10	2.29	2.39
Medium Hospitals (n=9)		2.21	2.44	2.18	2.31
Large Hospitals (n=7)		1.95	2.13	2.32	2.70
EU's in:					
Church Operated Hospitals (n=9)		2.01	2.38	2.29	2.88
Osteopathic Hospitals (n=3)		2.42	2.47	2.33	2.33
All Other Hospitals (n=18)		1.95	2.08	2.24	2.26
EU's Located in:					
SMSA (urban) Areas (n=21)		2.07	2.11	2.27	2.49
Non-SMSA Areas (n=9)		1.88	2.45	2.24	2.30
EU's in Hospitals Having:					
Medical Teaching Affiliations (n=17)		2.09	2.19	2.38	2.53
No Medical Teaching Affiliations (n=13)		1.92	2.24	2.11	2.29
EU's in Hospitals Having:					
Emergency Personnel Training Programs (n=15)		2.01	2.19	2.28	2.60
No Training Programs (n=15)		2.02	2.23	2.24	2.25

[a] The results, reported here in the form of mean scores, are based on the <u>combined</u> answers of hospital administrator (HAS) and supervising nurse (SRNS) respondents from each institution to the following multiple-part question: "Considering all the work-related contacts that the staff of the emergency unit have with..., <u>how satisfactory</u> would you say are their contacts from the standpoint of accomplishing the work of this emergency unit?" The response alternatives ranged from "(1) Completely satisfactory,"... to "(5) Not satisfactory at all." Thus, the lower the mean score the more adequate the work contacts.

have somewhat less satisfactory work contacts with health systems agencies than do the EU's of hospitals without such affiliations or programs. Second, and probably understandably, work contacts with ambulance personnel tend to be less satisfactory for EU's in non-urban than in urban areas. In addition, they tend to be less satisfactory in the case of osteopathic compared to non-osteopathic institutions. The work contacts of the former with ambulance personnel also are less satisfactory than they are for other not church operated institutions. This is not the case, however, regarding contacts with local health departments. And contacts with health systems agencies are more satisfactory for the units of not church operated hospitals, including osteopathic, than for the units of church operated hospitals. Finally, the emergency units of large hospitals have less satisfactory contacts with health systems agencies than do the units of small or medium size hospitals. On the other hand, the EU's of medium-size hospitals have less satisfactory contacts with ambulance personnel than do the EU's of either small or large hospitals.

Medical Control. Certain additional data concerning contacts with ambulance personnel are also interesting. These data (not shown in Table 63) were obtained from the physicians (MDS) working in the various EU's in response to a specific question about the amount of medical control exercised over the activities of ambulance personnel and emergency medical technicians who bring patients to each unit. On the average, the physicians from the 30 EU's in the study indicate that the medical control exercised is "moderate." As for most other measures, however, the amount of control varies greatly from one emergency unit to another, from more than "considerable" to "little."

Patient Transfer Arrangements. Potentially, some of the more important contacts with other organizations in the community concern inter-institutional transfers of patients. Most emergency units, and/or their parent hospitals, apparently have either formal or informal arrangements for accepting transfer patients from other institutions. In response to a specific question, at least half of the physicians (MDS) working in each EU report this to be the case of 26 (or 87%) of the 30 EU's in the study. In addition, almost half of the units (14 of the 30) have similar arrangements for transferring some of their patients into other institutions for care, again as reported by at least half of the MDS from each unit.

Emergency units with a high patient volume are the most likely ones to have arrangements for accepting patients from other institutions and units with a low patient volume are the least likely (100% vs. 70%). The same is true concerning arrangements for transferring EU patients to outside care facilities (60% of the high-volume but only 30% of the low-volume units report such arrangements). The emergency units of institutions with teaching affiliations, and institutions in urban areas, also are somewhat more likely than those of other institutions to have both types of patient transfer arrangements.

The above findings (not reported in table form) provide the base for the results presented in Table 64 concerning the relative adequacy of reported patient transfer arrangements. More specifically, Table 64 summarizes the responses of emergency unit physicians (MDS), separately for transfers-in and transfers-out, to the question: "Overall, how satisfactorily are these transfer arrangements working out from your point of view?"

It is obvious from Table 64 that the scores on the two measures are quite similar. In fact, there are no differences between how satisfactory the two types of transfer arrangements are for any of the hospital groupings shown, with the sole exception that in the case of osteopathic hospitals arrangements for accepting transfer patients are more satisfactory on the average than are

TABLE 64. THE ADEQUACY OF INSTITUTIONAL ARRANGEMENTS FOR RELEVANT PATIENT TRANSFERS, AS REPORTED BY PHYSICIANS (MDS) WORKING IN THE EMERGENCY UNITS[a]

Hospital Emergency Units (EU's) Involved		Adequacy of Arrangements for	
		Accepting Transfer Patients Into the EU	Transferring EU Patients Elsewhere (Out)
ALL EU'S IN THE STUDY SAMPLE	Mean:	2.53	2.51
	Range:	(1.00-3.50)	(1.60-3.80)
YOUR HOSPITAL'S EU			
EU's with:			
Low Patient Volume		2.51	2.40
Medium Pat. Volume		2.56	2.64
High Patient Volume		2.59	2.46
EU's in:			
Church Operated Hospitals		2.56	2.35
Osteopathic Hospitals		2.67	3.13
All Other Hospitals		2.54	2.48
EU's Located in:			
SMSA (urban) Areas		2.65	2.53
Non-SMSA Areas		2.33	2.44
EU's in Hospitals Having:			
Medical Teaching Affiliations		2.67	2.55
No Medical Teaching Affiliations		2.42	2.45
EU's in Hospitals Having:			
Emergency Personnel Training Programs		2.65	2.60
No Training Programs		2.46	2.42

[a] The results, reported here in the form of mean scores, are based on the responses of MDS from the various emergency units to a series of interview items dealing with patient transfer arrangements. These items first established the existence of transfer arrangements (whether written or informal agreements), and then asked: "Overall, how satisfactorily are these transfer arrangements working out from your point of view?" This open-ended question was asked separately for transfers-in and transfers-out. The responses given by MDS were coded on a five-point scale, ranging from "(1) Completely satisfactorily,"... to "(5) Not satisfactorily at all." Thus, the lower the mean score the more adequate the transfer arrangements.

those for transferring patients out (a reverse tendency is slightly evident in church operated hospitals). Considering all of the EU's for which data are available, the physicians indicate that both kinds of transfer arrangements are working out equally satisfactorily (on the average) in their respective emergency units. The overall mean score is almost exactly half-way between "very satisfactorily" and "fairly satisfactorily" for both.

On both measures, however, inter-unit variability is high, the transfer arrangements working out much more satisfactorily for some of the EU's than for others. Transfer-out arrangements are apparently less satisfactory in osteopathic than non-osteopathic hospitals. There is also a very weak trend for both transfer-in and transfer-out arrangements to be slightly less satisfactory in hospitals which are located in urban areas, which have medical teaching affiliations, or which have emergency personnel training programs than hospitals which do not have these characteristics. Overall, however, the important thing is that for institutions having either transfer-in or transfer-out arrangements, such arrangements are on the average working out at least "fairly" satisfactorily, though not "very satisfactorily." Half of the institutions in the study, moreover, apparently have neither formal nor informal arrangements for transferring some of their emergency unit patients to outside institutions for care.

Overall Tension with the Community

A general indicator of how satisfactory relations with the community are is the tension that the staff experience in their work relations with relevant people in the community. For this reason, hospital administrator respondents (HAS) and the physicians (MDS) and registered nurses (RNS) working in the various emergency units were asked the following question: "All things considered, how much <u>tension</u> (friction, strain, or conflict) would you say is there between... emergency unit staff <u>and</u> the community outside?" The obtained data are summarized in Table 65.

All three groups report relatively little tension in this area. However, MDS and RNS perceive even less tension, both reporting "very low" tension on the average, than do HAS, who report a level of tension midway between "low" and "very low." In addition, the level of tension reported by HAS varies more, across individual hospitals (from "high" to "no tension at all") than that reported by the other two groups (in the case of the data from MDS, for example, it varies from low to practically none at all). Inter-institutional variability exists regardless of the source of data, but since the overall tension is quite low on the average (according to every group) most emergency units seem to experience no major problem in this area.

Still a few trends are suggested by the findings. According to all three respondent groups, the level of tension between emergency unit staff and the community tends to be slightly lower on the average for the EU's of hospitals in urban than non-urban areas, and hospitals having either medical teaching affiliations or emergency personnel training programs compared to those which do not. According to the data from HAS, and possibly also RNS but not MDS, the level of tension is also lower in the case of osteopathic compared to non-osteopathic institutions. Finally, also according to the data from HAS, but not MDS or RNS, tension is higher on the average for medium-size hospitals than for either small or large hospitals (although the difference is not statistically significant in the latter case). Overall, however, the results show that relations with the community generally are not strained.

TABLE 65. TENSION BETWEEN EMERGENCY UNIT STAFF AND THE COMMUNITY OUTSIDE, AS REPORTED BY CERTAIN GROUPS OF RESPONDENTS[a]

Hospital Emergency Units (EU's) Involved		Level of Tension, According to		
		HAS	MDS	RNS
ALL EU'S IN THE STUDY SAMPLE (N=30 Hospital EU's)	*Mean:*	3.64	4.01	3.93
	Range:	(1.00-5.00)	(3.25-4.80)	(3.00-4.50)
YOUR HOSPITAL'S EU		--		
EU's in:				
Small Hospitals (n=14)		3.79	3.87	3.98
Medium Hospitals (n=9)		3.39	4.15	3.80
Large Hospitals (n=7)		3.67	4.09	3.99
EU's in:				
Church Operated Hospitals (n=9)		3.46	3.86	3.93
Osteopathic Hospitals (n=3)		4.17	4.00	4.26
All Other Hospitals (n=18)		3.64	4.09	3.87
EU's Located in:				
SMSA (urban) Areas (n=21)		3.75	4.08	3.98
Non-SMSA Areas (n=9)		3.39	3.84	3.81
EU's in Hospitals Having:				
Medical Teaching Affiliations (n=17)		3.75	4.15	3.95
No Medical Teaching Affiliations (n=13)		3.50	3.83	3.90
EU's in Hospitals Having:				
Emergency Personnel Training Programs (n=15)		3.73	4.14	4.04
No Training Programs (n=15)		3.54	3.87	3.82

[a] The results, reported here in the form of mean scores, are based on the responses of HAS, MDS, and RNS from each institution to the following question: "All things considered, how much tension (friction, strain, or conflict) would you say is there between... emergency unit staff and the community outside?" The response alternatives ranged from "(1) A high level of tension,"... to "(5) No tension at all." Thus, the lower the score the higher the level of tension; and, conversely, the higher the score the lower the level of tension.

Work Contacts with Key Individuals from the Community

So far, work relations between emergency unit staff and people from various organizations in the community, or the community considered as a whole, have been discussed from the perspective of respondents working within each unit or its parent hospital. The perspective of respondents from the outside community is introduced in the present section. Specifically, the selected community respondents (CRS) who participated in the study were asked about their own work contacts with the staff of the emergency units with which they have such contacts.

Interestingly, and somewhat surprisingly, the selected community respondents report having work contacts with the various units that average a period of 12 years for the 30 EU's in the study, the range being from a minimum of 6.5 years to a high of 20.5 years. Apparently, the CRS involved have had very considerable personal association with the emergency units. In terms of the organizations that they represent, considering all 30 EU's together, these respondents are distributed as follows: police departments, 26.5%; fire departments, 20.0%; ambulance companies, 10.5%; emergency medical service systems, 8.5%; coroner's or medical examiner's offices, 8.5%; local health departments, 8.0%; health systems agencies, 2.5%; and "all other" organizations, 15.5%.

These respondents were asked to indicate (a) "how satisfactory" their recent work contacts with each emergency unit were, and (b) the extent to which the staff of the unit generally "take into account" the work problems and needs of these particular respondents and their associates. The obtained data, summarized in Table 66, are very favorable to the emergency units.

First, for all 30 EU's in the study, CRS as a group regard their recent contacts with the emergency unit as "very satisfactory" on the average. The range across individual units on this measure is from midway between "completely"

TABLE 66. THE QUALITY OF WORK RELATIONS BETWEEN SELECTED COMMUNITY RESPONDENTS (CRS) AND STAFF WORKING IN THE EMERGENCY UNIT, AS REPORTED BY CRS[a]

Hospital Emergency Units (EU's) Involved		The Overall Adequacy of CRS Work Contacts With the EU Staff[b]	Extent EU Staff Take Into Account the Work Needs of CRS[c]
ALL EU'S IN THE STUDY SAMPLE (N=30 Hospital EU's)	Mean:	2.15	2.31
	Range:	(1.40-3.60)	(1.60-3.00)
YOUR HOSPITAL'S EU			
EU's in:			
Small Hospitals (n=14)		2.18	2.36
Medium Hospitals (n=9)		2.04	2.36
Large Hospitals (n=7)		2.20	2.15
EU's in:			
Church Operated Hospitals (n=9)		2.31	2.30
Osteopathic Hospitals (n=3)		2.28	2.21
All Other Hospitals (n=18)		2.05	2.33
EU's Located in:			
SMSA (urban) Areas (n=21)		2.11	2.31
Non-SMSA Areas (n=9)		2.22	2.32
EU's in Hospitals Having:			
Medical Teaching Affiliations (n=17)		2.08	2.22
No Medical Teaching Affiliations (n=13)		2.24	2.44
EU's in Hospitals Having:			
Emergency Personnel Training Programs (n=15)		2.15	2.27
No Training Programs (n=15)		2.15	2.35

Table 66 Continues

TABLE 66
(Continued)

---

[a] The results, reported here in the form of mean scores, are based on the answers of the selected community respondents (CRS) associated with each institution to two questions about their work relations with staff in the emergency unit.

[b] The question was: "Overall, how satisfactory, would you say, were your (recent work) contacts (with the emergency unit staff) from your point of view?" The responses of CRS to the open-ended question were coded on a five-point scale, ranging from "(1) Completely satisfactory,"... to "(5) Not satisfactory at all." Thus, the lower the mean score the better the quality of work relations.

[c] The question was: "Generally, in their work relations with you and your associates, to what extent do you feel that the people who work in this emergency unit take into account your own work problems and needs?" The response alternatives ranged from "(1) To a very great extent,"... to "(5) To a very small extent or not at all." Thus, the lower the mean score the better the quality of work relations.

and "very" satisfactory, at the one extreme, to midway between "fairly satisfactory" and "not so satisfactory" at the other. (The overall mean score is 2.15, while unit mean scores range from 1.40 to 3.60.) The selected community respondents also report that, on the average, the staff of the various units take into account the work problems and needs of these respondents and their associates almost "to a great extent." (On this measure, the overall mean score is 2.31, while the mean scores of individual units range from 1.60, which corresponds to midway between "to a very great extent" and "to a great extent," and 3.00 which corresponds exactly to "to a fair extent.")

Obviously, there is considerable (though not very high) inter-unit variability on both measures, particularly on the former, but the overall picture is very favorable on the average for the emergency units studied. Equally important, the findings show no significant differences whatsoever, on either measure, between units in one grouping and units in another, when the various groupings based on hospital size, location, control, medical teaching affiliation, and the presence/absence of training programs are properly compared. The overall picture is equally positive in all cases.

Problem-Causing Aspects of the Community

The medical and nursing staff from each emergency unit, key administrative and medical staff from each unit's parent hospital, and the selected community respondents were finally asked whether any particular aspects, or features, of the community are causing special problems or difficulties for the unit. These data were obtained with open-ended questions asked in the personal interviews completed by the respondents. Because of overall similarity in the patterns of findings, and in order both to conserve space and not to burden the reader unduly, only the data from registered nurses (RNS), hospital administrators

(HAS), and community respondents (CRS) are here presented in detail, respectively in Tables 67, 68, and 69. The data from emergency unit physicians (MDS) which are very similar to the data from RNS, and the data from other hospital physicians (HMDS) are only briefly discussed. In the tables presented, the results are summarized by showing the three most frequently mentioned aspects of the community which tend to cause special problems according to the respondents.

Before considering the findings, it is important to note that a substantial number of respondents from each group involved indicated either that no particular aspect of the community is causing any special problems for the emergency unit or that they did not know. More specifically, 26% of all the registered nurses and 56% of all the physicians from the emergency units in the study fall into this category. The corresponding figures for hospital administrators and selected hospital physicians are 35% and 48% respectively. Of the selected community respondents, 45% said there were no such problem-causing aspects and another 10% said they did not know.

Thus, the percent of respondents from each group who mentioned at least one particular aspect of the community is: 74% in the case of RNS, 44% in the case of MDS, 65% in the case of HAS, 52% in the case of HMDS, and 45% in the case of CRS. Of those who mentioned at least one aspect, however, some mentioned two or even three aspects (e.g., 52% of the RNS and 40% of the HAS mentioned at least two aspects, and about 20% of them in each case mentioned three aspects). The percentage figures shown in Tables 67, 68, and 69 are based on the total number of mentions given by all responding group members in each case.

For presentation purposes, the aspects mentioned by the respondents have been grouped into the following seven categories:

(1) <u>population characteristics</u>, such as mobility, income, education level, language barriers, etc.;

(2) <u>high utilization</u> of the emergency unit by "nonemergency" patients;

(3) <u>the characteristics of individual patients</u>, such as severity of condition, particular illnesses or injuries, drug abuse, industrial injury, etc.;

(4) <u>inadequate health care resources in the community</u>, such as a limited work force pool in the health care sector, shortage of family care practitioners, competition with other facilities for limited resources, etc.;

(5) <u>problems with various organizations</u> with which the emergency unit interacts, including federal or other health agencies, insurance providers, and organizations bringing patients into the emergency unit;

(6) <u>the physical environment</u>, including such aspects as distance, poor geographic location, congested or unsafe area, the size of the area being served, etc.; and

(7) <u>all other aspects</u> of the community mentioned that could not be grouped into the preceding categories.

Considering first the data from the registered nurses (RNS) working in the emergency units, Table 67, the results show that the more frequently mentioned of all aspects (as an aspect that causes special problems or difficulties for the emergency unit) is "the characteristics of patients." Almost 27% of all mentions given by the RNS from all the EU's in the study fall into this category. Even more significantly, perhaps, this is true for every one of the hospital groupings examined in the present report.

TABLE 67. ASPECTS OF THE COMMUNITY WHICH CREATE SPECIAL PROBLEMS FOR THE EMERGENCY UNIT, ACCORDING TO THE REGISTERED NURSES (RNS) WHO WORK IN THE UNIT[a]

Hospital Emergency Units (EU's) Involved	Total Mentions[b]	The Three Aspects Most Frequently Mentioned by RNS		
		First	Second	Third
ALL EU'S IN THE STUDY SAMPLE (N=30 Hospital EU's)	409	The characteristics of patients (26.7%)	High utilization by non-emergency patients (22.2%)	Population characteristics (19.6%)
YOUR HOSPITAL'S EU				
EU's in:				
Small Hospitals (n=14)	161	The characteristics of patients (26.1%)	High utilization by non-emergency patients (20.5%)	Problems with various organizations (19.9%)
Medium Hospitals (n=9)	140	The characteristics of patients (27.1%)	Population characteristics (22.1%)	High utilization by nonemergency patients (20.7%)
Large Hospitals (n=7)	108	The characteristics of patients (26.9%)	High utilization by non-emergency patients (26.9%)	Inadequate health care resources (14.8%)
EU's in:				
Church Operated Hospitals (n=9)	108	The characteristics of patients (27.8%)	Population characteristics (25.9%)	High utilization by nonemergency patients (19.4%)
Osteopathic Hospitals (n=3)	31	The characteristics of patients (25.8%)	High utilization by non-emergency patients (25.8%)	Problems with various organizations (25.8%)
All Other Hospitals (n=18)	270	The characteristics of patients (26.3%)	High utilization by non-emergency patients (23.0%)	Population characteristics (18.5%)
EU's Located in:				
SMSA (urban) Areas (n=21)	295	The characteristics of patients (26.8%)	Population characteristics (21.7%)	High utilization by nonemergency patients (21.4%)
Non-SMSA Areas (n=9)	114	The characteristics of patients (26.3%)	High utilization by non-emergency patients (24.6%)	Problems with various organizations (19.3%)
EU's in Hospitals Having:				
Medical Teaching Affiliations (n=17)	254	The characteristics of patients (26.0%)	High utilization by non-emergency patients (24.0%)	Population characteristics (18.9%)
No Medical Teaching Affiliations (n=13)	155	The characteristics of patients (27.7%)	Population characteristics (20.6%)	High utilization by nonemergency patients (19.4%)
EU's in Hospitals Having:				
Emergency Personnel Training Programs (n=15)	217	The characteristics of patients (22.6%)	High utilization by non-emergency patients (22.6%)	Population characteristics (21.7%)
No Training Programs (n=15)	192	The characteristics of patients (31.3%)	High utilization by non-emergency patients (21.9%)	Population characteristics (17.2%)

[a] The results are based on the responses of RNS from the various emergency units to the following open-ended question: "Is there anything about the community outside or about the population being served by the emergency unit that creates special problems or difficulties for this emergency unit?" Their responses were first coded into a large number of specific categories and then collapsed into the following seven general categories: (1) Population characteristics (e.g., income level, stability, etc.), (2) High utilization of EU by nonemergency patients, (3) The characteristics of patients (e.g., condition as they arrive, nonpaying patients, etc.), (4) Inadequate health care resources in the community (e.g., staff recruitment pool, etc.), (5) Problems with various organizations in the community, (6) Physical environment characteristics (e.g., geographic location), and (7) All other.

[b] The mentions indicated for each grouping of EU's represent the sum of mentions for all hospital EU's in the grouping combined. The percentages enclosed in parentheses after each particular aspect were computed using the summed mentions as a base. Of all the RNS in the study 75% mentioned at least one problematic aspect, 52% mentioned at least two, and 21% mentioned three.

The second most frequently mentioned aspect is "high utilization by non-emergency patients," accounting for 22% of all the mentions given by RNS. This holds both for the total sample and for most of the groupings (excepting the EU's of medium-size hospitals, church operated hospitals, hospitals in urban areas, and hospitals with no medical teaching affiliations -- in all of which cases "population characteristics" is the second most frequently mentioned item). The third most frequently mentioned aspect by RNS is "population characteristics," accounting for 20% of all the mentions given by these respondents. This pattern again applies to most hospital/EU groupings as well, with the following exceptions: for small hospitals, osteopathic hospitals, and hospitals in non-urban areas, "problems with various organizations" is the third most frequently mentioned aspect, while "inadequate health care resources" is third in the case of large hospitals.

The corresponding data from emergency unit physicians (MDS), not presented in table form, parallel those from RNS rather closely, with a few exceptions. Like RNS, the MDS mention "the characteristics of patients" more often -- in fact significantly more often -- than any of the other aspects. This item accounts for 32% of all the mentions given by MDS, and is mentioned most often in all but two of the various hospital/EU groupings ("problems with outside organizations" is the most mentioned in the case of osteopathic hospitals, and "population characteristics" is the most mentioned in the case of hospitals with emergency personnel training programs). The second and third most frequently mentioned aspects by MDS are the same as those mentioned by RNS, but in reverse order -- "population characteristics," which accounts for 23% of all the mentions given by MDS, and "high utilization by nonemergency patients," which accounts for 13% of all such mentions. Moreover, "population characteristics" is the second most frequently mentioned aspect in all hospital groupings except hospitals with training programs for which the "characteristics of patients" is second. Finally, in those groupings for which "high utilization" is not the third most frequently mentioned aspect, MDS mention either "problems with various organizations" or "inadequate health care resources" in its place.

In the case of selected hospital physicians (HMDS), the results are only in part similar to the preceding; in part, they parallel the data from hospital administrators (HAS), discussed below, more than they parallel the data from MDS and RNS, discussed above. Very briefly, the HMDS from the 30 institutions in the study mention "population characteristics" (accounts for 30% of their mentions), "the characteristics of patients" (accounts for 21% of their mentions), and "problems with outside organizations," first, second, and third most frequently, respectively. Only in a few of the various hospital groupings, moreover, do these respondents mention either "high utilization" or "inadequate health care resources" among the top three items, in place of one or another of the above aspects.

The results based on the data from hospital administrators (HAS) are shown in Table 68. The three top items according to these respondents are, in order of overall frequency: "problems with various organizations" (accounts for 26% of all the mentions given by HAS), "the characteristics of patients" (accounts for 22% of all mentions) and "population characteristics" (accounts for 17% of all mentions). The pattern varies a great deal from one hospital grouping to another, however, and the reader may wish to examine Table 68 in greater detail.

Finally, the corresponding findings based on the data provided by the selected community respondents (CRS), as to aspects of the community that tend to create problems or difficulties for the various emergency units, are

TABLE 68. ASPECTS OF THE COMMUNITY WHICH CREATE SPECIAL PROBLEMS FOR THE EMERGENCY UNIT, ACCORDING TO HOSPITAL ADMINISTRATOR RESPONDENTS (HAS)[a]

Hospital Emergency Units (EU's) Involved	Total Mentions[b]	The Three Aspects Most Frequently Mentioned by HAS		
		First	Second	Third
ALL EU'S IN THE STUDY SAMPLE (N=30 Hospital EU's)	86	Problems with various organizations (25.6%)	The characteristics of patients (22.1%)	Population characteristics (17.4%)
YOUR HOSPITAL'S EU		--	--	--
EU's in:				
Small Hospitals (n=14)	35	Problems with various organizations (25.7%)	The characteristics of patients (22.9%)	Population characteristics (17.1%)
Medium Hospitals (n=9)	26	Problems with various organizations (30.8%)	The characteristics of patients (26.9%)	Population characteristics (15.4%)
Large Hospitals (n=7)	25	Inadequate health care resources (24.0%)	Population characteristics (20.0%)	The characteristics of patients (16.0%)
EU's in:				
Church Operated Hospitals (n=9)	26	The characteristics of patients (30.8%)	Population characteristics (26.9%)	Problems with various organizations (19.2%)
Osteopathic Hospitals (n=3)	4	Problems with various organizations (75.0%)	Inadequate health care resources (25.0%)	--------
All Other Hospitals (n=18)	56	Problems with various organizations (25.0%)	The characteristics of patients (19.6%)	Inadequate health care resources (17.9%)
EU's Located in:				
SMSA (urban) Areas (n=21)	65	Problems with various organizations (24.6%)	The characteristics of patients (18.5%)	Inadequate health care resources (16.9%)
Non-SMSA Areas (n=9)	21	The characteristics of patients (33.3%)	Problems with various organizations (28.6%)	Population characteristics (23.8%)
EU's in Hospitals Having:				
Medical Teaching Affiliations (n=17)	56	Problems with various organizations (28.6%)	Population characteristics (19.6%)	Patient characteristics (17.9%)
No Medical Teaching Affiliations (n=13)	30	The characteristics of patients (30.0%)	Problems with various organizations (20.0%)	Population characteristics (13.3%); High utilization by nonemergency patients (13.3%)
EU's in Hospitals Having:				
Emergency Personnel Training Programs (n=15)	43	Problems with various organizations (30.2%)	The characteristics of patients (23.3%)	Inadequate health care resources (16.3%)
No Training Programs (n=15)	43	Problems with various organizations (20.9%)	The characteristics of patients (20.9%)	Population characteristics (20.9%)

[a] The results are based on the responses of HAS from the various hospitals to the following open-ended question: "Is there anything about the community outside or about the population being served by the emergency unit that creates special problems or difficulties for this emergency unit?" Their responses were first coded into a large number of categories and then collapsed into the following seven general categories: (1) Population characteristics (e.g., income level, stability, etc.), (2) High utilization of EU by nonemergency patients, (3) The characteristics of patients (e.g., condition as they arrive, nonpaying patients, etc.), (4) Inadequate health care resources in the community (e.g., staff recruitment pool, etc.), (5) Problems with various organizations in the community, (6) Physical environment characteristics (e.g., geographic location), and (7) All other.

[b] The mentions indicated for each grouping of EU's represent the sum of mentions for all hospital EU's in the grouping combined. The percentages enclosed in parentheses after each particular aspect were computed using the summed mentions as a base. Of all HAS respondents in the study, 65% mentioned at least one problematic aspect, 41% mentioned at least two, and 22% mentioned three.

summarized in Table 69. It is rather interesting that, like the HMDS, the CRS mention "population characteristics" in first place (this item accounts for 33% of all mentions given by CRS). In second place, they mention "high utilization by nonemergency patients" (this accounts for 20% of their mentions). And in third place, unlike any of the other respondent groups, they mention "the physical environment" (this accounts for 13% of their mentions) -- an aspect that places among the top three items only once in the entire series of findings about problem-causing aspects of the community.

The overall pattern of findings based on the data from each particular group of respondents, of course, may be also compared to the corresponding pattern based on the data from the remaining groups. Comparisons of this kind reveal a number of interesting differences concerning those aspects of the community that may be causing problems for the emergency units studied. Thus, for example, while emergency unit staff (RNS and MDS respondents) mention "the characteristics of patients" most frequently among all such aspects, other hospital staff (HAS and HMDS respondents) mention the same aspect second most frequently, and the community respondents (CRS) do not even include it among their three most frequently mentioned aspects.

On the other hand, both the community respondents (CRS) and the emergency staff (RNS as well as MDS) include among their three most frequently mentioned aspects "high utilization by nonemergency patients," while the hospital administrators (HAS) and selected hospital physicians (HMDS) do not. Both of the latter groups, however, unlike any of the other respondent groups, mention "problems with various organizations" in the community as one of the top three problem-causing aspects. For the selected physicians (HMDS) and the community respondents (CRS), but not the other three groups, "population characteristics" is the most frequently mentioned item of all. Unlike any of the other groups,

TABLE 69. ASPECTS OF THE COMMUNITY WHICH TEND TO CREATE PROBLEMS OR DIFFICULTIES FOR THE EMERGENCY UNIT, ACCORDING TO THE SELECTED COMMUNITY RESPONDENTS (CRS) ASSOCIATED WITH EACH UNIT[a]

Hospital Emergency Units (EU's) Involved	Total Mentions[b]	The Three Aspects Most Frequently Mentioned by CRS		
		First	Second	Third
ALL EU'S IN THE STUDY SAMPLE (N=30 Hospital EU's)	253	Population characteristics (33.2%)	High utilization by non-emergency patients (20.2%)	The physical environment (13.0%)
YOUR HOSPITAL'S EU				
EU's in:				
Small Hospitals (n=14)	133	Population characteristics (29.3%)	High utilization by non-emergency patients (18.0%)	The physical environment (14.3%)
Medium Hospitals (n=9)	63	Population characteristics (33.3%)	High utilization by non-emergency patients (27.0%)	The physical environment (14.3%)
Large Hospitals (n=7)	57	Population characteristics (42.1%)	High utilization by non-emergency patients (17.0%)	Problems with various organizations (10.5%)
EU's in:				
Church Operated Hospitals (n=9)	71	Population characteristics (39.4%)	Inadequate health care resources (16.9%)	High utilization by nonemergency patients (12.7%); The physical environment (12.7%)
Osteopathic Hospitals (n=3)	20	Population characteristics (25.0%)	Problems with various organizations (25.0%)	High utilization by nonemergency patients (20.0%); Inadequate health care resources (20.0%)
All Other Hospitals (n=18)	162	Population characteristics (31.5%)	High utilization by non-emergency patients (23.5%)	The physical environment (14.8%)
EU's Located in:				
SMSA (urban) Areas (n=21)	163	Population characteristics (34.4%)	High utilization by non-emergency patients (18.4%)	Problems with various organizations (12.9%)
Non-SMSA Areas (n=9)	90	Population characteristics (31.1%)	High utilization by non-emergency patients (23.3%)	The physical environment (13.0%)
EU's in Hospitals Having:				
Medical Teaching Affiliations (n=17)	135	Population characteristics (41.5%)	High utilization by non-emergency patients (20.7%)	Problems with various organizations (9.6%); The physical environment (9.6%)
No Medical Teaching Affiliations (n=13)	118	Population characteristics (23.7%)	High utilization by non-emergency patients (19.5%)	The physical environment (16.9%)
EU's in Hospitals Having:				
Emergency Personnel Training Programs (n=15)	127	Population characteristics (34.6%)	High utilization by non-emergency patients (20.5%)	The physical environment (14.2%)
No Training Programs (n=15)	126	Population characteristics (31.7%)	High utilization by non-emergency patients (19.8%)	Inadequate health care resources (12.7%)

[a] The results are based on the answers of the selected community respondents (CRS) connected with various emergency units to the following open-ended question: "Is there anything about the community here or about the population being served by this particular emergency unit that tends to create problems or difficulties for this emergency unit?" Their answers were first coded into a large number of categories and then collapsed into the following seven general categories: (1) Population characteristics (e.g., income level, stability, etc.), (2) High utilization of EU by nonemergency patients, (3) The characteristics of patients (e.g., condition as they arrive, nonpaying patients, etc.), (4) Inadequate health care resources in the community (e.g., staff recruitment pool, etc.), (5) Problems with various organizations in the community, (6) Physical environment characteristics (e.g., geographic location), and (7) All other.

[b] The mentions indicated for each grouping of EU's represent the sum of mentions for all hospital EU's in the grouping combined. The percentages enclosed in parentheses after each particular aspect were computed using the summed mentions as a base. Of all the CRS in the study, 45% mentioned at least one problematic aspect and 19% mentioned two. (Of the CRS respondents 45% said there were no problematic aspects and 10% did not know.)

moreover, the community respondents (CRS) include "the physical environment" among their three most frequently mentioned aspects. Similar additional comparisons can be readily made on the basis of the findings presented in this section.

Summary

In this chapter, the work relations of emergency units with the community were discussed, using a variety of measures and taking into account not only the perspective of the staff working in the units but also the views of key staff from the rest of the hospital, and the views of respondents from the community. Overall, according to most measures, relations with the community are quite favorable, on the average, for the emergency units studied. At the same time, there is considerable room for improvement in certain particular areas, such as inter-institutional patient transfer arrangements (especially transfer-out arrangements), the extent of inter-institutional collaboration for the purpose of improving emergency medical services in the community, or the adequacy of information that staff have about relevant outside health agencies and regulatory bodies.

Equally important, on most of the measures, there is a great deal of variability across individual emergency units, or hospitals, indicating that relations with the community are very favorable in the case of some of the institutions but very deficient in the case of others (even though the general picture for the total sample may be favorable). The results also show certain differences for the various groupings of hospitals/EU's examined. Emergency units with a high patient volume, for example, on the average have more adequate information about outside health agencies and regulatory bodies than do other units. In addition, they apparently collaborate more with other institutions in the community on emergency care matters.

The findings also show that the emergency units studied have more satisfactory work contacts with police departments than with health systems agencies; that tension between emergency unit staff and the community is generally low to very low (although hospital administrators report slightly more tension in this area than do emergency unit nurses or physicians); that only half of the hospitals have either formal or informal arrangements for transferring some of their emergency unit patients to other care institutions; that the community respondents associated with the various emergency units (for a period that averages 12 years) view their work relations with the units very favorably; etc.

With this chapter, discussion of the results of the study concerning the various work relations in which the emergency units engage -- internally, with the parent hospital, and with the community outside -- has been concluded. Having also discussed, in the earlier chapters, the inputs and organizational characteristics of emergency units, the report next turns to consider patient satisfaction, in Chapter 8, and the social, economic, and clinical efficiency of the units -- in Chapters 9, 10, and 11, respectively.

Chapter 8

REPUTATION IN THE COMMUNITY AND PATIENT SATISFACTION

Thus far, the report has concentrated on input variables and on the internal organizational situation of emergency units. The rest of the report focuses on various "outcomes," or on the output side. In the present chapter, the reputation of emergency units in their respective communities, responsiveness to community expectations, and the satisfaction of patients with their emergency visits are discussed.

Good relations with the community, such as described in Chapter 7, and high patient satisfaction probably also mean, or lead to, a good reputation for an emergency unit (and possibly also the parent hospital). The emergency unit occupies a rather unique and strategically important organizational position within the hospital. It not only provides care to a significant number and variety of patients but it also continuously interacts with the outside community directly, more than any of the hospital's other patient units. A considerable number of the patients admitted to the hospital enter through the emergency unit, and an even greater number are treated and released by the unit itself. The care given to these patients, therefore, may greatly affect the reputation of both the emergency unit and the hospital, as well as patient satisfaction. In this light, it is not surprising that "providing comprehensive emergency services" and "maintaining a high level of patient satisfaction" are high goal priorities (see Chapter 2) for many emergency units.

The Reputation and Responsiveness of Emergency Units

Evaluations of the reputation of emergency units were obtained from the physicians (MDS) and registered nurses (RNS) working in each EU, the selected key physicians from the rest of the hospital (HMDS), and the selected community respondents (CRS) associated with each institution. (The patients who participated in the study were asked about the hospital's reputation only.) The findings from these data are presented in Table 70.

On the average, the reputation of the emergency units studied, as assessed by all four groups of respondents, is "good" to "very good." The community respondents and emergency unit physicians evaluate it almost as "very good" and somewhat more favorably, on the average, than do the selected hospital physicians or the registered nurses, both of whom evaluate it as half-way between "good" and "very good." The reputation attributed to individual emergency units by the four groups of respondents varies, however, from a level exactly midway between "excellent" and "very good" (data from MDS and from RNS), at the positive end of the scale, to a level approaching "a fair reputation" only (data from HMDS) at the other end.

The results also show a number of significant differences between emergency unit groupings. First, according to every group of respondents involved, the EU's of the large hospitals have (on the average) the best reputation in the community, followed by the EU's of the medium-size hospitals, and then the EU's of the small hospitals (these last units still have a better than "good" reputation, however). The differences between large and small hospitals on this measure are all significant; the differences between large and medium-size hospitals are significant according to the data from MDS and RNS,

TABLE 70. THE EMERGENCY UNIT'S REPUTATION IN THE COMMUNITY,
AS PERCEIVED BY VARIOUS GROUPS OF RESPONDENTS[a]

		EU Reputation, According to			
Hospital Emergency Units (EU's) Involved		CRS	HMDS	MDS	RNS
ALL EU'S IN THE STUDY SAMPLE (N=30 Hospital EU's)	Mean: Range:	2.26 (1.60-3.20)	2.49 (1.89-3.80)	2.27 (1.50-3.29)	2.55 (1.50-3.71)
YOUR HOSPITAL'S EU					
EU's in:					
Small Hospitals (n=14)		2.43	2.69	2.57	2.74
Medium Hospitals (n=9)		2.22	2.44	2.14	2.54
Large Hospitals (n=7)		1.97	2.16	1.84	2.16
EU's in:					
Church Operated Hospitals (n=9)		2.29	2.71	2.33	2.61
Osteopathic Hospitals (n=3)		2.35	2.16	2.68	2.99
All Other Hospitals (n=18)		2.23	2.44	2.17	2.44
EU's Located in:					
SMSA (urban) Areas (n=21)		2.26	2.39	2.22	2.55
Non-SMSA Areas (n=9)		2.25	2.72	2.38	2.55
EU's in Hospitals Having:					
Medical Teaching Affiliations (n=17)		2.07	2.32	2.06	2.43
No Medical Teaching Affiliations (n=13)		2.51	2.71	2.54	2.69
EU's in Hospitals Having:					
Emergency Personnel Training Programs (n=15)		2.08	2.34	1.97	2.24
No Training Programs (n=15)		2.43	2.64	2.57	2.85

[a] The results, reported here in the form of mean scores, are based on the responses of the CRS, HMDS, MDS, and RNS associated with each institution to the following question: "At the present time, what kind of a reputation does this emergency unit have in the community outside?" The response alternatives were: (1) An excellent reputation, (2) a very good reputation, (3) a good reputation, (4) a fair reputation, and (5) a rather poor reputation. Thus, the lower the score the better the reputation. Mean scores were first computed separately for each EU and then averaged for the EU's in the different categories.

but not HMDS or CRS; and the differences between medium-size and small hospitals are not significant except in the case of the data from MDS. The reputation of emergency units, therefore, appears to correlate positively with the size of the parent hospitals.

Second, the emergency units of hospitals with emergency personnel training programs have a better reputation on the average than those of hospitals without such programs, according to all four of the respondent groups. And, similarly, the units of hospitals with medical teaching affiliations have a better reputation in the community than do those of hospitals without such affiliations.

Third, as evaluated by the RNS and MDS, but not the HMDS or CRS, the emergency units of the non-osteopathic hospitals (whether or not church operated) have a better reputation than those of the osteopathic hospitals. However, according to the HMDS (only) the latter have the best reputation, on the average. Obviously, the HMDS disagree with the other groups in this case.

Finally, when the emergency units of urban area hospitals are compared to those of non-urban area hospitals, the data from all but one of the respondent groups show no differences in the reputation of the units. The exception again involves the HMDS, according to whom the reputation of the former units is on the average better than the reputation of the latter.

The reputation of parent hospitals. As mentioned earlier, the patients (PATS) who completed questionnaires for the study -- representing 28 of the 30 EU's in the sample -- were asked about the hospital's reputation in the community. Their evaluations (not shown in table form) indicate that the reputation of the hospitals in which the EU's are located is "very good" on the average. At the same time, the reputation of individual hospitals ranges rather widely, from "excellent" to only "fair," based on the patients' evaluations.

As was the case above with the reputation of emergency units, moreover, the results show that, on the average, the large hospitals have a better reputation than do the small ones, and that those with either medical teaching affiliations or emergency personnel training programs also tend to have a better reputation than do those without such affiliations or training programs. These findings are consistent with those concerning the reputation of emergency units as assessed by respondents other than the patients.

Emergency unit responsiveness to community expectations. An emergency unit's reputation in the community is probably related to the perceived adequacy with which the unit is meeting current community expectations regarding the services it provides. Data on this variable were obtained from the selected community respondents (CRS), the hospital administrators (HAS), and the physicians (MDS) and registered nurses (RNS) working in the various EU's. They are summarized in Table 71.

Considering first all of the emergency units in the sample, the several groups of respondents are in agreement that, on the average, the EU's are meeting current community expectations almost "very adequately." Of the respondents, the MDS give the most favorable evaluation, followed by the RNS, the CRS, and finally the HAS -- in that order. The data from the HAS also show the greatest inter-unit variability on the present measure (the unit mean scores based on these data indicate that some of the EU's meet community expectations better than "very adequately" while others do so worse than "not so adequately"). The data from the RNS show the smallest inter-unit variability; and those from the MDS and CRS show moderate variability. On the whole, nevertheless, even though there is still room for improvement, it appears that the responsiveness of emergency units to community expectations

TABLE 71. ADEQUACY WITH WHICH THE EMERGENCY UNIT IS MEETING CURRENT COMMUNITY EXPECTATIONS, AS ASSESSED BY VARIOUS GROUPS OF RESPONDENTS[a]

Hospital Emergency Units (EU's) Involved		Adequacy of Meeting Expectations, According to			
		CRS	HAS	MDS	RNS
ALL EU'S IN THE STUDY SAMPLE (N=30 Hospital EU's)	Mean:	2.31	2.39	2.02	2.22
	Range:	(1.55-3.00)	(1.67-4.50)	(1.20-2.75)	(1.73-2.71)
YOUR HOSPITAL'S EU			--		
EU's in:					
Small Hospitals (n=14)		2.37	2.50	2.19	2.30
Medium Hospitals (n=9)		2.25	2.52	1.91	2.25
Large Hospitals (n=7)		2.28	2.00	1.83	2.01
EU's in:					
Church Operated Hospitals (n=9)		2.43	2.56	2.09	2.26
Osteopathic Hospitals (n=3)		2.35	2.67	2.29	2.43
All Other Hospitals (n=18)		2.25	2.26	1.94	2.16
EU's Located in:					
SMSA (urban) Areas (n=21)		2.34	2.18	1.98	2.25
Non-SMSA Areas (n=9)		2.25	2.89	2.11	2.14
EU's in Hospitals Having:					
Medical Teaching Affiliations (n=17)		2.22	2.10	1.89	2.16
No Medical Teaching Affiliations (n=13)		2.44	2.77	2.19	2.29
EU's in Hospitals Having:					
Emergency Personnel Training Programs (n=15)		2.23	2.28	1.85	2.10
No Training Programs (n=15)		2.40	2.50	2.19	2.33

[a]The results reported here in the form of mean scores are based on the responses of the CRS, HAS, MDS, and RNS associated with each institution to the following question: "On the whole, how adequately would you say is this emergency unit meeting current community expectations regarding the services it provides?" The response alternatives were: (1) Extremely adequately, (2) very adequately, (3) fairly adequately, (4) not so adequately, and (5) not adequately at all. Thus, the lower the mean scores the more adequately the emergency unit is meeting community expectations.

is generally quite good, and also congruent with the reputation that the various units appear to enjoy in their respective communities.

Differences between emergency unit groupings on the present measure are not as numerous or as marked as those concerning the reputation of the units. But, they are generally in the same direction. First, the emergency units of large hospitals again score the best (on the average) on meeting community expectations, according to the data from all the respondent groups except CRS. They score significantly better than the units of small hospitals based on the data from MDS, and significantly better than the units of either the medium-size or the small hospitals based on the data from HAS. The data from RNS show only a trend, but in the same direction, and those from the CRS show no differences associated with hospital size.

Second, the units of institutions with medical teaching affiliations, and also emergency personnel training programs, in varying degrees score better on the average than those of institutions without such affiliations or programs, according to the data from all four of the respondent groups. However, the differences are pronounced only in the data from emergency unit physicians and, with regard to teaching affiliations only, the data from hospital administrators.

Finally, as assessed by administrator respondents, the adequacy with which the emergency units are meeting community expectations is greater, on the average, for urban than non-urban units, and also for the units of hospitals which are not church operated (excluding osteopathic) than the units of either the osteopathic or the church operated institutions. And, as assessed by emergency unit physicians, it is greater for the units of the non-osteopathic hospitals which are not church operated than for the units of the osteopathic institutions.

Perceived realism of community expectations. An additional, follow-up question concerning community expectations was asked of the hospital administrators (HAS) and of the physicians (MDS) and registered nurses (RNS) working in the various units. The question was: "How realistic would you say are the community's expectations regarding the services provided by (this) emergency room?" The obtained data are summarized in Table 72.

On the average, the expectations of the communities involved are judged by each of the three groups to be close to, and slightly better than, just "fairly realistic" but not "very realistic." The overall mean scores for the 30 EU's in the sample are identical -- 2.92 -- in the case of the data from HAS and RNS; in the case of the data from MDS the overall mean score is 2.70, signifying somewhat more realistic expectations. Across individual EU's, the scores based on the data from the three groups range from around 2.00, signifying "very realistic" expectations, to between 3.33 and 3.50, signifying less than "fairly realistic" expectations. Thus, inter-unit variability on the present measure is moderate, regardless of the specific source of data. Apparently, the communities in which the emergency units operate do not differ very greatly with respect to the realism of their expectations, as perceived by those working in the institutions studied.

Finally, with only a very few and rather inconsistent exceptions, the findings show no differences between emergency unit groupings (or community groupings) on this measure. The exceptions are: (a) as viewed by the hospital administrators, community expectations are somewhat more realistic in the case of osteopathic hospitals than the other not church operated institutions; (b) in contrast, as viewed by the registered nurses, community expectations are somewhat less realistic in the case of osteopathic institutions than in the case of either the other not church operated institutions or the church

TABLE 72. DEGREE TO WHICH THE COMMUNITY'S EXPECTATIONS ABOUT THE EMERGENCY UNIT'S SERVICES ARE REALISTIC, ACCORDING TO CERTAIN GROUPS OF RESPONDENTS[a]

		Degree Expectations are Realistic, According to		
Hospital Emergency Units (EU's) Involved		HAS	MDS	RNS
ALL EU'S IN THE STUDY SAMPLE (N=30 Hospital EU's)	Mean: Range:	2.92 (2.00-3.50)	2.70 (2.17-3.33)	2.92 (2.18-3.35)
YOUR HOSPITAL'S EU		--		
EU's in:				
Small Hospitals (n=14)		2.96	2.81	3.01
Medium Hospitals (n=9)		2.85	2.58	2.87
Large Hospitals (n=7)		2.93	2.61	2.80
EU's in:				
Church Operated Hospitals (n=9)		2.87	2.72	2.87
Osteopathic Hospitals (n=3)		2.67	2.64	3.21
All Other Hospitals (n=18)		2.99	2.69	2.90
EU's Located in:				
SMSA (urban) Areas (n=21)		2.96	2.61	2.90
Non-SMSA Areas (n=9)		2.83	2.88	2.96
EU's in Hospitals Having:				
Medical Teaching Affiliations (n=17)		2.95	2.57	2.91
No Medical Teaching Affiliations (n=13)		2.89	2.86	2.93
EU's in Hospitals Having:				
Emergency Personnel Training Programs (n=15)		2.91	2.62	2.87
No Training Programs (n=15)		2.93	2.77	2.97

[a] The results, reported here in the form of mean scores, are based on the responses of HAS, MDS, and RNS from each institution to the following question: "All things considered, how realistic would you say are the community's expectations regarding the services provided by this emergency unit?" The response alternatives were: (1) Extremely realistic, (2) very realistic, (3) fairly realistic, (4) not so realistic, and (5) not realistic at all. Thus, the lower the mean scores the more realistic the community's expectations.

operated institutions; and (c) as viewed by the physicians, but not the nurses or the administrators, community expectations are somewhat more realistic in the case of institutions which have medical teaching affiliations than those which do not, and in the case of the urban than the non-urban area institutions.

Patient Satisfaction

The reputation of emergency units in the communities which they serve is probably affected very significantly by the reputation of the parent hospitals, and vice versa. But, in addition, it is probably related to, and affected by, the degree to which the units are perceived to be meeting relevant community expectations, and the satisfaction of their clients. Quite apart from its potential relationship to the reputation of a unit, of course, patient satisfaction is an important criterion in its own right, and certainly one criterion of the overall effectiveness of a unit.

The patients who participated in the study (certain recent patients from all but two of the thirty emergency units in the sample, as earlier described), therefore, were asked a number of questions about their emergency visit experience. Some of these questions focus on patient satisfaction directly, others reflect patient satisfaction or dissatisfaction indirectly, and still others pertain to areas other than satisfaction or are less relevant to satisfaction than they are to other aspects. For these reasons, some of the data provided by the patients (PATS) have been discussed in previous chapters or will be discussed in the chapters on economic and clinical efficiency which follow. Here, the data from one open-ended and several more specific questions concerning patient satisfaction will be examined.

First, in their questionnaires, the patients were asked the following open-ended question: "Thinking back to your visit, what aspects of your experience in the emergency room did you find the most satisfactory?" The patients were instructed to respond in their own words and were informed that they could indicate more than one aspect. Of the 388 patients from the 28 emergency units who completed questionnaires, 46% mentioned two aspects and 43% mentioned only one (yielding a combined total of 522 mentions), while the remaining 11% did not mention any aspect of their emergency visit as being particularly satisfactory.

The patients' responses were first coded into a large number of specific categories and then collapsed, for purposes of presentation and reporting, into the following seven general categories:

(1) Quality of care: all responses concerning the quality of care (medical, nursing) received by the patient at any stage of the emergency visit -- admission, triage, diagnosis, treatment, disposition, and follow-up;

(2) Emergency unit staff resources: all responses about the quality, adequacy, sufficiency, or quantity of the unit's staff, including medical and nursing staff;

(3) Emergency unit physicians (attitudes of, interaction with): all responses concerning communication received from the doctor(s), the attitudes of the doctors, or the quality of physician-patient interaction;

(4) Emergency unit nurses (attitudes of, interaction with): all responses concerning communication received from the nurse(s), the attitudes of the nurses, or the quality of nurse-patient interaction;

(5) Waiting time or length of visit: responses referring to waiting after arrival at the unit before being seen by a nurse or a doctor,

the amount of time required for diagnosis or treatment, or the total length (from time-in to time-out) of the emergency visit;

(6) <u>The staff's attitudes and/or actions</u>: any responses referring to the patient's interaction with staff of the unit, the communication received from staff, or the attitudes of staff which did not indicate the particular staff involved (i.e., which referred to the staff in general without any differentiation, and could not therefore be included in categories #4 or #5); and,

(7) <u>All other responses</u>: responses not included in any of the preceding categories, e.g., responses concerning the size or physical layout of the unit.

Table 73 presents the results concerning those aspects that the patients found "the most satisfactory." Considering first all of the data for all the emergency units combined, the most frequently mentioned aspects by patients as "the most satisfactory aspects" of their visits involve <u>waiting time or length of visit</u> (which accounts for 19% of all responses), followed closely in second place by <u>the staff's attitudes and actions</u> (which accounts for 18% of all responses). The <u>quality of care</u> was mentioned third most often (14% of all responses), followed by: <u>emergency unit staff resources</u> (10%), <u>emergency unit physicians</u> (8%), and <u>emergency unit nurses</u> (7%).

Apparently, as indicated by their explicit statements in response to the above question, the patients were <u>especially</u> satisfied more with respect to waiting time or the duration of their visit, and also with respect to the staff's attitudes and actions, than they were with the quality of care as such. This does not necessarily mean that the quality of care was not satisfactory, or even high, as viewed by the patients. It might be that the quality of care was more difficult for patients to judge (and therefore patients were reluctant to mention it) and/or less salient than were these other aspects.

TABLE 73. PARTICULAR ASPECTS OF THEIR EMERGENCY UNIT VISIT THAT THE PATIENTS FOUND THE MOST SATISFACTORY[a]

Hospital Emergency Units (EU's) Involved	Total Mentions[b]	The Three Aspects Most Frequently Mentioned by Patients as the Most Satisfactory		
		First	Second	Third
ALL EU'S IN THE STUDY SAMPLE (N=28 Hospital EU's)	522	Waiting time or length of visit (18.8%)	The staff's attitudes and actions (17.6%)	Quality of care (14.0%)
YOUR HOSPITAL'S EU				
EU's with:				
Low Patient Volume (n=9)	113	Waiting time or length of visit (20.4%)	The staff's attitudes and actions (15.9%)	Quality of care (14.2%)
Medium Pat. Volume (n=10)	160	The staff's attitudes and actions (18.8%)	Quality of care (15.0%)	Emergency unit staff resources (11.3%); the nurses (11.3%)
High Patient Volume (n=9)	249	Waiting time or length of visit (23.3%)	The staff's attitudes and actions (17.7%)	Quality of care (13.3%)
EU's in:				
Church Operated Hospitals (n=8)	80	Waiting time or length of visit (22.5%)	Quality of care (15.0%)	The staff's attitudes and actions (13.8%)
Osteopathic Hospitals (n=3)	67	Quality of care (17.9%)	The staff's attitudes and actions (14.9%)	Waiting time or length of visit (13.4%)
All Other Hospitals (n=17)	375	Waiting time or length of visit (18.9%)	The staff's attitudes and actions (18.9%)	Quality of care (13.1%)
EU's Located in:				
SMSA (urban) Areas (n=19)	334	Waiting time or length of visit (17.7%)	The staff's attitudes and actions (17.7%)	Quality of care (15.0%)
Non-SMSA Areas (n=9)	188	Waiting time or length of visit (20.7%)	The staff's attitudes and actions (17.6%)	Quality of care (12.2%)
EU's in Hospitals Having:				
Medical Teaching Affiliations (n=16)	317	The staff's attitudes and actions (19.9%)	Waiting time or length of visit (16.7%)	Quality of care (13.6%)
No Medical Teaching Affiliations (n=12)	205	Waiting time or length of visit (22.0%)	Quality of care (14.6%)	The staff's attitudes and actions (14.1%)
EU's in Hospitals Having:				
Emergency Personnel Training Programs (n=13)	264	The staff's attitudes and actions (18.9%)	Waiting time or length of visit (18.6%)	Quality of care (14.4%)
No Training Programs (n=15)	258	Waiting time or length of visit (19.0%)	The staff's attitudes and actions (16.3%)	Quality of care (13.6%)

[a] The results are based on the responses of patients (PATS) visiting the various emergency units to the following open-ended question: "Thinking back to your visit, what parts or aspects of your experience in the emergency room did you find <u>the most satisfactory</u>?" Relevant data were obtained from patients who had recently visited 28 of the 30 emergency units in the study (the other two institutions did not allow patient participation in the study). Patient responses were first coded into a large number of categories and then collapsed into the following seven general categories: (1) Quality of care, (2) Emergency unit staff resources, (3) the Doctors, (4) the Nurses, (5) Waiting time or length of visit, (6) the Attitudes and actions of the staff, and (7) All other.

[b] The mentions indicated for each grouping of EU's represent the sum of mentions for all hospital EU's in the grouping combined. The percentages enclosed in parentheses after each particular aspect were computed using the summed mentions as a base. Of the participating patient respondents 89% mentioned at least one aspect and 46% mentioned two.

When the data are examined separately for each of the various groupings of emergency units, Table 73 shows a number of differences. Waiting time or length of visit, for example, is mentioned much less frequently as one of the most satisfactory aspects by patients who visited emergency units with a medium, compared to either a low or a high, patient volume. It is also mentioned less frequently by patients who visited osteopathic hospital units than by patients who visited the units of other hospitals, whether church operated or not. (Certain additional data about waiting time are discussed in Chapter 11.)

Other differences concern the staff's attitudes and actions. Aspects in this category are mentioned more frequently by patients who visited the units of hospitals having medical teaching affiliations than by patients who visited the units of hospitals not having teaching affiliations. (The converse is true, however, concerning waiting time or length of visit.) Similarly, they are mentioned more frequently by patients who visited the units of the not church operated hospitals (excluding osteopathic) than the units of the church operated hospitals.

For most emergency unit groupings, as for the total sample, the quality of care is the third most frequently mentioned aspect. For some of the groupings, however, it is the second or first most frequently mentioned. But in all cases, the difference from one grouping of EU's to another, with respect to the frequency with which the quality of care is mentioned by patients as one of the most satisfactory aspects of their visit, is small.

The specific pattern of findings which characterize each particular grouping of emergency units may be seen in Table 73. Finally, it should be pointed out, the patterns shown in Table 73 do not necessarily apply to individual emergency units, which may differ substantially from one another as well as from the average situation of the particular groupings to which they belong.

Patient satisfaction with certain aspects of the care process. Two specific, and probably major, sources of patient satisfaction/dissatisfaction are the explanations given to the patient by the staff and the staff's understanding of the patient's problem, both as perceived by the patient. Accordingly, the patients in the study were asked: (a) "To what extent did the staff who took care of you make an effort to really understand your problem?", and (b) "On the whole, were you satisfied with the way the emergency room staff explained to you how your problem should be handled?" Their answers are summarized in Table 74.

Patient satisfaction in both of these areas is generally high. According to the data, the staff of the various emergency units involved on the average made an effort to understand the patients' problems to "a great extent." And, similarly, the patients in the different units on the average report that they are "very satisfied" with the explanations given to them by the staff. Across individual emergency units, the range in the mean scores with respect to the first measure is from 1.13 to 3.00, or from "a very great extent" to "a fair extent"; and with respect to the second measure, it is from 1.00 to 2.67 or from "extremely satisfied" to slightly better than "fairly satisfied." In both cases, the inter-unit variability is moderate, indicating that some of the units are doing considerably better than others, although the overall situation is quite favorable.

When the results for particular groupings of emergency units are examined, the patterns which characterize the sample as a whole still apply with only minor deviations. Moreover, the various groupings differ little from one another, on either of the two measures. There are only two small exceptions in this connection. First, the patients who visited the emergency units of church operated hospitals were, on the average, more satisfied with the

TABLE 74. STAFF'S UNDERSTANDING AND EXPLANATION TO THE PATIENTS OF THEIR MEDICAL PROBLEMS[a]

Hospital Emergency Units (EU's) Involved		Extent of Staff Effort to Understand the Patient's Problem[b]	Patient Satisfaction With Staff's Explanation of the Problem[c]
ALL EU'S IN THE STUDY SAMPLE (N=28 Hospital EU's)	Mean: Range:	2.07 (1.13-3.00)	2.04 (1.00-2.67)
YOUR HOSPITAL'S EU			
EU's with:			
Low Patient Volume (n=9)		2.00	2.07
Medium Pat. Volume (n=10)		2.18	2.03
High Patient Volume (n=9)		2.03	2.03
EU's in:			
Church Operated Hospitals (n=8)		2.05	1.87
Osteopathic Hospitals (n=3)		2.28	2.22
All Other Hospitals (n=17)		2.05	2.09
EU's Located in:			
SMSA (urban) Areas (n=19)		2.10	2.00
Non-SMSA Areas (n=9)		2.01	2.14
EU's in Hospitals Having:			
Medical Teaching Affiliations (n=16)		2.01	2.04
No Medical Teaching Affiliations (n=12)		2.16	2.05
EU's in Hospitals Having:			
Emergency Personnel Training Programs (n=13)		1.92	1.98
No Training Programs (n=15)		2.21	2.10

Table 74 Continues

TABLE 74
(Continued)

---

^aThe results, reported here in the form of mean scores, are based on the responses of recent emergency unit patients (PATS visiting 28 EU's) to two questionnaire items.

^bThe question was: "To what extent did the staff who took care of you make an effort to really understand your problem?" The response alternatives were: (1) To a very great extent, (2) to a great extent, (3) to a fair extent, (4) to a small extent, and (5) to a very small extent or not at all. Thus, the lower the mean scores, the greater the staff's efforts to understand their patients' problems. (Of the participating patient respondents, 12% chose a special response option, namely "There was no need for the staff to make such an effort," and are therefore excluded from the computations.)

^cThe question was: "On the whole, were you satisfied with the way the emergency room staff explained to you how your problem should be handled?" The response alternatives were: (1) I was extremely satisfied, (2) very satisfied, (3) fairly satisfied, (4) not so satisfied, and (5) I was not satisfied at all. Thus, the lower the mean score the greater the patient satisfaction with the staff's explanation.

explanations given to them by the staff than were those who visited the units of osteopathic hospitals. And, second, the staff in the units of hospitals which have emergency personnel training programs on the average made a slightly greater effort than their counterparts in hospitals which do not have such programs to understand the patients' problems.

Patients' assessments of how well the doctors and nurses "took care" of them. The last table in this section, Table 75, shows how the patients from the various emergency units evaluate the overall care given to them by the physicians and by the nurses. The specific question asked of the patients was: "Overall, how well would you say did the doctor (or doctors) who treated you in the emergency room take care of you?" A parallel question was asked about the nurses. These evaluations, of course, may be indicative of perceived (by the patients) clinical efficiency as well as patient satisfaction. (Data from the patients about other aspects of clinical efficiency are discussed in Chapter 11.)

On the average, the doctors in the various emergency units took care of the patients "very well," in fact slightly better than "very well," according to the patients (PATS) in the study. The same is true about the nurses who, according to the same respondents, took care of the patients even slightly better than did the doctors. The situation of individual emergency units, however, is far from uniform. The mean scores of individual units show an identical range for both measures, from 1.00 (which corresponds to "extremely well") to 3.00 (which corresponds to only "fairly well"). This is a substantial range, suggesting that the patients of some of the units are considerably more satisfied than those of other units with how well they were taken care of by the physicians, and by the nurses, who cared for them during their emergency visit.

TABLE 75. PATIENTS' ASSESSMENTS OF THE CARE THEY RECEIVED FROM THE DOCTORS AND FROM THE NURSES IN THE EMERGENCY UNIT[a]

Hospital Emergency Units (EU's) Involved		How Well the Doctors Took Care of the Patients[b]	How Well the Nurses Took Care of the Patients[c]
ALL EU'S IN THE STUDY SAMPLE (N=28 Hospital EU's)	*Mean:* *Range:*	1.86 (1.00-3.00)	1.73 (1.00-3.00)
YOUR HOSPITAL'S EU			
EU's with:			
Low Patient Volume (n=9)		1.79	1.61
Medium Pat. Volume (n=10)		1.89	1.84
High Patient Volume (n=9)		1.89	1.72
EU's in:			
Church Operated Hospitals (n=8)		1.85	1.78
Osteopathic Hospitals (n=3)		1.85	1.70
All Other Hospitals (n=17)		1.87	1.70
EU's Located in:			
SMSA (urban) Areas (n=19)		1.94	1.74
Non-SMSA Areas (n=9)		1.70	1.70
EU's in Hospitals Having:			
Medical Teaching Affiliations (n=16)		1.73	1.70
No Medical Teaching Affiliations (n=12)		2.03	1.77
EU's in Hospitals Having:			
Emergency Personnel Training Programs (n=13)		1.77	1.67
No Training Programs (n=15)		1.94	1.77

Table 75 Continues

TABLE 75
(Continued)

---

^aThe results, reported here in the form of mean scores, are based on the responses of recent emergency unit patients (PATS visiting 28 EU's) to a pair of questionnaire items.

^bThe question was: "Overall, how <u>well</u> would you say did the doctor (or doctors) who treated you in the emergency unit <u>take care of you</u>?" The response alternatives ranged from "(1) Extremely well,"... to "(5) Not well at all." Thus, the <u>lower</u> the mean score the more favorable the assessment by the patients.

^cThe question was: "And how about the nurse (or nurses) who took care of you in the emergency unit? Overall, how <u>well</u> did they <u>take care of you</u>?" The response alternatives were the same as for the preceding question. Thus, the <u>lower</u> the mean score the more favorable the assessment by the patients.

The results in Table 75 also show that, according to the patients, the physicians in the emergency units of hospitals which have medical teaching affiliations did a better job, on the average, than did their counterparts in the units of hospitals which do not have such affiliations. There are no other significant differences between emergency unit groupings with respect to either of the two measures.

Finally, patient respondents were also asked about the number of physicians who treated them and whether "there seemed to be enough doctors" in the unit (these data are not presented in table form). Very briefly, as expected, the large majority of the patients were treated by a single physician. However, 9% of all the patients report that they were not seen by a physician. Of those who were seen, 88% were treated by one physician and the remaining 12% were treated by two or, in some cases, three physicians. Individual emergency units, however, show some deviation from this pattern. The patients from the various units further report that, on the average, there were "enough doctors on hand to take care of all the patients in the emergency room within a reasonable amount of time." None of the units were seen as having "more than enough doctors," but some were seen as having "not enough doctors."

Summary

The data reviewed in this chapter indicate that the emergency units studied have been quite successful, on the average, in maintaining a generally high level of patient satisfaction as well as a good reputation in their respective communities. Various groups of respondents, from within as well as outside the units, judge the reputation of the units to be midway between "good" and "very good." Most of the same respondents also believe that the emergency units are generally meeting community expectations almost "very adequately," on the average, even though these expectations are perceived by them as being only "fairly realistic" in most cases. Additionally, patients who recently visited the various emergency units for care report that the doctors, and also the nurses, took care of them "very well," and made considerable effort to understand their problems and explain to them their care requirements adequately.

Differences among emergency unit groupings on the same measures also exist, however. The emergency units of large hospitals (and the hospitals themselves), for example, have a better reputation in the community, on the average, than do the units of small and medium-size hospitals, according to the respondents. The former units also are seen as meeting community expectations more adequately than the latter. Similarly, the emergency units of hospitals with medical teaching affiliations are seen as having a better reputation, and as meeting community expectations more adequately, than are the units of hospitals without such affiliations. Patients also appear to be more satisfied with various aspects of their visit in the former than in the latter units, except for waiting time or the length of their visit. Some of the same trends characterize the emergency units of institutions which have emergency personnel training programs compared to those which do not. A few differences in the areas of reputation and patient satisfaction associated with the units' location and institutional control were also found and discussed.

Finally, the results show that the situation of individual emergency units in the areas of reputation and patient satisfaction is not uniformly favorable. Inter-unit variability on most of the measures examined is moderate to moderately high, suggesting that some of the emergency units are doing a considerably better job than others.

Chapter 9

STAFF ATTITUDES AND SATISFACTION: SOCIAL EFFICIENCY

Another important criterion of the overall effectiveness of emergency units has to do with social efficiency -- the integration, commitment, and personal goal attainment of the various staff who do the work. The attitudes of staff members toward the job and the unit and the satisfactions which they derive from their work, in return for their efforts, are important not only to the individuals involved but also to the unit as an organizational entity. They are important to an emergency unit because, among other things, they can significantly affect the quality and efficiency of staff performance, and therefore also patient satisfaction and the economic and clinical efficiency of the unit.

The emergency units studied apparently do not emphasize highly the goal priority of improving working conditions for the staff (see Chapter 3). Yet, the satisfaction of staff members depends on such things as working conditions, the nature of the job, and the rewards associated with working in the unit. To a considerable degree, these factors determine a person's motivation to perform at a particular level and his or her feelings of being an integrated and valued member of the emergency unit and the hospital. This chapter, therefore, focuses on the way in which staff members appraise various aspects of their jobs and work situation. More specifically, the chapter examines the attitudes and satisfaction of the physicians (MDS), registered nurses (RNS), and full-time licensed practical nurses (LPNS) who are working in the various emergency units.

Discussed first are staff evaluations of the emergency unit as a place to work. Then, the identification of staff members with their respective unit, or their commitment to the unit, is examined. Considered next are the perceptions of the staff concerning certain aspects of their job, including the experience of "unreasonable pressure for better performance," the appropriateness/inappropriateness of work responsibilities, and variety on the job for the nurses. Finally, the satisfaction of staff members with both the financial/monetary and non-financial rewards that they derive from working in the unit is reviewed. (Certain additional data about the characteristics of the staff were included in the chapter on staff resources, Chapter 2, and supplementary background information is presented in the Appendix.) These findings may be personally important to emergency unit staff members, since they describe the psychological and economic "returns" accrued to them for their performance.

The Emergency Unit as a Place to Work

The physicians (MDS), registered nurses (RNS), and practical nurses (LPNS) working in the various EU's were asked the following question: "On the whole, what do you think of this emergency unit as a place to work?" Their responses are summarized in Table 76.

On the average, the emergency units studied are regarded by their respective staff as "very good" places to work. The practical nurses involved (those working full-time in a number, but not all, of the 30 EU's) give somewhat more favorable evaluations than the registered nurses and the physicians, but all three groups generally agree that the units are very good places to work. At the same time, the data show a good deal of variability across individual emergency units (see the ranges of unit mean scores), some of which

TABLE 76. EVALUATION BY THE STAFF OF THE EMERGENCY UNIT AS A PLACE TO WORK[a]

		Quality of EU as a Place to Work, According to		
Hospital Emergency Units (EU's) Involved		MDS	RNS	LPNS
ALL EU'S IN THE STUDY SAMPLE (N=30 Hospital EU's)	Mean: Range:	2.18 (1.33-3.00)	2.04 (1.27-3.00)	1.72 (1.00-3.00)
YOUR HOSPITAL'S EU				
EU's with:				
Low Patient Volume (n=10)		2.37	2.07	1.73
Medium Pat. Volume (n=10)		2.20	2.21	2.12
High Patient Volume (n=10)		1.98	1.86	1.41
EU's in:				
Church Operated Hospitals (n=9)		2.37	2.08	1.29
Osteopathic Hospitals (n=3)		2.30	2.07	2.00
All Other Hospitals (n=18)		2.07	2.02	1.79
EU's Located in:				
SMSA (urban) Areas (n=21)		2.10	2.04	1.74
Non-SMSA Areas (n=9)		2.38	2.05	1.67
EU's in Hospitals Having:				
Medical Teaching Affiliations (n=17)		2.13	1.97	1.84
No Medical Teaching Affiliations (n=13)		2.25	2.14	1.50
EU's in Hospitals Having:				
Emergency Personnel Training Programs (n=15)		2.04	1.84	1.58
No Training Programs (n=15)		2.32	2.24	1.88

[a] The results, presented here in the form of mean scores, are based on the responses of MDS, RNS, and LPNS from the various emergency units to the question: "On the whole, what do you think of this Emergency Unit as a place to work?" The response alternatives were: (1) It is an excellent place to work, (2) a very good place, (3) a good place, (4) a fair place, and (5) a rather poor place to work. Thus, the <u>lower</u> the mean score the more favorable the evaluation of the EU as a place to work. Mean scores were first computed separately for each EU and then averaged for the EU's in the different groupings.

are viewed by their staff as "excellent," or almost excellent, places to work, or as "very good" places, while others are seen only as "a good place" to work.

There are also some differences between emergency unit groupings. First, units with a high patient volume receive the most favorable evaluations on the present measure by all three of the respondent groups -- MDS, RNS, and LPNS. Moreover, according to the physicians, these units are on the average better places to work than are those with a low patient volume. The evaluations of the nurses are in the same direction, although the differences are not significant in their case. However, according to the data from both registered and practical nurses, the emergency units with a high patient volume are better places to work, on the average, than are those with a medium patient volume. The evaluations by physicians are in the same direction.

Second, according to the RNS, the emergency units of hospitals with emergency personnel training programs are on the average better places to work than are those of hospitals without such programs. The data from LPNS and MDS show a similar trend. Concerning medical teaching affiliation, on the other hand, the differences are neither significant nor clear cut. The MDS and RNS tend to evaluate the units of hospitals with teaching affiliations somewhat more favorably while the LPNS tend to evaluate the units of hospitals without such affiliations somewhat more favorably.

Finally, according to the physicians, the units of hospitals which are not church operated, excluding osteopathic institutions, are on the average better places to work than are those of church operated hospitals. In contrast, from the perspective of the practical nurses, the latter units are better places to work than are those of the osteopathic and other not church operated institutions. The data from the registered nurses show no differences whatsoever in this connection. And the same is true when comparing urban to non-urban area institutions, regardless of whose staff's evaluations are considered.

Staff Identification with the Units

The same three groups of respondents in each emergency unit studied were asked the following question: "Personally, how strongly identified with, or how strongly committed do you feel you are to, ...this emergency unit?" The obtained data are summarized in Table 77.

First, it is clear that the level of identification/commitment varies substantially among the three groups. On the average, the full-time practical nurses are more strongly identified with their respective units (midway between "extremely strongly" and "very strongly") than are the registered nurses (identified almost "very strongly") who, in turn, are more strongly identified with their units than are the physicians (the MDS are identified with the units at a level midway between "very" and "moderately" strongly, on the average). Obviously, in the case of physicians, identification with the units may be lower than desirable in many institutions.

It is also interesting that while the variability across individual emergency units concerning staff identification is very small in the case of practical nurses, and small to moderate in the case of registered nurses, it is very high in the case of physicians. The unit mean scores based on the data from physicians range from 1.50 (indicating a level of identification exactly midway between "extremely strong" and "very strong") to 3.83 (indicating that the physicians are less than "moderately strongly" identified with the unit -- in fact only "fairly strongly").

Concerning the identification of practical nurses, the results show no differences from one grouping of emergency units to another; identification

TABLE 77. STAFF IDENTIFICATION WITH THEIR RESPECTIVE EMERGENCY UNITS[a]

Hospital Emergency Units (EU's) Involved		Degree of Identification with the EU on the Part of		
		MDS	RNS	LPNS
ALL EU'S IN THE STUDY SAMPLE (N=30 Hospital EU's)	Mean: Range:	2.58 (1.50-3.83)	2.12 (1.40-2.83)	1.58 (1.00-2.00)
YOUR HOSPITAL'S EU				
EU's with:				
Low Patient Volume (n=10)		2.76	2.35	1.63
Medium Pat. Volume (n=10)		2.61	2.10	1.60
High Patient Volume (n=10)		2.35	1.89	1.54
EU's in:				
Church Operated Hospitals (n=9)		2.69	2.20	1.58
Osteopathic Hospitals (n=3)		2.63	2.21	1.50
All Other Hospitals (n=18)		2.51	2.06	1.60
EU's Located in:				
SMSA (urban) Areas (n=21)		2.49	2.13	1.58
Non-SMSA Areas (n=9)		2.78	2.08	1.58
EU's in Hospitals Having:				
Medical Teaching Affiliations (n=17)		2.34	2.00	1.56
No Medical Teaching Affiliations (n=13)		2.89	2.27	1.62
EU's in Hospitals Having:				
Emergency Personnel Training Programs (n=15)		2.56	2.12	1.61
No Training Programs (n=15)		2.60	2.12	1.55

[a] The results, presented here in the form of mean scores, are based on the responses of MDS, RNS, and LPNS from the various EU's to the question: "Personally, how strongly identified with or how strongly committed do you feel you are to... this emergency unit?" The response alternatives were: (1) Extremely strongly, (2) very strongly, (3) moderately strongly, (4) fairly strongly, and (5) not strongly. Thus, the lower the mean score, the higher the identification with the unit.

with the units is uniformly high. The identification of registered nurses is stronger, on the average, in units with a high than in units with a low patient volume. The same is true about physician identification. In addition, the identification of physicians is on the average stronger in the EU's of hospitals with teaching affiliations than in the EU's of hospitals without such affiliations. And a similar, though less pronounced, trend emerges when comparing urban and non-urban area units; physician identification tends to be stronger in the urban units.

Staff Perceptions of Certain Job Characteristics

Favorable attitudes about one's job often depend on such things as task variety, appropriate division of work responsibilities, and freedom from undue pressure. These types of variables, moreover, have been found in past organizational research to correlate with job performance. Certain data on these variables, therefore, were also collected in the present study and will be discussed in this section.

The physicians and nurses working in the various emergency units were asked, among other things, if, while working in the unit, they feel "any pressure for better performance over and above what (they) think is reasonable." Their responses are summarized in Table 78, which shows the amount of unreasonable pressure experienced by each group of respondents.

Based on their own reports, the full-time practical nurses working in the units generally feel the least amount of unreasonable pressure (between "a very small amount" and "no pressure at all," on the average), followed by the physicians, and then the registered nurses (who report barely more than just "a very small amount" of unreasonable pressure). Overall, then, the situation in the emergency units studied is very favorable, on the average, with respect

TABLE 78. STAFF'S PERCEPTION OF UNREASONABLE PRESSURE
FOR "BETTER PERFORMANCE"[a]

Hospital Emergency Units (EU's) Involved		Amount of Pressure Perceived by		
		MDS	RNS	LPNS
ALL EU'S IN THE STUDY SAMPLE (N=30 Hospital EU's)	Mean: Range:	1.83 (1.00-2.86)	2.15 (1.25-3.14)	1.54 (1.00-4.00)
YOUR HOSPITAL'S EU				
EU's with:				
Low Patient Volume (n=10)		1.76	1.90	1.40
Medium Pat. Volume (n=10)		1.70	2.22	1.61
High Patient Volume (n=10)		2.02	2.33	1.56
EU's in:				
Church Operated Hospitals (n=9)		1.83	2.23	2.00
Osteopathic Hospitals (n=3)		1.67	1.68	1.58
All Other Hospitals (n=18)		1.85	2.19	1.39
EU's Located in:				
SMSA (urban) Areas (n=21)		1.82	2.09	1.54
Non-SMSA Areas (n=9)		1.86	2.30	1.50
EU's in Hospitals Having:				
Medical Teaching Affiliations (n=17)		1.87	2.19	1.59
No Medical Teaching Affiliations (n=13)		1.77	2.10	1.43
EU's in Hospitals Having:				
Emergency Personnel Training Programs (n=15)		1.86	2.02	1.50
No Training Programs (n=15)		1.80	2.29	1.57

[a]The results, presented here in the form of mean scores, are based on the responses of MDS, RNS, and LPNS from the various EU's to the following question: "When working in the emergency unit, do you feel any pressure for better performance over and above what you think is reasonable?" The response alternatives were: (1) I feel no pressure at all over and above what is reasonable, (2) a very small amount, (3) a small amount of pressure, (4) a moderate amount of pressure, and (5) a great or very great amount of pressure. Thus, the lower the mean score, the smaller the amount of unreasonable pressure experienced by the staff.

to the relative freedom of their medical and nursing staff from undue pressure.

Across individual emergency units, nevertheless, there is considerable variability on the pressure measure, especially based on the data from practical nurses. Very briefly, regardless of the specific group involved, in some of the units the staff report virtually no pressure at all over and above what they consider reasonable. In some other units, however, the physicians and registered nurses report more than a very small amount of such pressure, and the practical nurses report a moderate amount. The significance of this variability is difficult to estimate without more detailed analysis of the data. What is clear at this point, and this may prove more important, is that the overall situation of the units does not appear to be problematic with respect to the pressure experienced by their staff.

Among emergency unit groupings, only a few differences are suggested by the data. On the average, the practical nurses working in the units of church operated hospitals report somewhat more unreasonable pressure than their counterparts in other hospitals, and the registered nurses report less pressure in osteopathic hospital units compared to the units of other hospitals, including those which are church operated. In addition, the registered nurses and the physicians tend to report somewhat more pressure, on the average, in emergency units which have a high patient volume than in other units. No differences in reported pressure are found with reference to urban/non-urban location, medical teaching affiliation, or emergency personnel training programs.

Those of the respondents who reported at least some unreasonable pressure were also asked to indicate the main source of the pressure (data not shown in table form). Of the physicians falling into this category, slightly more than one-third pointed to themselves as the main source of pressure, and an additional one-fifth attributed the pressure to professional colleagues (the remaining indicated a variety of sources). Of the registered nurses, one-quarter mentioned themselves as the main source, and another quarter (slightly less) attributed the pressure to their work load; an additional 15% attributed the pressure to the doctors, and 12% attributed it to the supervising nurses. Finally, the few practical nurses who reported some unreasonable pressure typically pointed to the work load or to themselves as the main sources of the pressure.

Next, the nurses were asked about the appropriateness/inappropriateness of work responsibilities in the unit. The specific question was: "To what extent do you find that you have to do things on your job that you feel should be the responsibility of other people in the emergency unit?" The data from this question are summarized in Table 79.

In general, both the registered and the practical nurses feel that they must take on inappropriate responsibilities, in their respective units, only to slightly more than "a small extent." Across individual emergency units, however, there is high variability in the data from practical nurses (unit mean scores range from 1.00, which corresponds to "a very great extent," to 5.00, which corresponds to "a very small extent or not at all"). The data from registered nurses show much smaller, but still considerable, inter-unit variability. Apparently, in some of the units nurses perceive a good deal of inappropriateness in work responsibilities while in others the situation in this respect is virtually unproblematic.

It is also interesting that the data from registered nurses do not show any significant differences between one grouping of emergency units and another with respect to reported inappropriateness of work responsibilities. The data from practical nurses, on the other hand, show several differences. On the average,

TABLE 79. INAPPROPRIATENESS OF WORK RESPONSIBILITIES IN THE EMERGENCY UNIT, AS REPORTED BY THE NURSES (RNS, LPNS)[a]

		Extent of Inappropriateness According to	
Hospital Emergency Units (EU's) Involved		RNS	LPNS
ALL EU'S IN THE STUDY SAMPLE (N=30 Hospital EU's)	Mean: Range:	3.69 (2.71-4.25)	3.86 (1.00-5.00)
YOUR HOSPITAL'S EU			
EU's with:			
Low Patient Volume (n=10)		3.75	4.13
Medium Pat. Volume (n=10)		3.62	3.67
High Patient Volume (n=10)		3.69	3.86
EU's in:			
Church Operated Hospitals (n=9)		3.56	4.17
Osteopathic Hospitals (n=3)		3.71	3.83
All Other Hospitals (n=18)		3.74	3.78
EU's Located in:			
SMSA (urban) Areas (n=21)		3.65	4.06
Non-SMSA Areas (n=9)		3.77	3.00
EU's in Hospitals Having:			
Medical Teaching Affiliations (n=17)		3.70	3.65
No Medical Teaching Affiliations (n=13)		3.67	4.29
EU's in Hospitals Having:			
Emergency Personnel Training Programs (n=15)		3.79	3.99
No Training Programs (n=15)		3.58	3.72

[a] The results, presented here in the form of mean scores, are based on the responses of RNS and LPNS from the various EU's to the following question: "To what extent do you find that you have to do things on your job that you feel should be the responsibility of other people in the emergency unit?" The response alternatives were: (1) To a very great extent, (2) a great extent, (3) a fair extent, (4) a small extent, and (5) to a very small extent or not at all. Thus, the lower the mean score the greater the inappropriateness; and, conversely, the higher the score the smaller the extent of inappropriate responsibilities on the job.

these respondents report more inappropriateness in the units of hospitals which have medical teaching affiliations, and in the units which are located in non-urban areas, than they do in the remaining units in each case. The same respondents report somewhat less inappropriateness, on the average, in the units of church operated hospitals compared to other hospitals, and in units which have a low patient volume compared to the rest of the emergency units.

Finally, the nurses were asked about the amount of variety that characterizes the activities which they perform. The results on this measure are presented in Table 80. Both the registered and the practical nurses report that, on the average, there is "considerable" variety in the activities which they perform in their respective units. Inter-unit variability on this measure is moderate; the range is from "very considerable" or nearly very considerable variety, depending upon the nursing group involved, to "moderate" or somewhat better than moderate variety. Once again, therefore, the overall situation of the emergency units studied is quite good on the average from the perspective of the nurses.

Some differences among emergency unit groupings apparently also exist, however, as they do among individual units. Specifically, both the registered and the practical nurses report more variety on the average in units which have a high patient volume than in units which have either a medium or a small patient volume (between the latter two groupings there is no difference). Similarly, registered and practical nurses alike report more variety, on the average, in the units of the church operated hospitals than in the units of the osteopathic hospitals. They also report less variety in the units of the latter hospitals than in the units of non-osteopathic hospitals which are not church operated. Finally, unlike the registered nurses, the practical nurses report more variety on the average in the units of hospitals which

TABLE 80. AMOUNT OF VARIETY ON THE JOB FOR EMERGENCY UNIT NURSES (RNS, LPNS)[a]

Hospital Emergency Units (EU's) Involved		Amount of Variety According to	
		RNS	LPNS
ALL EU'S IN THE STUDY SAMPLE (N=30 Hospital EU's)	Mean: Range:	2.05 (1.40-2.75)	1.83 (1.00-3.00)
YOUR HOSPITAL'S EU			
EU's with:			
Low Patient Volume (n=10)		2.11	2.03
Medium Pat. Volume (n=10)		2.27	2.10
High Patient Volume (n=10)		1.75	1.50
EU's in:			
Church Operated Hospitals (n=9)		1.98	1.67
Osteopathic Hospitals (n=3)		2.52	2.50
All Other Hospitals (n=18)		2.00	1.73
EU's Located in:			
SMSA (urban) Areas (n=21)		2.12	1.81
Non-SMSA Areas (n=9)		1.88	1.92
EU's in Hospitals Having:			
Medical Teaching Affiliations (n=17)		2.03	1.83
No Medical Teaching Affiliations (n=13)		2.07	1.81
EU's in Hospitals Having:			
Emergency Personnel Training Programs (n=15)		1.91	1.59
No Training Programs (n=15)		2.18	2.08

[a] The results, presented here in the form of mean scores, are based on the responses of RNS and LPNS from the various EU's to the following question: "Generally, how much variety would you say is there in the activities which you perform on the job in this emergency unit?" The response alternatives were: (1) Very considerable variety, (2) considerable variety, (3) moderate variety, (4) some variety, and (5) little or very little variety. Thus, the lower the mean score, the greater the variety of activities.

have emergency personnel training programs, than in the units of hospitals which do not have such programs.

Staff Satisfaction with Financial and Non-financial Rewards

In this area, the emergency unit physicians (MDS), registered nurses (RNS), and practical nurses (LPNS) participating in the study were asked a pair of questions. First, they were asked: "Considering your work efforts and contributions here, how satisfied are you with the <u>financial or monetary rewards</u> that you derive from your work in this emergency unit?" Then, they were asked a similar question concerning <u>non-financial rewards</u>. The results are presented in Tables 81 and 82, respectively.

Compared to the other findings in this chapter, the findings regarding staff satisfaction with financial rewards are less favorable. Interestingly, moreover, the overall level of satisfaction expressed by the three groups is virtually the same when the data from all the emergency units in the sample are considered (see Table 81). On the average, the MDS, RNS, and LPNS from the various units are better than just "fairly satisfied" but not "very satisfied" with the financial rewards of their work. The overall mean scores for all the EU's in the sample based on the data from the three groups are between 2.55 and 2.65, indicating that the staff of the various units are closer to "fairly satisfied" than to "very satisfied" on the average.

Equally important, for the physicians as well as the nurses, the variability on this measure across individual EU's is very high, indicating major inter-unit differences in staff satisfaction with financial rewards. The unit mean scores show that in some of the units the staff are better than "very satisfied" (midway between "very" and "completely" satisfied or better, depending on the particular staff considered) while in other units they are

TABLE 81. EMERGENCY UNIT STAFF SATISFACTION WITH THE FINANCIAL REWARDS OF THEIR WORK[a]

Hospital Emergency Units (EU's) Involved		Satisfaction with Financial Rewards on the Part of		
		MDS	RNS	LPNS
ALL EU'S IN THE STUDY SAMPLE (N=30 Hospital EU's)	Mean:	2.56	2.65	2.55
	Range:	(1.50-3.56)	(1.40-3.67)	(1.00-3.67)
YOUR HOSPITAL'S EU				
EU's in:				
Small Hospitals (n=14)		2.81	2.74	2.98
Medium Hospitals (n=9)		2.39	2.62	2.25
Large Hospitals (n=7)		2.28	2.51	2.44
EU's in:				
Church Operated Hospitals (n=9)		2.73	2.72	2.00
Osteopathic Hospitals (n=3)		2.67	2.18	2.83
All Other Hospitals (n=18)		2.46	2.69	2.64
EU's Located in:				
SMSA (urban) Areas (n=21)		2.53	2.58	2.52
Non-SMSA Areas (n=9)		2.64	2.82	2.67
EU's in Hospitals Having:				
Medical Teaching Affiliations (n=17)		2.41	2.62	2.63
No Medical Teaching Affiliations (n=13)		2.77	2.69	2.38
EU's in Hospitals Having:				
Emergency Personnel Training Programs (n=15)		2.52	2.68	2.51
No Training Programs (n=15)		2.61	2.63	2.58

[a] The results, presented here in the form of mean scores, are based on the responses of MDS, RNS, and LPNS from the various EU's to the following question: "Considering your work efforts and contributions here, how satisfied are you with the financial or monetary rewards that you derive from your work in this emergency unit?" The response alternatives were: (1) Completely satisfied, (2) very satisfied, (3) fairly satisfied, (4) not so satisfied, and (5) not satisfied at all. Thus, the lower the mean score, the greater the staff satisfaction with the financial rewards of their job.

less than only "fairly satisfied" (close to "not so satisfied" in some cases). Improvements in some of the units would therefore appear necessary for the social efficiency of the unit to be adequate.

The results in Table 81 are also interesting when the various groupings of EU's are examined. First, the physicians in the units of large hospitals are significantly more satisfied, on the average, than are those in the units of small hospitals. The same holds true for practical nurses (these nurses, however, are most satisfied in the units of medium-size hospitals) and, to a lesser extent, for registered nurses as well (though in their case the difference is not significant). All three groups -- MDS, RNS, and LPNS -- are least satisfied with financial rewards in the emergency units of small hospitals.

Physicians are also more satisfied, on the average, in the units of hospitals which have medical teaching affiliations than in the units of other institutions. (The data from nurses show no comparable differences.) In addition, they tend to be somewhat more satisfied in the units of the not church operated hospitals (excluding osteopathic) than in the units of osteopathic and church operated hospitals. The registered nurses, in contrast, are more satisfied in the units of osteopathic compared to non-osteopathic hospitals. The practical nurses, on the other hand, are least satisfied in the units of osteopathic hospitals and most satisfied in the units of church operated hospitals. Finally, the data show no differences in staff satisfaction with financial rewards associated either with the location of emergency units or with the presence/absence of emergency personnel training programs.

Staff satisfaction with non-financial rewards. The final data in this chapter, summarized in Table 82, concern the satisfaction of MDS, RNS, and LPNS with the non-financial, or social-psychological, rewards of their work. On

TABLE 82. EMERGENCY UNIT STAFF SATISFACTION WITH THE NON-FINANCIAL REWARDS OF THEIR WORK[a]

		Satisfaction with Non-Financial Rewards on the Part of		
Hospital Emergency Units (EU's) Involved		MDS	RNS	LPNS
ALL EU'S IN THE STUDY SAMPLE (N=30 Hospital EU's)	Mean: Range:	2.52 (1.80-3.33)	2.39 (1.60-3.00)	1.81 (1.00-3.00)
YOUR HOSPITAL'S EU				
EU's in:				
Small Hospitals (n=14)		2.69	2.43	1.93
Medium Hospitals (n=9)		2.38	2.36	1.63
Large Hospitals (n=7)		2.38	2.33	1.91
EU's in:				
Church Operated Hospitals (n=9)		2.52	2.43	1.71
Osteopathic Hospitals (n=3)		3.02	2.47	2.00
All Other Hospitals (n=18)		2.44	2.35	1.80
EU's Located in:				
SMSA (urban) Areas (n=21)		2.52	2.37	1.84
Non-SMSA Areas (n=9)		2.54	2.42	1.67
EU's in Hospitals Having:				
Medical Teaching Affiliations (n=17)		2.44	2.40	1.75
No Medical Teaching Affiliations (n=13)		2.63	2.37	1.93
EU's in Hospitals Having:				
Emergency Personnel Training Programs (n=15)		2.42	2.42	1.91
No Training Programs (n=15)		2.63	2.36	1.70

[a] The results, presented here in the form of mean scores, are based on the responses of MDS, RNS, and LPNS from the various EU's to the following question: "Considering your work efforts and contributions here, how satisfied are you with all of the non-financial rewards that you derive from working in this emergency unit?" The response alternatives were: (1) Completely satisfied, (2) very satisfied, (3) fairly satisfied, (4) not so satisfied, and (5) not satisfied at all. Thus, the lower the mean score, the greater the satisfaction of the staff with the non-financial rewards of their work.

this measure of staff satisfaction, compared to the above measure, the situation of emergency units is more favorable from the perspective of the nurses but not from the perspective of the physicians.

Overall, the LPNS are the most satisfied group with the non-financial rewards of their work (slightly better than "very satisfied," on the average), followed by the RNS (who are somewhat less than "very satisfied"), and then the MDS (who are almost exactly midway between "very" and "fairly" satisfied). The registered nurses are closer to the physicians than they are to the practical nurses on the present measure (on the financial rewards measure, it will be recalled, the three groups expressed the same level of satisfaction). Across individual emergency units, for all three groups, the variability in staff satisfaction is considerably smaller than it was for financial rewards, but not especially small. In some of the units, the staff are just "fairly satisfied" (even less in the case of MDS) while in other units they are better than "very satisfied" with non-financial rewards.

When examining the various groupings of EU's, the data from nurses, RNS as well as LPNS, show no significant differences from one grouping to another in the average level of staff satisfaction with non-financial rewards. The data from physicians, however, indicate a higher level of satisfaction, on the average, in the emergency units of large and also medium-size hospitals than in the units of small hospitals. In addition, they indicate a higher level of satisfaction in the units of both the church operated and the non-osteopathic hospitals than in the units of osteopathic hospitals. No comparable difference is found in relation to medical teaching affiliation (unlike the case with financial rewards), although a weak trend in the data directionally favors the units of institutions with such an affiliation.

Summary

In this chapter, the findings of the study concerning various aspects of the social efficiency of emergency units were presented and discussed. On the whole, the social efficiency of the units in the sample, as reflected in the attitudes of the staff toward their respective jobs and work situation, in staff identification with the units, and in staff satisfaction with financial and non-financial rewards, appears to be adequate on the average but not particularly high.

Individual emergency units differ considerably from one another on many of the measures examined in the present area. Additionally, staff attitudes, identification, and satisfaction are not uniformly favorable according to the three groups of respondents involved -- MDS, RNS, and LPNS -- either when the total sample or when particular groupings of units are examined. In most cases, the situation of emergency units is more satisfactory on the average from the perspective of the nurses, particularly the practical nurses, than from the perspective of the physicians. The difference is especially pronounced with respect to staff identification with, or commitment to, the units. All three groups of respondents appear to be least satisfied (at about the same level) with the financial rewards of their work. On the other hand, all of them evaluate the units as "very good" places to work, on the average. Differences among emergency unit groupings on the measures studied also exist, particularly in relation to hospital size and/or emergency unit patient volume, and in relation to medical teaching affiliation (especially in the data from physicians) and to the presence/absence of emergency personnel training programs (in the data from nurses).

Chapter 10

FINANCIAL ASPECTS AND ECONOMIC EFFICIENCY

The resources, particularly staff resources, of the emergency units studied were discussed in detail in Chapter 2, with emphasis on their organization, relative adequacy and stability, and overall work capability, following the description of some of the facilities and work inputs of the units in Chapter 1. The financial situation and economic efficiency of the units, which (along with clinical effiency) reflect how well the available resources are being utilized, are considered in the present chapter. Revenues in relation to expenditures, fees charged in relation to expenditures and costs incurred, and professional work hours invested in relation to number of patient visits processed by the various units are the principal concerns of this chapter.

Economic aspects were rarely mentioned by respondents, from within as well as outside the unit, as major problems facing the emergency units in the sample; nor were they mentioned among the major strengths of the units (see Chapter 3). Furthermore, while "maintaining high standards of patient care" is one of the foremost goal priorities of the units, "keeping the costs of service down" is not (see Chapter 3). Nor is "providing care at the lowest cost possible" especially emphasized, as indicated by the appropriateness and performance of clinical procedures in the various units (see Chapter 11). These findings may well suggest that the financial condition of the units is a healthy one, but they do not also mean that the economic efficiency of the units is high, or even acceptable.

Nevertheless, economic efficiency is an important criterion to consider in assessing an emergency unit's organizational effectiveness. Further, economic efficiency/inefficiency is likely to have a significant impact not only on staff performance and satisfaction within the unit, but also on the unit's relations with the parent hospital and with the community. From the perspective of the hospital, an emergency unit must use its financial and staff resources in a productive and efficient way, if it is not to drain resources from the larger organization. From the perspective of the patients and the community, service charges must be kept sufficiently low to make emergency care available to all those who need it or request it. High costs and economic inefficiency, moreover, are likely to invite both public criticism and government interference.

In any event, the findings in the present chapter show consistently large differences among emergency units in the area of economic efficiency. Some of the variation on some of the measures (most of which are based on data from hospital records, and many of which are expressed in the form of "output" to "input" ratios) conceivably might be due to inconsistency or insufficiently high uniformity in accounting and record-keeping practices among the institutions involved. But, given the data collection techniques used (data were provided by each hospital in "raw" form and in the simplest way possible, following detailed instructions and a standardized and pretested procedure, and using an identical data collection instrument), and based upon our knowledge and examination of the data, this is unlikely to be a significant source of the variation found. (Incidentally, when incomplete data were available the institution(s) involved were not included in the computations.) For most of the measures, most of the variation undoubtedly reflects true differences among the emergency units studied.

These differences in economic efficiency may be the result of multiple factors, including staff motivation and performance, the adequacy with which work problems are resolved, the quality of work relations within the unit and between it and its parent hospital, the goal priorities emphasized by the unit, the adequacy and utilization of available resources, the composition of patient inputs and the quality of service provided, etc. -- and generally the variables discussed in the preceding chapters, Chapters 1-9. In the forthcoming analyses of the study, the most important of these variables will be examined in detail to ascertain their relationship to the measures included in the present chapter, and thus specify the factors which may explain the differences in the economic efficiency of emergency units. In addition, the relationship between economic and clinical efficiency will be similarly ascertained.

In the meantime, we return to the concerns of the present chapter. First, using data for the "most recent quarter," the operating budgets and expenditures of emergency units will be considered, both by themselves and in relation to the parent hospital's budget. Second, average revenue per patient visit, total "cost to the hospital" of an average visit, and the ratio of emergency unit revenues to emergency unit expenditures will be examined. Third, "basic fee" charges, charges additional to the basic fee, and total charges per patient visit will be considered, along with the reactions to patient charges by various groups of respondents, including the patients and selected community respondents who participated in the study. Finally, the ratio of the number of patient visits to the number of professional hours worked (by physicians, and by registered nurses) will be examined.

The Operating Budgets and Expenditures of Emergency Units

Based on data supplied from hospital records (RECS), covering "the most recent quarter" (usually the quarter ending in September 1977), the total operating budgets and total operating expenditures of the emergency units studied are shown in Table 83. The operating budgets (for payroll and other requirements) of the units for the most recent quarter average $69,262, and their total operating expenditures average $69,730. The range of operating expenditures across individual emergency units is somewhat greater ($9,516-$194,060) than is the range of operating budgets ($12,220-$172,800). In both respects, however, inter-unit variability obviously is very great.

As would be expected, the higher the patient volume the larger the budgets and the higher the expenditures of the units, on the average. The emergency units of urban area hospitals also have larger budgets and expenditures (at least twice as large), on the average, than do their counterparts in non-urban area hospitals. Furthermore, the units of hospitals with medical teaching affiliations, as well as those of hospitals with emergency personnel training programs, have substantially larger operating budgets and expenditures, on the average, than do the units of the remaining institutions in each case. The church operated and osteopathic hospital units have smaller budgets and expenditures than do the units of the remaining hospitals (but the latter are also generally larger units than the former).

The results also show that, on the average, expenditures are fairly close to the budgets for the different groupings of emergency units. In half of the groupings, average operating budgets exceed average operating expenditures while in the other half the reverse is true. (Included among the former are: the emergency units in the medium patient volume category, the units of church operated hospitals and osteopathic hospitals, urban area units, and the units

TABLE 83. THE EMERGENCY UNIT'S OPERATING BUDGET AND EXPENDITURES FOR THE MOST RECENT QUARTER[a]

Hospital Emergency Units (EU's) Involved		Total Operating Budget[b]	Total Operating Expenditures[c]
ALL EU'S IN THE STUDY SAMPLE (N=29 Hospital EU's)	Mean:	$69,262	$69,730
	Range:	($12,220 - $172,800)	($9,516 - $194,060)
YOUR HOSPITAL'S EU			
EU's with:			
Low Patient Volume (n=10)		$33,724	$34,203
Medium Pat. Volume (n=9)		$70,474	$66,326
High Patient Volume (n=10)		$100,150	$108,320
EU's in:			
Church Operated Hospitals (n=9)		$59,095	$54,348
Osteopathic Hospitals (n=2)		$59,149	$44,781
All Other Hospitals (n=18)		$74,904	$80,193
EU's Located in:			
SMSA (urban) Areas (n=20)		$86,045	$84,783
Non-SMSA Areas (n=9)		$33,830	$36,279
EU's in Hospitals Having:			
Medical Teaching Affiliations (n=16)		$84,790	$90,374
No Medical Teaching Affiliations (n=13)		$48,558	$44,321
EU's in Hospitals Having:			
Emergency Personnel Training Programs (n=14)		$85,811	$86,587
No Training Programs (n=15)		$54,919	$53,997

[a] These findings are based on data from hospital records (RECS) supplied by the participating institutions.

[b] Includes budgeted amount for payroll and other operating requirements. The operating budgets of the emergency units in the study were first summed and then averaged for the EU's in each particular grouping shown. (Two of the 30 institutions did not specify the quarterly budget for their emergency unit, and are therefore excluded.)

[c] Includes total expenditures for payroll and other operating requirements. The expenditures of emergency units in the study were first summed and then averaged for the EU's in each particular grouping shown. (One of the 30 institutions did not specify quarterly expenditures for its emergency unit and is therefore excluded.)

of hospitals which do not have medical teaching affiliations or emergency personnel training programs.) With only a single exception, however, for none of the groupings is the excess in question greater than ten percent (over the base figure). (The exception involves the osteopathic hospital units, which average a much larger operating budget than expenditures for the most recent quarter.) The situation of individual emergency units, however, is much more variable with respect to the difference between operating budget and operating expenditures.

The next table, Table 84, shows (a) the payroll budget of emergency units as a percentage of the payroll budget of their parent hospitals, and (b) the total operating budget of the units as a percentage of the total operating budget of their parent hospitals. In both cases, the data again cover the most recent quarter (and are averaged for the emergency units in the total sample, as they are for the units in each grouping).*

On the average, the payroll budgets of the emergency units studied represent only 2.94% of their parent hospitals' payroll budgets. For individual units, however, this figure varies widely, from a low of 1.30% to a high of 8.19%. When the total operating budgets are similarly considered, instead of the payroll budgets, the inter-unit variability is smaller but still very great, from 0.79% to 5.92%; on the average, the total operating budgets of the emergency units represent 2.54% of the operating budgets of their parent hospitals. Clearly, some of the units are allocated a much higher proportion of their parent hospital's budget (payroll as well as total) than are other

---

*Incidentally, when the quarterly data are extrapolated to cover an entire year, resulting figures are consistent, but almost always larger, than the comparable figures provided by the various hospitals for "the most recent year." The quarterly data are used since they are not only sufficiently stable but are also the most recent data available.

TABLE 84. THE EMERGENCY UNIT'S BUDGET AS A PERCENTAGE OF THE HOSPITAL'S BUDGET, FOR THE MOST RECENT QUARTER[a]

Hospital Emergency Units (EU's) Involved		EU Payroll Budget as a Percentage of the Hospital's Payroll Budget[b]	EU Operating Budget as a Percentage of the Hospital's Total Operating Budget[c]
ALL EU'S IN THE STUDY SAMPLE (N=28 Hospital EU's)	Mean: Range:	2.94% (1.30%-8.19%)	2.54% (0.79%-5.92%)
YOUR HOSPITAL'S EU			
EU's with:			
Low Patient Volume (n=9)		2.12	2.05
Medium Pat. Volume (n=9)		3.06	2.85
High Patient Volume (n=10)		3.58	2.70
EU's in:			
Church Operated Hospitals (n=8)		2.45	2.11
Osteopathic Hospitals (n=2)		3.24	3.02
All Other Hospitals (n=18)		3.13	2.68
EU's Located in:			
SMSA (urban) Areas (n=19)		2.91	2.69
Non-SMSA Areas (n=9)		3.01	2.22
EU's in Hospitals Having:			
Medical Teaching Affiliations (n=16)		2.38	2.45
No Medical Teaching Affiliations (n=12)		3.70	2.66
EU's in Hospitals Having:			
Emergency Personnel Training Programs (n=13)		2.94	2.58
No Training Programs (n=15)		2.94	2.51

[a] These findings are based on data from hospital records (RECS) supplied by the participating institutions. (Two of the 30 hospitals in the study did not provide the necessary data and are therefore excluded.)

[b] Based on budgeted amounts for payrolls only. The budgeted payroll of each emergency unit was divided by the parent hospital's budgeted payroll. Then, the resulting products were averaged for the EU's in each particular grouping.

[c] Based on budgeted amounts for payroll plus other operating requirements. The total operating budget of each EU was divided by the parent hospital's total operating budget. Then, the resulting products were averaged for the EU's in each particular grouping.

units. The figures under discussion also indicate that emergency units receive a greater proportion of the hospitals' payroll budgets than of the hospitals' total operating budgets (or of the hospitals' budgets for operating requirements other than payroll).

The payroll, and also total operating, budgets of emergency units with a high or medium patient volume, as compared to units with a low patient volume, represent a significantly greater proportion of the hospitals' corresponding budgets (on the average). The same pattern characterizes the emergency units of hospitals which are not, as compared to those which are, church operated. With respect to total operating budget only, the units of urban area hospitals also claim a larger share of their parent hospitals' operating budgets than do the units of non-urban area hospitals. And with respect to payroll budget only, the units of hospitals which have no medical teaching affiliations claim a larger share than do the units of hospitals which have such affiliations. Between the units of hospitals which have and those which do not have emergency personnel training programs, there are no differences -- either with respect to the payroll budget or with respect to the total operating budget.

Revenues in Relation to Costs and Expenditures

Data on realized revenues from patient visits to each emergency unit during the most recent quarter, and on the current "total cost to the hospital" of an average patient visit are summarized in Table 85. On the whole, for the institutions in the sample, the average revenue per patient visit to the emergency units ($28.09) is greater than the "total cost" of the average visit to the hospitals ($24.29), by almost 16%. These, however, are average figures for the 28 units in the sample (sufficient data were not provided by two hospitals). Across individual emergency units, average revenue per patient

TABLE 85. AVERAGE HOSPITAL REVENUE PER PATIENT VISIT TO THE EMERGENCY UNIT AND TOTAL COST TO THE HOSPITAL PER VISIT[a]

Hospital Emergency Units (EU's) Involved		Average Revenue Per Patient Visit to the Emergency Unit[b]	Total "Cost to the Hospital" of an Average Patient Visit to the Emergency Unit[c]
ALL EU'S IN THE STUDY SAMPLE (N=28 Hospital EU's)	Mean:	$28.09	$24.29
	Range:	($9.78 - $54.64)	($0.50 - $63.00)
YOUR HOSPITAL'S EU			
EU's with:			
Low Patient Volume (n=9)		$29.61	$26.44
Medium Pat. Volume (n=9)		$26.10	$29.33
High Patient Volume (n=10)		$28.50	$17.80
EU's in:			
Church Operated Hospitals (n=8)		$33.59	$19.11
Osteopathic Hospitals (n=2)		$24.61	$48.00
All Other Hospitals (n=18)		$26.03	$24.23
EU's Located in:			
SMSA (urban) Areas (n=20)		$30.63	$27.11
Non-SMSA Areas (n=8)		$21.73	$18.33
EU's in Hospitals Having:			
Medical Teaching Affiliations (n=16)		$26.41	$24.31
No Medical Teaching Affiliations (n=12)		$30.33	$24.25
EU's in Hospitals Having:			
Emergency Personnel Training Programs (n=14)		$29.67	$19.69
No Training Programs (n=14)		$26.50	$28.27

Table 85 Continues

TABLE 85
(Continued)

---

[a] These findings are based on data from hospital records (RECS) supplied by the participating institutions. (Two of the 30 hospitals in the study did not provide the necessary data and are therefore excluded.)

[b] Data on revenues (exclude physician fees) are for the most recent quarter. For each hospital EU, total revenues from all patient visits during this period were divided by the total number of visits. Then, the resulting products were averaged for the EU's in each particular grouping.

[c] These cost figures were provided by the hospitals for "the present time" rather than for the most recent quarter. The data provided were averaged for the EU's in each particular grouping shown. The cost figures specified include both "direct" and "indirect" costs combined. However, for 24 or more of the 28 institutions involved these total cost figures do not include costs for any of the following services: X-ray, EKG, laboratory, anesthesiology, social services, respiratory therapy, and ambulance service. (The number of hospitals, from among the 28 involved, which included costs in their "total cost" figures for one or another of those particular services is very small, ranging up to a maximum of only 3.)

visit varies widely, from a low of $9.78 to a high of $54.64, and the range is even greater for total cost to the hospital ($0.50-$63.00). In some of the units, the revenue-cost difference is very high while in others it is only moderate or even low.

The results are also interesting when the different groupings of emergency units are compared. First, revenues per patient visit are significantly higher, on the average, for urban than non-urban area units. They are also considerably higher for the units of church operated hospitals than those of other institutions. And they are somewhat higher for: emergency units with a low patient volume compared to the rest of the units; the units of hospitals which have no medical teaching affiliations compared to those which do; and the units of hospitals which have emergency personnel training programs compared to those which do not.

Second, total costs to the hospital per visit are again significantly higher, on the average, for urban than non-urban area units. But, they are lower for the units of church operated hospitals than the units of other hospitals, and for the units of institutions which have emergency personnel training programs compared to those which do not (in both cases, the reverse pattern holds true with regard to revenues). Costs to the hospital per visit, moreover, are significantly lower for emergency units with a high patient volume than for units with either a medium or a low patient volume (between the latter two groupings the difference, which favors the low over the medium volume units, is small).

Finally, on the average, revenue per visit exceeds total cost to the hospital by at least 20% in the following groupings of emergency units: EU's with a high patient volume; the EU's of church operated hospitals; the EU's of hospitals which have no medical teaching affiliations; and the EU's of hospitals which have emergency personnel training programs. The excess of revenue over cost is especially large for EU's with a high patient volume and for the EU's of church operated hospitals. In contrast, costs to the hospital exceed revenues per visit by at least 20% in one grouping only -- the EU's of osteopathic hospitals (data from only two institutions are involved in this particular grouping, however).

Emergency unit revenues in relation to emergency unit expenditures. The results from still another measure of economic efficiency, one that relates revenues to expenditures, are presented in Table 86. The figures shown represent the ratio of total emergency unit revenues to total emergency unit expenditures during the most recent quarter. (Incidentally, all but two of the units which are participating in the study are considered as separate "cost centers" in their respective institutions.)

The ratio of revenues to expenditures for the emergency units in the sample during the most recent quarter averages 1.89, indicating 89% more revenues than expenditures on the average. Equally important, this ratio varies greatly among individual units (but, from about 1.00 on upwards). At the one extreme of the distribution of these ratios, one of the emergency units shows a ratio of 0.97 (indicating that revenues did not quite match expenditures), while at the other extreme one of the units shows a ratio of 5.68 (indicating that the unit's revenues were more than five times greater than its expenditures). In short, inter-unit variability on the present measure is extremely great; some of the units probably just break even while others realize revenues equivalent to two, three, or even five times the amount of their expenditures.

TABLE 86. EMERGENCY UNIT REVENUES IN RELATION TO EMERGENCY UNIT EXPENDITURES DURING THE MOST RECENT QUARTER[a]

Hospital Emergency Units (EU's) Involved	The Ratio of Total EU Revenues to Total EU Expenditures[b]
ALL EU'S IN THE STUDY SAMPLE (N=29 Hospital EU's)	Mean: 1.89 Range: (0.97-5.68)
YOUR HOSPITAL'S EU	
EU's with:	
Low Patient Volume (n=10)	1.68
Medium Pat. Volume (n=9)	1.53
High Patient Volume (n=10)	2.41
EU's in:	
Church Operated Hospitals (n=9)	1.91
Osteopathic Hospitals (n=2)	1.66
All Other Hospitals (n=18)	1.90
EU's Located in:	
SMSA (urban) Areas (n=20)	1.93
Non-SMSA Areas (n=9)	1.80
EU's in Hospitals Having:	
Medical Teaching Affiliations (n=16)	1.85
No Medical Teaching Affiliations (n=13)	1.93
EU's in Hospitals Having:	
Emergency Personnel Training Programs (n=14)	2.12
No Training Programs (n=15)	1.67

[a] These findings are based on data from hospital records (RECS) supplied by the participating institutions.

[b] For each emergency unit, total hospital revenues (excluding physician fees) from all patient visits to the EU during the most recent quarter were divided by total expenditures for EU payroll _and_ other requirements during the same period. Then, the obtained ratios were averaged for the EU's in each particular grouping. (Data are missing for one of the 30 EU's in the study.)

Considering next the various groupings of emergency units, the findings show especially high ratios for EU's with a high patient volume (the average revenues to expenditures ratio for these units is 2.41), and for the EU's of hospitals which have emergency personnel training programs (these units show an average ratio of 2.12). The lowest average ratio for any of the groupings is found in the case of EU's which have a medium patient volume (the specific ratio is 1.53, indicating about 50% more revenues than expenditures on the average). The next lowest (1.66) is found in the case of the osteopathic hospital units.

Other findings in Table 86 show that, on the average, the ratio of revenues to expenditures is considerably greater for EU's with a high patient volume than those with either a medium or a low patient volume (between the latter two groupings the difference is small). Similarly, it is considerably greater for the EU's of hospitals which have emergency personnel training programs than those of hospitals which do not. And, to a lesser extent, the average ratio is also greater for the EU's of non-osteopathic hospitals (both church operated and other) than the EU's of osteopathic hospitals; the ratio is almost identical for the units of non-osteopathic hospitals which are church operated and those which are not. Finally, the average ratio of revenues to expenditures is only slightly higher for urban area units than it is for non-urban area units (1.93 vs. 1.80).

Emergency Unit Service Charges

Data on hospital charges to patients for their emergency visits during the most recent quarter are summarized in Table 87. These include: (a) the "basic fee" charged by the hospital per visit (exclusive of physician fees); (b) average hospital charges <u>additional</u> to the basic fee per patient visit (exclusive of physician fees); and (c) average "total charges" per patient visit (again exclusive of physician fees). The number of emergency units in the sample for which data are available on these three measures is 29, 25, and 24, respectively.

The "basic fee" charged by the institutions in the study for an emergency visit averages $17.28 (based on data for "the most recent quarter"). Across individual emergency units, however, the basic fee ranges from a low of $7.00 to a high of $30.00 -- once more indicating great inter-unit variability. The basic fee is substantially higher, on the average, in urban compared to non-urban area units, and in the units of osteopathic compared to non-osteopathic hospitals. It is highest, on the average, in the units of osteopathic hospitals, and lowest in the units located in non-urban (i.e., non-SMSA) areas (and next lowest in the units of church operated hospitals). Other differences may be seen in Table 87.

Hospital charges <u>additional</u> to the "basic fee" average $11.32 per emergency visit (for the 25 EU's in the sample for which these data are available), and range across institutions from a low of $1.00 to a high of $48.00 per patient visit. Thus, average additional charges amount to about 64% of the basic fee charged by the hospitals for an average emergency unit visit, but there is great variability among individual institutions in this respect. These additional charges are lowest, on the average, in the non-urban area units, and next lowest in emergency units having a high patient volume; they are highest in the osteopathic hospital units, and next highest in units having a low patient volume. Further, the additional charges are significantly lower, on the average, in emergency units with a high compared to either a medium or a low patient volume, in non-urban area compared to urban area units, and in non-osteopathic compared to osteopathic hospital units.

Finally, Table 87 shows comparable findings for average <u>total charges</u> (exclusive of physician fees) per emergency unit visit by the various insti-

TABLE 87. HOSPITAL CHARGES TO PATIENTS FOR THEIR EMERGENCY UNIT VISITS (EXCLUSIVE OF PHYSICIAN FEES), FOR THE MOST RECENT QUARTER[a]

		Average Charges per Patient Visit		
Hospital Emergency Units (EU's) Involved		"Basic Fee"[b]	"Additional Charges"[c]	Total Charges[d]
ALL EU'S IN THE STUDY SAMPLE (N=29 Hospital EU's)	Mean: Range:	$17.28 ($7.00-$30.00)	$11.32 ($1.00-$48.00)	$27.08 ($13.00-$74.00)
YOUR HOSPITAL'S EU				
EU's with:				
Low Patient Volume (n=10)		$15.60	$13.80	$29.40
Medium Pat. Volume (n=9)		$19.11	$12.17	$24.80
High Patient Volume (n=10)		$17.30	$8.00	$25.78
EU's in:				
Church Operated Hospitals (n=8)		$14.13	$11.63	$23.14
Osteopathic Hospitals (n=3)		$22.00	$34.00	$54.50
All Other Hospitals (n=18)		$17.89	$8.13	$25.27
EU's Located in:				
SMSA (urban) Areas (n=20)		$19.15	$13.59	$30.94
Non-SMSA Areas (n=9)		$13.11	$6.50	$19.37
EU's in Hospitals Having:				
Medical Teaching Affiliations (n=17)		$18.23	$10.69	$27.77
No Medical Teaching Affiliations (n=12)		$15.92	$12.00	$26.27
EU's in Hospitals Having:				
Emergency Personnel Training Programs (n=15)		$17.80	$10.42	$28.25
No Training Programs (n=14)		$16.71	$12.15	$25.92

Table 87 Continues

TABLE 87
(Continued)

---

[a] These findings are based on data from hospital records (RECS) supplied by the participating institutions.

[b] This is the "basic fee" charged by a hospital for a patient visit to the emergency unit. The data provided by the various institutions in the study were averaged for the EU's in the particular groupings shown. (One hospital did not indicate its "basic fee.")

[c] These are charges for the average patient visit to the emergency unit <u>additional</u> to the "basic fee." They are hospital charges exclusive of physician fees. The "additional charges" specified by the various institutions were averaged for the EU's in the particular groupings shown. (Five of the 30 institutions in the study did not indicate their charges additional to the "basic fee," and are therefore excluded from the computations.)

[d] These "total charges" per patient visit were computed by summing the "basic fee" and the "additional charges." separately for each of the 24 institutions which provided complete data for this purpose. (The other six institutions are excluded from the computations.) Then, the resulting products were averaged for the EU's in each particular grouping shown.

tutions. Data on this measure are available for 24 of the 30 EU's in the study sample. The results show that total hospital charges per patient visit average $27.08 for the institutions studied, based on data for the most recent quarter. Across individual institutions, however, average total charges range widely, from a low of $13.00 to a high of $74.00 per patient visit.

On the average, total charges are highest in the emergency units of osteopathic hospitals, and next highest in the urban area units. They are lowest in the non-urban area EU's, and next lowest in the EU's of church operated hospitals. The findings also show that total charges are higher in EU's with a low than either a medium or a high patient volume. They are also somewhat higher in the EU's of hospitals which have emergency personnel training programs than those which do not, and slightly higher in the EU's of hospitals which have medical teaching affiliations compared to those which do not. (It also follows that total charges are much higher, on the average, in the EU's of osteopathic compared to non-osteopathic hospitals, and in the urban compared to the non-urban area EU's.)

Respondent reactions to patient charges. Those of the recent emergency unit patients (PATS) in the study who already knew what the charges for their visits were (a total of 51% of the patients who completed questionnaires) were asked how they felt about the charges. The selected community respondents (CRS) and the selected hospital physicians (HMDS) who participated in the study also were asked their views concerning patient charges for emergency service by the institutions with which they were associated. And the physicians (MDS) and registered nurses (RNS) working in the various emergency units were likewise asked their reactions to patient charges. The obtained data are all summarized in Table 88.

TABLE 88. REACTION TO PATIENT CHARGES FOR CARE IN THE EMERGENCY UNIT ON THE PART OF VARIOUS GROUPS

Hospital Emergency Units (EU's) Involved		Patient Charges as Evaluated by				
		MDS[a]	RNS[a]	HMDS[a]	CRS[a]	PATS[b]
ALL EU'S IN THE STUDY SAMPLE (N=30 Hospital EU's)	Mean:	3.04	3.19	3.46	3.37	3.74
	Range:	(2.25-3.83)	(2.19-4.00)	(2.33-4.29)	(3.00-4.33)	(3.00-5.00)
YOUR HOSPITAL'S EU						
EU's with:						
Low Patient Volume (n=10)		3.22	2.87	3.57	3.28	3.68
Medium Pat. Volume (n=10)		3.01	3.37	3.14	3.55	3.69
High Patient Volume (n=10)		2.88	3.33	3.67	3.31	3.84
EU's in:						
Church Operated Hospitals (n=9)		3.16	2.94	3.49	3.17	3.61
Osteopathic Hospitals (n=3)		3.11	3.13	3.43	3.00	3.73
All Other Hospitals (n=18)		2.96	3.32	3.45	3.53	3.79
EU's Located in:						
SMSA (urban) Areas (n=21)		3.06	3.17	3.50	3.41	3.93
Non-SMSA Areas (n=9)		2.98	2.23	3.38	3.30	3.55
EU's in Hospitals Having:						
Medical Teaching Affiliations (n=17)		2.91	2.30	3.49	3.43	3.76
No Medical Teaching Affiliations (n=13)		3.19	3.04	3.42	3.30	3.70
EU's in Hospitals Having:						
Emergency Personnel Training Programs (n=15)		3.01	3.25	3.72	3.39	3.68
No Training Programs (n=15)		3.06	3.12	3.20	3.36	3.79

[a] These results, presented here in the form of mean scores, are based on the responses of the RNS, MDS, HMDS, and CRS associated with the various institutions to the following question: "Considering the kind of service that this emergency unit provides to its patients, how do you feel about what it charges the patients (or their insurance) for their care?" The response alternatives were: (1) Patient charges are too low..., (2) they are rather low, (3) they are about right, (4) they are rather high, (5) they are very high, and (6) patient charges are extremely high. Using the data from each group of respondents, mean scores were first computed separately for each EU and then averaged for the EU's in the different categories. The lower the mean scores, the lower the charges from the perspective of the respondents.

[b] These results, reported in the form of mean scores, are based on the responses of recent patients (PATS) from the various emergency units to the question: "How do you feel about the charges for your visit?" The response alternatives were the same as those in the question about patient charges which was asked of RNS, MDS, HMDS, and CRS. Thus, the lower the mean score, the lower the charges from the perspective of patients. Only patients who indicated knowledge of the charges for their emergency visit (a total of 51% of all the patients in the study) were asked to answer this question. (Two of the 30 institutions did not allow patient participation in the study and are therefore excluded.)

On the average, all five groups of respondents evaluate patient charges fairly favorably. The overall mean scores for the emergency units in the sample based on the data from the five groups are between 3.04 (data from MDS) and 3.74 (data from PATS). On the scale used, a value of 3.00 signifies that patient charges are "about right," and a value of 4.00 signifies that patient charges are "rather high" (5.00 would correspond to "very high" and 2.00 to "rather low").

Of the five groups, however, the patients are the most critical, i.e., give the least favorable evaluation; and the emergency unit physicians give the most favorable evaluation, followed closely by the registered nurses. The community respondents and the selected hospital physicians (whose evaluations are very similar) occupy intermediate positions. On the average, the emergency unit physicians evaluate patient charges significantly more favorably than any other group except the registered nurses, and the patients evaluate the charges significantly less favorably than any other group, including the community respondents, except the selected hospital physicians (who, next to the patients, are the most critical of the five groups). In an absolute sense, of course, patient charges are not regarded as excessively high on the average by any of the respondent groups -- in all cases they are regarded as being somewhere between "about right" and "rather high."

On the present measure of economic efficiency, therefore, the emergency units in the study as a group come out probably better than might have been expected. The situation of particular units, however, is another matter. The ranges of the mean scores (based on the data from the five groups of respondents) shown in Table 88 indicate moderately high inter-unit variability. For some of the units, for example, the patients evaluate the charges as "about right," at the positive end of the spectrum, while for others they evaluate them as "rather high" or even "very high," at the other end of the spectrum. The selected hospital physicians evaluate the charges almost as "rather low" for some of the units, as "about right" for others, and as "rather high" or higher for still other units. The data from the other groups show somewhat smaller, but not much smaller, inter-unit variability.

With reference to the various groupings of units, the results show the following main differences: (a) the patients evaluate the charges more favorably in the non-urban than the urban area EU's; (b) the community respondents evaluate patient charges more favorably in the case of church operated and osteopathic hospital EU's than in the case of non-osteopathic hospitals which are not church operated; (c) the selected hospital physicians evaluate emergency unit charges more favorably for EU's with a medium compared to either a low or a high patient volume, and for the EU's of hospitals which do not have emergency personnel training programs compared to those which do; (d) the emergency unit physicians evaluate the charges more favorably in EU's with a high than a low patient volume; and, (e) the registered nurses evaluate the charges more favorably in EU's with a low compared to either a medium or a high patient volume (contrary to the physicians), in the EU's of church operated hospitals than those of other hospitals (excluding osteopathic), and in the EU's of hospitals which have medical teaching affiliations compared to those which do not.

Professional Staff Hours Worked in Relation to Patient Visits Processed

The final table in this chapter, Table 89, summarizes certain data indicating the output of the emergency units in relation to the staff resources used. More specifically, Table 89 shows the ratio of the number of patient visits to (a) the number of physician hours worked, and (b) the number of registered nurse hours worked.

TABLE 89. NUMBER OF PATIENT VISITS TO THE EMERGENCY UNIT IN RELATION TO THE NUMBER OF HOURS WORKED BY THE REGISTERED NURSES (RNS) AND BY THE PHYSICIANS (MDS) IN THE UNIT

Hospital Emergency Units (EU's) Involved		Ratio of Patient Visits to		Ratio of Patient Visits to	
		Number of RN Hours Worked According to Hospital Records[a]	Number of RN Hours Worked as Reported by the RNS[b]	Number of Physician Hours Worked According to Hospital Records[c]	Number of Physician Hours Worked as Reported by the MDS[d]
ALL EU'S IN THE STUDY SAMPLE (N=29 Hospital EU's)	Mean: Range:	1.56 (0.57-5.25)	1.49 (0.52-4.06)	2.48 (0.59-4.57)	3.26 (0.53-12.17)
YOUR HOSPITAL'S EU					
EU's with:					
Low Patient Volume (n=10)		1.30	1.17	2.23	3.07
Medium Pat. Volume (n=10)		1.55	1.50	1.73	2.57
High Patient Volume (n=9)		1.85	1.84	3.33	4.23
EU's in:					
Church Operated Hospitals (n=9)		1.61	1.43	2.90	4.00
Osteopathic Hospitals (n=3)		1.31	1.29	1.46	1.56
All Other Hospitals (n=17)		1.57	1.56	2.48	3.17
EU's Located in:					
SMSA (urban) Areas (n=20)		1.41	1.50	2.42	2.85
Non-SMSA Areas (n=9)		1.87	1.48	2.65	4.17
EU's in Hospitals Having:					
Medical Teaching Affiliations (n=17)		1.57	1.63	2.67	3.17
No Medical Teaching Affiliations (n=12)		1.54	1.29	2.15	3.38
EU's in Hospitals Having:					
Emergency Personnel Training Programs (n=14)		1.69	1.64	2.93	4.41
No Training Programs (n=15)		1.43	1.35	2.03	2.19

[a] This ratio was computed separately for each emergency unit by dividing the number of patient visits during the "most recent week" by the total number of hours worked during the same week by all registered nurses (whether full-time or part-time, and including supervisory RN's) in the unit. The resulting ratios were then averaged for the EU's in each particular grouping shown. The data for computing these ratios were obtained from hospital records (RECS) supplied by the participating institutions. (One of the 30 hospitals did not provide the necessary data and is therefore excluded.)

[b] These ratios were computed in exactly the same manner as those described in footnote "a", except that the denominator in each case consisted of: total RN hours worked in "a typical week" as reported by the RNS from each emergency unit in the questionnaires that they completed for the study. (Again, one hospital is excluded.)

[c] These ratios were computed in exactly the same manner as those described in footnote "a", except that physician hours instead of RN hours were used in the computations. The necessary data from hospital records (RECS) were available for 24 of the 30 institutions in the sample.

[d] These ratios were computed in exactly the same manner as those described in footnote "b", except that physician hours were used (instead of RN hours) as reported in the questionnaires completed by the MDS from each emergency unit. (Data are missing for one of the 30 hospitals.)

The number of patient visits to each emergency unit is for "the most recent week," for which records were available (in most cases, the same week during which staff were interviewed at each institution). Data on staff hours worked were supplied from hospital records (RECS) for the same week as the data concerning patient visits, separately for physician hours and for registered nurse hours. In addition, the physicians (MDS) and registered nurses (RNS) working in the various emergency units who completed interviews and questionnaires for the study also provided relevant data by reporting the total number of hours each was working in the emergency unit in a "typical week." In all cases, the data for each emergency unit involved represent the total number of patient visits and the total number of hours worked by all of the doctors, and all of the registered nurses, working in each emergency unit.

Because both self-reported work hours and hours based on hospital records are available for each staff, two different but comparable ratios are shown in Table 89 for patient visits to physician hours worked, as well as for patient visits to registered nurse hours worked. The ratios shown for the total sample are averaged ratios for the emergency units involved, and the same applies with reference to each particular grouping of units included in the table.

In all cases, the higher the ratio shown, the larger the number of patients treated in the emergency unit per staff hour worked. A high ratio probably indicates that staff resources are being used efficiently; but, it could also indicate, at least for some of the units, a heavy workload for the staff or insufficient staffing. Conversely, a low ratio may be indicative either of inefficiency or of a particularly complex workload (e.g., a higher proportion of unusually demanding cases). The findings, therefore, will be subjected to more intensive scrutiny in the forthcoming analyses of the study. In the meantime, individual institutions and their staffs should interpret the ratios in the light of their own experience and situation.

Considering first the total sample, the findings show that the ratio of patient visits to registered nurse hours worked averages about 1.50 for the emergency units studied, whether the data about hours are from hospital records or self-reported. But, this ratio varies greatly across individual units, ranging from 0.57 to 5.25 (when using hours from records) and from 0.52 to 4.06 (when using self-reported hours in the denominator). For some of the units, in other words, the ratio in question is at least several times higher than the corresponding ratio for other units. It is doubtful that such a high inter-unit variability could be accounted for, even for the most part, by differences in workload and/or patient composition among the units (the latter differences would have to be exceedingly great, and none of the data from the study support such a pattern). What is more probable is that the units differ very substantially in the work efficiency of their registered nurses, and that efficiency differences account for much if not most of the observed variability across individual emergency units in the ratios under consideration.

The findings also show that, on the average, the ratio of patient visits to registered nurse hours worked is greater in units with a high patient volume, than units with a medium patient volume, than units with a low patient volume -- both when self-reported hours and hours from records are used for its computation. It is similarly higher in the units of hospitals which have emergency personnel training programs than in the units of hospitals which do not, in the units of the non-osteopathic compared to osteopathic hospitals, and (to a less pronounced extent) in the units of hospitals which have medical teaching affiliations compared to those which do not. For urban vs. non-urban units, the results are mixed.

Considering next the corresponding data regarding the ratio of patient visits to physician hours worked, the findings are equally interesting. First, this ratio averages 2.48 for the emergency units in the sample when physician hours based on hospital records are used, and 3.26 when self-reported physician hours are used in the computations.* Across individual emergency units, the former figure ranges from 0.59 to 4.57, and the latter from 0.53 to 12.17. While inter-unit variability is considerably larger in the latter case, the important point is that in both cases it is very great. As with the findings concerning the ratios involving the data about registered nurses, here too it appears that the work efficiency of the medical staff is highly variable from one emergency unit to another.

The findings involving the medical staff, moreover, are very similar for the most part to those involving the nursing staff when the different groupings of emergency units are examined. First, on the average, the ratio of patient visits to physician hours worked is greater for units with a high patient volume, than units with a low patient volume, than units with a medium patient volume (in that order). Second, it is greater on the average for the units of church operated hospitals, than the units of other non-osteopathic hospitals, than the units of osteopathic hospitals (in that order). Third, it is similarly greater for the units of hospitals which have than those which do not have emergency personnel training programs. And, fourth, the ratio in question is greater for non-urban than for urban area units. In all of these cases, moreover, the difference between the average ratios compared holds as specified whether the data on physician hours are from records or self-reported. (For the remaining grouping of units, the one based on medical teaching affiliation, the results are mixed.)

---

*The discrepancy between the two figures is due, probably for the most part, to the fact that the time base for hours worked is similar but not identical, and the fact that the individual physicians involved are not all the same, in the data used for computing the two ratios for each emergency unit.

Finally, the findings for the various groupings of units show that, on the average, the ratios of patient visits to physician hours worked are highest for emergency units which have a high patient volume, and for the units of hospitals which have emergency personnel training programs. Overall, the results in Table 89 suggest that the work efficiency of the professional staff varies greatly among the emergency units studied. (These results, of course, have little to say about clinical efficiency, or the quality of care provided by the staff, which is the subject of Chapter 11).

Summary

The findings of the study concerning various aspects of the economic situation of emergency units were presented and discussed in this chapter. On most of the measures, major differences were found between particular groupings of units. More important, the range of scores of the individual units on these measures indicates that inter-unit variability in the present area is extremely high. This suggests that the level of economic efficiency characterizing the emergency units in the sample varies greatly from one unit to another. These differences, along with differences in the other criteria of organizational effectiveness (clinical efficiency, patient satisfaction, and social efficiency) studied, will be examined thoroughly and intensively in the forthcoming analyses of the project, as will the correlates of these differences and the inter-relationships among the various criterion measures. We now turn to consider the clinical efficiency of the emergency units.

Chapter 11

CLINICAL EFFICIENCY: CARE PROCEDURES, STAFF PERFORMANCE, AND QUALITY OF CARE

This, the final, chapter of the report focuses on the last and probably most important aspect of organizational effectiveness considered in the present study -- that of clinical efficiency. An emergency unit may be financially healthy and economically efficient but clinically inefficient, and vice versa, it may be both economically and clinically efficient, or it may be neither -- whether in an absolute sense or by comparison to other emergency units.

Very briefly, clinical efficiency involves the excellence of staff performance and the quality of patient care provided, given the current state of medical knowledge and technology and contemporary clinical standards in medicine, nursing, and the other health professions. The quality of care, as the main outcome and principal output of staff performance, is the core component of clinical efficiency. High quality care, of course, also presupposes sufficient quantity (which, in turn, presupposes adequate staffing), but it is the quality of care itself that constitutes the principal criterion of clinical efficiency -- the quality of care provided by the clinical staff to the patients of the unit at all stages of the care process, from the point of patient entry into the unit to the point of patient exit.

Controlling for patient requirements and condition (i.e., for the composition of the unit's patient workload), clinical efficiency depends directly on the appropriateness (vis-à-vis standards) of clinical practices and procedures, both diagnostic and therapeutic, the prompt implementation of clinical measures, and the continual excellence of professional performance, by both the medical and the nursing staff. It is essentially these critical determinants of the quality of care that are responsible for the level of clinical efficiency which may characterize an emergency unit.

These important determinants, in turn, depend on such things as the qualifications and experience (i.e., competence), the quantity and stability, and the organization of the staff (see Chapter 2), the goal priorities of the unit (see Chapter 3), the facilities, structure, and internal organizational situation of the unit (see Chapter 1 and Chapter 4), and the nature of problem solving and work relations within the unit and between it and its parent hospital as well as the outside community (see Chapters 5-7). The correlates of clinical efficiency also may be many and varied. Clinical efficiency may well be found to correlate positively, at least in some institutions, with such other favorable outcomes as the acceptability of care and patient satisfaction (Chapter 8), staff satisfaction (Chapter 9), and even cost effectiveness (Chapter 10), but this is not necessarily the case for all or even most emergency units at all or even most times. Whether such relationships exist for the emergency units studied is one of the major questions to be addressed in the forthcoming analyses of the data.

In the meantime, the purpose of this chapter is to present the preliminary findings of the study about the appropriateness of clinical procedures, the quality of medical and nursing staff performance, and the quality of patient care provided in the various emergency units -- about clinical efficiency. The importance of these aspects of clinical efficiency to the emergency units, as well as to their parent hospitals, is reflected in the great emphasis placed by the units on the goal priority of "maintaining high standards of patient care" (see Chapter 3). Consistent with their importance, moreover, these key aspects were measured in the present study using several different techniques and several sources of data (from the performers themselves, i.e., the nurses and physicians working in each unit, qualified peers from the rest of the hospital, and patients) representing different legitimate perspectives. The obtained results from most of these data and techniques (certain measures, e.g., measures based on data from the patients' medical records, are not included because they require sophisticated technical analysis before they can be constructed) are summarized in this chapter.

In the first section, findings concerning the appropriateness and performance of clinical procedures (medical treatment and nursing care procedures) used in the various emergency units are presented. Included in the second section are findings about patient waiting time and the promptness of medical attention, and about patient "processing" time, or the length of patient visits. In the next section, assessments by patients (PATS) and selected community respondents (CRS) of certain aspects of care process (staff competence/performance) and care outcome are presented. Reported in the fourth section is information about patient death rates, based on data supplied from hospital records (RECS). Summarized in the fifth section are evaluations of the quality of medical management and nursing care provided to patients with certain conditions (in five particular categories).

In the final section of the chapter, findings are presented concerning: (a) the quality of overall medical care and overall nursing care in the various emergency units, as rated by qualified respondents other than the performers; and (b) assessments of the quality of medical care by the physicians (MDS), and of the quality of nursing care by the registered nurses (RNS), provided in their respective units as compared to the quality of care provided in the emergency units of other hospitals with which the respondents are familiar.

The Appropriateness and Performance of Care Procedures

The physicians (MDS) and supervising nurses (SRNS) of the emergency units in the study, and also the hospital administrator (HAS) respondents, were asked to provide their evaluations of the medical treatment and nursing care procedures used in their respective units. More specifically, they were asked to assess these procedures from the standpoint of "enabling the staff of the unit to provide care": (a) of the highest quality possible, (b) as promptly as it should be provided, and (c) at the lowest cost possible. (This last criterion was used for comparison purposes although, strictly speaking, it reflects economic rather than clinical efficiency.) The evaluations provided by the MDS are summarized in Table 90; those provided by the SRNS and the HAS are not presented in table form but will be briefly discussed as well.

The results in Table 90 show that more of the clinical procedures used in the emergency units are regarded (by the physicians) as "very appropriate" with respect to the quality than with respect to the promptness or the cost of care. Overall, in fact, these procedures are evaluated by the MDS significantly more favorably with respect to the quality of care than with respect to the promptness of care, and significantly more favorably with respect to promptness than with respect to cost. The corresponding mean scores for the 30 EU's in the sample are 1.75, 2.09, and 2.46 (on the scale used, 1.00 represents the most favorable and 5.00 the least favorable evaluation possible). In addition, the data show very limited inter-unit variability with reference to the quality of care criterion (unit mean scores range from 1.33 to 2.00), suggesting a good deal of uniformity among emergency units in this respect, but considerably more variability with reference to promptness and to cost.

The corresponding evaluations by the supervising nurses and hospital administrators (data not shown), moreover, agree with these evaluations by

TABLE 90. APPROPRIATENESS OF THE MEDICAL TREATMENT AND NURSING CARE PROCEDURES USED IN THE VARIOUS EMERGENCY UNITS, AS ASSESSED BY THE PHYSICIANS (MDS) WHO WORK THERE[a]

Hospital Emergency Units (EU's) Involved		Level of Appropriateness of Procedures With Respect to Enabling the Staff to Provide Care:		
		of the Highest Quality Possible	as Promptly as it Should be Provided	at the Lowest Cost Possible
ALL EU'S IN THE STUDY SAMPLE (N=30 Hospital EU's)	*Mean:* *Range:*	1.75 (1.33-2.00)	2.09 (1.20-3.00)	2.46 (1.50-3.17)
YOUR HOSPITAL'S EU				
EU's in:				
Small Hospitals (n=14)		1.84	2.19	2.57
Medium Hospitals (n=9)		1.67	1.94	2.41
Large Hospitals (n=7)		1.68	2.10	2.31
EU's in:				
Church Operated Hospitals (n=9)		1.82	2.21	2.45
Osteopathic Hospitals (n=3)		1.89	1.99	2.63
All Other Hospitals (n=18)		1.69	2.05	2.43
EU's Located in:				
SMSA (urban) Areas (n=21)		1.74	2.04	2.44
Non-SMSA Areas (n=9)		1.78	2.21	2.50
EU's in Hospitals Having:				
Medical Teaching Affiliations (n=17)		1.71	2.05	2.47
No Medical Teaching Affiliations (n=13)		1.80	2.15	2.45
EU's in Hospitals Having:				
Emergency Personnel Training Programs (n=15)		1.69	2.02	2.39
No Training Programs (n=15)		1.81	2.17	2.52

Table 90 Continues

TABLE 90
(Continued)

---

^aThe results, presented here in the form of mean scores, are based on the responses of MDS from the various emergency units to the following set of questions: "Please think of the various medical treatment and nursing care procedures used in this emergency unit. On the whole, are most of them appropriate from the standpoint of enabling the staff to provide care of the highest quality possible?" The identical question was then repeated with reference to "care at the lowest cost possible," and with reference to "care as promptly as it should be provided." The response alternatives for these questions were: (1) All or almost all of (these) procedures are very appropriate, (2) the large majority of them are, (3) the majority of them are, (4) about half of them are, and (5) fewer than half of them are very appropriate. Mean scores were first computed separately for each emergency unit and then averaged for the EU's in the particular categories shown. The lower the mean scores, the more procedures are seen as "very appropriate" (i.e., the higher the overall level of appropriateness) by the MDS.

physicians (except that inter-unit variability with reference to each of the three criteria is greater in the data from SRNS and from HAS than it is in the data from MDS). According to all three groups, the procedures in the various units are the most appropriate with respect to enabling the staff to provide care of the highest quality possible, and are the least appropriate with respect to cost. The findings from the present series also suggest that, on the average, clinical efficiency probably surpasses the economic efficiency of the emergency units studied. The situation of individual units, however, may not conform to the general pattern.

It is also interesting that the above pattern (that more of the procedures are regarded as "very appropriate" with reference to quality than to promptness than to cost) also holds for each of the various groupings of emergency units considered separately, without exception. When the various groupings are properly compared to each other, moreover, there are no significant differences between groupings in the evaluations provided by physicians with reference to any of the three criteria (see Table 90). Some weak trends, however, are apparent. First, regardless of the referent criterion, the procedures are on the average evaluated least favorably by the physicians in the emergency units of small (rather than medium-size or large) hospitals. They are also evaluated slightly more favorably in urban than in non-urban area units, and in the units of hospitals which have emergency personnel training programs compared to hospitals which do not. The same is true, but with reference to quality and promptness only, in the units of hospitals which have medical teaching affiliations compared to those which do not (with reference to cost, there is no difference).

The data from hospital administrators (not shown) indicate no differences between emergency unit groupings in the evaluation of procedures with respect to the quality of care criterion. With respect to the cost of care, administrators evaluate the procedures more favorably, on the average, in the EU's of hospitals which are not church operated (excluding the osteopathic institutions) than in the EU's of either the church operated or the osteopathic hospitals. And with respect to the promptness of care, they evaluate the procedures more favorably, on the average, in: the urban than the non-urban area EU's; the EU's of hospitals which have medical teaching affiliations compared to those which do not; the EU's of hospitals which are not church operated compared to those which are; and in the EU's of large compared to medium-size hospitals.

Finally, the corresponding data from the supervising nurses indicate that, with reference to the quality of care, the procedures are evaluated more favorably in the emergency units of large than of medium-size hospitals (procedures in the latter are also evaluated somewhat less favorably than they are for the units of small hospitals). With reference to the promptness of care, the procedures are evaluated more favorably in the EU's of large than in the EU's of either the medium-size or the small hospitals (between the latter two groupings there is no difference). And with reference to the cost of care, they are evaluated more favorably in the EU's of both large and small hospitals than in the EU's of medium-size hospitals, and in the EU's of church operated hospitals than the EU's of hospitals which are not church operated (both osteopathic and non-osteopathic).

<u>The performance of care procedures</u>. Just as the physicians (MDS) were asked their evaluations of the <u>appropriateness</u> of clinical procedures, the registered nurses (RNS) working in the various units were asked their evaluations of <u>how well the same procedures are being performed</u> with reference to the same three

criteria -- the quality, promptness, and cost of care. The findings from these data about the quality of performance of medical treatment and nursing care procedures are presented in Table 91. Overall, the results concerning the performance of procedures parallel those about the appropriateness of procedures very closely.

Considering first all of the 30 EU's in the sample, the results show that clinical procedures are performed slightly better than "very well" (the overall mean score is 1.81), on the average, from the standpoint of providing care of the <u>highest quality possible</u>. The same procedures are performed almost "very well" (2.27), on the average, from the standpoint of providing care <u>as promptly as it should be provided</u>. And they are performed at a level midway between "very well" and "fairly well" (2.57) from the standpoint of providing care <u>at the lowest cost possible</u>.

Again, in other words, the procedures are performed best with respect to the quality of care and least well with respect to the cost of care. Moreover, on the average, they are performed significantly better with reference to quality than to promptness, and significantly better with reference to promptness than with reference to cost. These patterns are the same as those previously found concerning the appropriateness of procedures. Appropriateness and quality of performance are thus mutually reinforcing.

Across individual emergency units, the range of mean scores concerning the quality of the performance of procedures is relatively high when promptness is the referent criterion (1.40-3.17), suggesting major differences among the units, moderate when cost is the referent criterion (2.00-3.20), and relatively low when the quality of care is the referent criterion (1.50-2.40). In some of the units, the procedures are performed even more poorly than just "fairly well," both with respect to the promptness and to the cost of

TABLE 91. THE QUALITY OF PERFORMANCE OF THE MEDICAL TREATMENT AND NURSING CARE PROCEDURES USED IN EMERGENCY UNITS, AS EVALUATED BY THE REGISTERED NURSES (RNS) WHO WORK THERE[a]

Hospital Emergency Units (EU's) Involved		How Well the Procedures are Performed With Respect to Providing Patient Care:		
		of the Highest Quality Possible	as Promptly as it Should be Provided	at the Lowest Cost Possible
ALL EU'S IN THE STUDY SAMPLE (N=30 Hospital EU's)	Mean: Range:	1.81 (1.50-2.40)	2.27 (1.40-3.17)	2.57 (2.00-3.20)
YOUR HOSPITAL'S EU				
EU's in:				
Small Hospitals (n=14)		1.84	2.41	2.49
Medium Hospitals (n=9)		1.79	2.21	2.73
Large Hospitals (n=7)		1.78	2.06	2.52
EU's in:				
Church Operated Hospitals (n=9)		1.95	2.59	2.40
Osteopathic Hospitals (n=3)		1.74	1.96	2.53
All Other Hospitals (n=18)		1.76	2.16	2.65
EU's Located in:				
SMSA (urban) Areas (n=21)		1.82	2.15	2.59
Non-SMSA Areas (n=9)		1.80	2.56	2.52
EU's in Hospitals Having:				
Medical Teaching Affiliations (n=17)		1.78	2.20	2.65
No Medical Teaching Affiliations (n=13)		1.85	2.36	2.46
EU's in Hospitals Having:				
Emergency Personnel Training Programs (n=15)		1.83	2.21	2.57
No Training Programs (n=15)		1.80	2.33	2.56

Table 91 Continues

TABLE 91
(Continued)

---

^aThe results, presented here in the form of mean scores, are based on the responses of RNS from the various emergency units to the following set of questions: "On the whole, in this emergency unit, how well performed (or how well carried out) are the medical treatment and nursing care procedures from the standpoint of providing patient care of the highest quality possible?" The identical question was then repeated with reference to "care at the lowest cost possible," and with reference to "care as promptly as it should be provided." The response alternatives for these questions were: (1) The large majority of these procedures are extremely well performed, (2) very well performed, (3) fairly well performed, (4) not so well performed, and (5) not performed well at all. Mean scores were first computed separately for each emergency unit and then averaged for the EU's in the particular categories shown. The lower the mean scores, the better the procedures are performed according to the RNS.

care, while in others they are performed "very well" or better. With respect to the quality of care, however, performance is generally better and more uniform across the EU's.

The results in Table 91 also show that the general pattern of findings which characterizes the total sample, as discussed above, also characterizes each of the various groupings of emergency units considered separately, with only two very minor deviations. (In the EU's of church operated hospitals, the procedures tend to be performed slightly better with respect to cost than to promptness, and in the non-urban area EU's they tend to be performed equally well with respect to cost and promptness, but in neither case is the difference significant.) Finally, the results show no significant differences from one grouping of units to another, either when the quality or when the cost of care is the referent criterion. But from the standpoint of the promptness of care, they show that the procedures are on the average better performed in the EU's of large than the EU's of small hospitals, in the EU's of hospitals which are not vs. those which are church operated, and in the urban compared to the non-urban area EU's. Apart from these differences, there are only a few inconsequential trends among emergency unit groupings.

Overall, based upon the measures examined in this section, when both the quality and the promptness of care are taken into account, the clinical efficiency of the emergency units studied appears to be moderately high on the average. It also appears to be higher than the economic efficiency of the units. The situation of individual units, however, may differ considerably from the general pattern.

Promptness of Medical Attention, Patient Waiting Time, and the Length of Patient Visits

The physicians (MDS) and registered nurses (RNS) working in the emergency units were also asked to estimate (a) the percent of patients visiting their respective units who were seen by a doctor within 15 minutes after arrival, and (b) the average length of patient visits ("from time-in to time-out") in a typical day. Similarly, the patients (PATS) included in the study were asked about their own waiting time and length of visit. The data from these questions are discussed in the present section.

Table 92 shows the estimates by MDS and RNS of the percent of patients seen by a doctor within 15 minutes after arriving at the emergency unit. On the average, of the patients visiting the 30 EU's in the study, 60% were seen by a doctor within 15 minutes according to the data from MDS; but the figure varies widely across individual units, from a low of 30% to a high of 95%. Based on the data from RNS, the inter-unit variability is even greater, from 10% to 97%, while the average figure for all of the units is 53%. Thus, to the extent that promptness of medical attention is an indicator of clinical efficiency, the emergency units studied differ greatly from one another in their efficiency level according to these data.

Compared to the nurses, the physicians overestimate the percent of patients seen by a doctor within 15 minutes after arrival, both in the total sample and in each of the various groupings of emergency units (except in units with a high patient volume and the few osteopathic hospital units). The difference between the average estimates provided by the two groups is especially high (greater than 15%) in the case of EU's with a low patient volume, the EU's of church operated hospitals, and the non-urban area EU's. In all these cases, the MDS report the higher percentage figure, as they do when the total sample

TABLE 92. PERCENT OF THE PATIENTS VISITING THE VARIOUS EMERGENCY UNITS WHO WERE SEEN BY A DOCTOR WITHIN 15 MINUTES AFTER ARRIVAL[a]

Hospital Emergency Units (EU's) Involved	Percent of Patients Seen, According to	
	MDS	RNS
ALL EU'S IN THE STUDY SAMPLE (N=30 Hospital EU's) *Mean:* *Range:*	59.6% (30.3%-95.5%)	53.2% (10.2%-97.0%)
YOUR HOSPITAL'S EU		
EU's with:		
Low Patient Volume (n=10)	70.3	50.4
Medium Pat. Volume (n=10)	56.5	55.5
High Patient Volume (n=10)	52.1	53.7
EU's in:		
Church Operated Hospitals (n=9)	57.3	39.5
Osteopathic Hospitals (n=3)	50.5	63.5
All Other Hospitals (n=18)	62.4	58.3
EU's Located in:		
SMSA (urban) Areas (n=21)	60.5	59.2
Non-SMSA Areas (n=9)	57.6	39.2
EU's in Hospitals Having:		
Medical Teaching Affiliations (n=17)	54.9	51.8
No Medical Teaching Affiliations (n=13)	65.8	55.0
EU's in Hospitals Having:		
Emergency Personnel Training Programs (n=15)	62.9	57.5
No Training Programs (n=15)	56.4	48.9

[a]These results are based on estimates provided by the physicians (MDS) and registered nurses (RNS) working in the various emergency units. Using these estimates, mean percentage figures were first computed separately for each emergency unit and then averaged for the EU's in the particular categories shown. The _higher_ the percentage figure, the _larger_ the proportion of patients who were seen by a doctor within 15 minutes after arriving at the emergency unit.

is considered, but in the latter case the difference between MDS and RNS amounts to just over 6%.

Based on the data from MDS (and as reflected in the present measure), the promptness of medical attention is greatest on the average in the EU's which have a low patient volume and least in the EU's of osteopathic hospitals (70.3% vs. 50.5%), with the other groupings of units occupying intermediate positions. But, based on the data from RNS, it is greatest in the EU's of osteopathic hospitals and least in the non-urban area EU's (63.5% vs. 39.2%). Obviously, nurses and physicians do not agree very well when some of the groupings of units are considered. On the other hand, they agree that (in varying degrees) a higher proportion of the patients were seen by a doctor within 15 minutes in the urban compared to the non-urban area EU's, in the EU's of hospitals with emergency personnel training programs compared to those without such programs, in the EU's of hospitals not having compared to those having medical teaching affiliations, and in the EU's of hospitals which are not church operated (excluding the osteopathic institutions) compared to those which are.

The average length of patient visit. The results on this measure, presented in Table 93, show that, compared to the nurses, the doctors consistently underestimate the average length of patient visits in their respective units, but the two groups of respondents are in remarkable agreement as to the groupings of units in which the length is longer or shorter. In this respect, the patterns of findings from the two sets of data are identical when the various groupings of units are properly compared to each other -- in spite of the fact that the estimates based on the data from MDS are lower than those based on the data from RNS for each and every grouping involved. As we will shortly see, moreover, the corresponding patterns of findings from the data provided

TABLE 93. AVERAGE LENGTH (IN MINUTES) OF PATIENT VISITS TO THE VARIOUS EMERGENCY UNITS IN A TYPICAL DAY[a]

Hospital Emergency Units (EU's) Involved		Average Visit Length, According to	
		MDS	RNS
ALL EU'S IN THE STUDY SAMPLE (N=30 Hospital EU's)	*Mean:* *Range:*	51 (35-109)	60 (42-121)
YOUR HOSPITAL'S EU			
EU's with:			
Low Patient Volume (n=10)		41	48
Medium Pat. Volume (n=10)		54	62
High Patient Volume (n=10)		58	68
EU's in:			
Church Operated Hospitals (n=9)		50	57
Osteopathic Hospitals (n=3)		53	67
All Other Hospitals (n=18)		51	60
EU's Located in:			
SMSA (urban) Areas (n=21)		54	61
Non-SMSA Areas (n=9)		45	57
EU's in Hospitals Having:			
Medical Teaching Affiliations (n=17)		57	66
No Medical Teaching Affiliations (n=13)		44	51
EU's in Hospitals Having:			
Emergency Personnel Training Programs (n=15)		53	64
No Training Programs (n=15)		50	56

[a] These results are based on estimates provided by the physicians (MDS) and registered nurses (RNS) working in the various emergency units. The estimates were given in number of minutes and were for the average duration ("from time-in to time-out") of all patient visits to the emergency unit in "a typical day." Using these estimates, mean numbers of minutes were first computed separately for each of the emergency units and then averaged for the EU's in the particular categories shown. The greater the mean number of minutes, the longer the patients had to stay from time of admission to time of discharge.

by the patients concerning the length of their visits (Table 94) are the same as those based on the data from the physicians and the nurses -- all three groups are in agreement.

The length of patient visits for the 30 EU's in the sample averages 51 minutes according to the MDS, and 60 minutes according to the RNS. The situation of individual emergency units differs greatly, however. The range across units is enormous, from 35 to 109 minutes based on the data from MDS and from 42 to 121 minutes based on the data from RNS (and the data from patients support the same conclusion). In either case, obviously there seems to be room for improvement in the situation of some of the units. This may be an important area for improvement, moreover, not only because the average length of patient visits may reflect the clinical efficiency of the units, but also because it is likely to have a significant impact on economic efficiency and on patient satisfaction (and probably also on social efficiency or staff satisfaction).

Yet, it should not be assumed that shorter average length is necessarily better than longer length, or vice versa, from the standpoint of high clinical efficiency. Unusually lengthy visits (e.g., visits averaging over 100 minutes in an emergency unit) in most cases probably reflect clinical inefficiency, but unusually short visits do not necessarily imply efficiency. More important, it may be that an "optimal length" range exists beyond which clinical efficiency suffers (i.e., technically, the relationship between length of visits and clinical efficiency may well be a curvilinear one), so that both very long and very short length could be equally undesirable from the standpoint of clinical efficiency. In the forthcoming analyses of the study, this hypothesis will be tested. In the meantime, due caution is required by all concerned when assessing the situation of an emergency unit based upon the average length of patient visits.

In any case, the results in Table 93 show that, according to both nurses and physicians, the average length of patient visits is significantly shorter in EU's with a low, compared to either a medium or a high, patient volume (between the latter two groupings the difference is small), and is longest in the high volume EU's. Similarly, it is significantly shorter, on the average, in the EU's of those hospitals which do not have medical teaching affiliations than those which do. And, in varying degrees, it tends to be shorter for non-urban than urban area EU's; for the EU's of hospitals which do not, compared to those which do, have emergency personnel training programs; and for the EU's of hospitals which are church operated compared to those which are not. For any one grouping of units, of course, the average length of patient visits is shorter based on the estimates provided by MDS than those provided by RNS, as already pointed out. (The difference between the two estimates is especially high in the case of the few osteopathic hospital units, and in the case of non-urban area units.)

The data from patients. The corresponding findings from the data provided by the patients (PATS) who completed questionnaires for the study (representing 28 of the 30 EU's in the sample) are presented in Table 94.

Very briefly, with respect to waiting time, the patients who had recently visited the various units report that, on the average, they had to wait 14 minutes after arrival before they were seen either by a nurse or by a doctor.[*] (The results in Table 92, it will be recalled, concerned waiting time before the patients were seen by a doctor.) Average waiting time, once again, varies enormously from one emergency unit to another, the range being from 1 minute

---

[*]The median of the mean scores of the 28 units on this measure is 9 minutes.

TABLE 94. WAITING TIME AFTER ARRIVAL AND THE TOTAL LENGTH OF THEIR EMERGENCY UNIT VISITS, AS REPORTED BY PATIENTS (PATS)[a]

Hospital Emergency Units (EU's) Involved		Average Waiting Time, in Minutes	Average Length of Patient Visits, in Minutes
ALL EU'S IN THE STUDY SAMPLE (N=28 Hospital EU's)	Mean: Range:	14 (1-41)	67 (30-120)
YOUR HOSPITAL'S EU			
EU's with:			
Low Patient Volume (n=9)		9	63
Medium Pat. Volume (n=10)		17	73
High Patient Volume (n=9)		15	67
EU's in:			
Church Operated Hospitals (n=8)		7	55
Osteopathic Hospitals (n=3)		18	75
All Other Hospitals (n=17)		16	73
EU's Located in:			
SMSA (urban) Areas (n=19)		15	67
Non-SMSA Areas (n=9)		12	67
EU's in Hospitals Having:			
Medical Teaching Affiliations (n=16)		17	72
No Medical Teaching Affiliations (n=12)		10	63
EU's in Hospitals Having:			
Emergency Personnel Training Programs (n=13)		14	71
No Training Programs (n=15)		14	65

Table 94 Continues

TABLE 94
(Continued)

---

[a]These results, reported here in the form of mean number of minutes, are based on the responses of patients (PATS) who had recently visited each emergency unit to a pair of questions. The first question was: "After arriving at the emergency room, about how long did you have to wait until you were seen by a nurse or a doctor? (Please write in the approximate number of minutes you had to wait.)" The second question was: "All in all, about how much time did you spend in the emergency room during your visit? In other words, how long did your visit last from the time you arrived there until you were discharged from the emergency room?" The response alternatives provided ranged from (1) about 15 minutes, (2) about 30 minutes,... to (9) about 3 hours, and (10) more than 3 hours. Using the data from each question (after conversion to number of minutes in the case of the second question), mean scores were first computed separately for each emergency unit and then averaged for the EU's in the particular categories shown. (Two of the 30 institutions did not allow patient participation in the study and are therefore excluded.)

to 41 minutes. Generally, however, patients report that they had to wait significantly longer (on the average) in: the EU's of hospitals with than without medical teaching affiliations (on this, PATS agree with the comparable estimates provided by MDS and by RNS); EU's with a medium or high, compared to a low, patient volume (again PATS, MDS, and RNS are in agreement); and the EU's of hospitals which are not, compared to those which are, church operated, (in this case the other two groups of respondents are not in agreement with the patients).

With respect to the total length of their visits, Table 94 shows that, as reported by the patients, the length of visits in the emergency units studied averages 67 minutes (compared to 60 minutes according to the nurses and 51 minutes according to the doctors, as discussed earlier). The range across individual units is again great, from 30 to 120 minutes (and fairly similar to the range based on the corresponding data from RNS and from MDS). Generally, the average length of emergency unit visits, as reported by patients, is significantly shorter in: the EU's of hospitals which do not have, compared to those which do, medical teaching affiliations; the EU's of hospitals which are, compared to those which are not, church operated; and in EU's which have a low, compared to a medium, patient volume. (In all of these cases, the patients again agree with the doctors and with the nurses.) A few more, but minor, differences concerning the average length of patient visits may be seen in Table 94.

Finally, viewed in their entirety, the findings on the measures included in the present section suggest considerable differences in clinical efficiency among the emergency units studied. The precise meaning of the particular differences found, however, can not be determined without further analysis of the data. Nor could it be determined independently of the other results included in the present chapter. Moreover, the meaning of these differences should be assessed in the context of the earlier findings (see Chapter 1) concerning the composition of patient in-puts, or workload, in the various units, the findings concerning available staff resources (see Chapter 2), and the findings concerning patient satisfaction (see Chapter 8). Even then, of course, readers should exercise prudence and caution in interpreting the results about patient waiting time and length of visit.

Assessment by Patients of Certain Aspects of Care Process and Outcome

One of the questions asked of the patients (PATS) who participated in the study was: "Thinking of the staff who took care of you in the emergency room, to what extent did they really seem to know what they were doing?" Moreover, a similar question ("As far as you can tell..., how well do the people who work in this emergency unit really seem to know what they are doing?") was asked of the community respondents (CRS) who participated in the study. The results summarizing the data from both of these questions are presented in Table 95. (Results concerning patient satisfaction, which may also relate to clinical efficiency, have been presented in Chapter 8.)

Based on these data from patients, the overall mean score for the 28 units involved is 1.83, indicating that the staff "really" seemed to know what they were doing "to a great extent" (in fact slightly better). And the corresponding mean score based on the data from the community respondents concerning all 30 units in the sample is almost as favorable, namely 2.05 (which indicates that the staff "really" knew what they were doing "very well"). In both cases, however, there is considerable inter-unit variability. In the case of the data from patients, unit mean scores range from 1.00 (or the staff knew "to a very great extent") to 2.50 (or the staff knew midway between "to a very

TABLE 95. ASSESSMENT BY EMERGENCY UNIT PATIENTS (PATS) AND COMMUNITY RESPONDENTS (CRS) OF CERTAIN ASPECTS OF STAFF COMPETENCE[a]

		Extent to Which the Staff "Know What They are Doing" According to	
Hospital Emergency Units (EU's) Involved		CRS[b]	PATS[c]
ALL EU'S IN THE STUDY SAMPLE (N=30 Hospital EU's)	*Mean:* *Range:*	2.05 (1.25-3.00)	1.83 (1.00-2.50)
YOUR HOSPITAL'S EU			
EU's with:			
Low Patient Volume (n=10)		1.97	1.85
Medium Pat. Volume (n=10)		2.02	1.87
High Patient Volume (n=10)		2.17	1.78
EU's in:			
Church Operated Hospitals (n=9)		2.18	1.78
Osteopathic Hospitals (n=3)		2.06	1.96
All Other Hospitals (n=18)		1.99	1.83
EU's Located in:			
SMSA (urban) Areas (n=21)		2.11	1.87
Non-SMSA Areas (n=9)		1.91	1.76
EU's in Hospitals Having:			
Medical Teaching Affiliations (n=17)		2.02	1.78
No Medical Teaching Affiliations (n=13)		2.09	1.91
EU's in Hospitals Having:			
Emergency Personnel Training Programs (n=15)		2.05	1.70
No Training Programs (n=15)		2.05	1.95

Table 95 Continues

TABLE 95
(Continued)

---

^aThe results, presented here in the form of mean scores, are based on data obtained from patients (PATS) who had recently visited the various emergency units and from selected community respondents (CRS) associated with each unit.

^bThese respondents were asked the following open-ended question: "As far as you can tell from your work contacts with them, how well do the people who work in this emergency unit really seem to know what they are doing?" Their responses were coded on a five-point scale ranging from "(1) Extremely well,"... to "(5) not well at all."

^cThese respondents were asked: "...Thinking of the staff who took care of you in the emergency room, to what extent did they really seem to know what they were doing?" The response alternatives ranged from "(1) To a very great extent," ... to "(5) to a very small extent or not at all." (Two of the 30 institutions did not allow patient participation and are therefore excluded.)

great extent" and "to a fair extent"). And in the case of the data from community respondents, they range from 1.25 (or almost "extremely well") to 3.00 (or exactly "fairly well"). On the present measure, therefore, some of the emergency units are doing considerably better than others according to either group of respondents.

The results in Table 95 also show that, regardless of which group of respondents is assessing the situation, the various groupings of emergency units do not differ significantly from one another when properly compared. On the average, the mean score of the units in each grouping does not differ much from the corresponding score of the units in the comparison groupings, or from the overall mean score of all the units in the sample. Therefore, the situation is equally favorable among groupings, although it varies from one individual emergency unit to another.

The next table, Table 96, summarizes the data from patients (PATS) to an even more interesting, and perhaps more important, question. The question was: "In your opinion, are there any things that the (emergency unit) staff could have done, but did not do, to give you better care?" Table 96 shows the percent of the patients from the various units who responded "yes" (as opposed to either "no" or "I don't know") to this particular question.

It is rather interesting, and perhaps disconcerting, that on the average 26% of the patients visiting the various emergency units believe that the staff could have done more to give them better care (but did not do so). Even more remarkable, the percent of patients who believe this to be the case ranges phenomenally across individual units from a low of 0% to a high of 100% -- the range could not possibly be any greater. According to this measure of clinical efficiency, therefore, there seems to be enormous room for improvement in a great many of the emergency units studied.

TABLE 96. PERCENT OF EMERGENCY UNIT PATIENTS (PATS) REPORTING THAT THE STAFF COULD HAVE DONE MORE FOR THEM, AND PERCENT REPORTING POST-VISIT "COMPLICATIONS"[a]

Hospital Emergency Units (EU's) Involved		Percent of Patients (PATS) Reporting That	
		The EU Staff Could Have Done More for Them[b]	They Experienced Post-Visit "Complications"[c]
ALL EU'S IN THE STUDY SAMPLE (N=28 Hospital EU's)	Mean: Range:	26.3% (0%-100.0%)	25.6% (0%-57.9%)
YOUR HOSPITAL'S EU			
EU's with:			
Low Patient Volume (n=9)		36.5	25.4
Medium Pat. Volume (n=10)		23.1	27.9
High Patient Volume (n=9)		19.6	23.2
EU's in:			
Church Operated Hospitals (n=8)		30.6	16.9
Osteopathic Hospitals (n=3)		36.8	36.9
All Other Hospitals (n=17)		22.4	27.6
EU's Located in:			
SMSA (urban) Areas (n=19)		28.9	25.0
Non-SMSA Areas (n=9)		20.9	26.9
EU's in Hospitals Having:			
Medical Teaching Affiliations (n=16)		21.6	28.3
No Medical Teaching Affiliations (n=12)		32.6	22.0
EU's in Hospitals Having:			
Emergency Personnel Training Programs (n=13)		23.0	25.5
No Training Programs (n=15)		29.2	25.6

Table 96 Continues

TABLE 96
(Continued)

---

^{a}The results are here presented in the form of mean percentages. Percentage figures were first computed separately for each emergency unit and then averaged for the EU's in the particular categories shown. (Two of the 30 institutions did not allow patient participation and are therefore excluded.)

^{b}These results are based on the responses of recent patients (PATS) to the following question: "In your opinion, are there any things the emergency unit staff could have done, but did not do, to give you better care? The percent of each unit's patients responding Yes (as opposed to "no" or "I don't know") was used in performing the computations described in footnote "a."

^{c}These results are based on the responses of recent patients (PATS) to the following question: "During the first week after you returned home following your visit to the emergency room, did you have any difficulties or complications related to the problem for which you had gone there in the first place?" The percent of each unit's patients responding Yes was used in performing the computations described in footnote "a."

On the average, significantly more of the patients who visited the EU's of osteopathic and (to a lesser extent) church operated hospitals believe that the staff could have done more for them, compared to the patients who visited the EU's of other hospitals. Similarly, significantly more of the patients who visited EU's with a low patient volume, compared to EU's with either a medium or a high patient volume, believe that the staff could have done more to give them better care. Further, a significantly greater proportion of the patients who visited the urban, compared to the non-urban area units believe the same thing, and the same applies to patients who visited the EU's of hospitals with no medical teaching affiliations compared to hospitals with such affiliations. Finally, a similar trend is evident when comparing the patients visiting the EU's of hospitals with no emergency personnel training programs vs. the EU's of hospitals having such programs. Accordingly, the item under discussion seems to be a very discriminating measure not only among individual emergency units but also between groupings of units.

Table 96 also summarizes the data from an additional, and equally interesting question. Specifically, these data were provided by the patients (PATS) in response to the following question: "During the <u>first week</u> after you returned home following your visit to the emergency room did you have any difficulties or complications related to the problem for which you had gone there in the first place?"

On the average, again 26% of the patients visiting the various emergency units in the sample report that they experienced post-visit complications or difficulties. This figure ranges across individual units from a low of 0% to a high of 58%, suggesting that the outcome may have been much less favorable, on the average, for the patients visiting some of the units than for the patients visiting other of the units in the sample.

The results in Table 96 also show that, on the average, a higher proportion of the patients visiting the EU's of osteopathic hospitals than the EU's of other not church operated hospitals report post-visit difficulties, and a higher proportion of those visiting the EU's of the latter hospitals report such difficulties compared to patients visiting the EU's of church operated hospitals. Similarly, a higher proportion of the patients visiting the EU's of hospitals having medical teaching affiliations report post-visit difficulties compared to the patients visiting the EU's of hospitals not having such affiliations. Interestingly, however, no differences on the present measure are found in relation to the patient volume of the units, the location of the units, or the presence/absence of emergency personnel training programs.

The most important findings, in Table 96, of course, concern the extremely great variability among individual emergency units with respect to the percent of patients reporting post-visit difficulties or complications, and also with respect to the percent of patients who believe that the staff <u>could</u> have done, but did not do, more to give them better care. In both respects, there are apparently major differences in the clinical efficiency of the emergency units studied.

Patient Death Rates

Although deaths among people who visit hospital emergency units for care, or are taken there for medical attention, are a relatively infrequent phenomenon, and although they do not necessarily mean poor care when they occur, it was thought advisable at least to examine patient death rates. Possible differences in this area among the emergency units studied, it was decided, should be at least interesting to ascertain. And, if found to exist, their implications with regard to the clinical efficiency of the units also should be traced out eventually (e.g., by studying these differences in relation to differences among the units on other pertinent measures such as those included in the present chapter and the measures on patient composition included in Chapter 1).

Accordingly, data on death rates were collected. Only 23 of the 30 institutions in the study, however, were able to provide the necessary information from their records (RECS). The information was supplied in terms of numbers of deaths and then was converted by the research staff, for purposes of reporting, into death rates per thousand patient visits. Death rates were computed separately based on the number of patients who were pronounced "dead on arrival" and on the number of patients who died "while in the emergency unit." In both cases, the data are for "the most recent quarter."

The death rates for the 23 emergency units for which data were made available are summarized in Table 97. The results show that, during the most recent quarter, the number of patients who were classified as dead on arrival averages 2.59 per thousand patient visits for the 23 EU's involved. Across individual emergency units, the figure ranges from 0 to 11.5 deaths per thousand patient visits, indicating very substantial inter-unit variability on this measure.

With reference to the various groupings of emergency units, the results show that, on the average, this particular death rate is greater for EU's with a low patient volume, than it is for EU's with a medium patient volume, than it is for EU's with a high patient volume. It is also greater for the EU's of the non-osteopathic hospitals, both church operated and not church operated (between these two groupings there is no difference), than for the EU's of osteopathic hospitals, and for the EU's of hospitals which have compared to those which do not have medical teaching affiliations. And it is just slightly greater for the EU's of hospitals which do not have emergency personnel training programs compared to those which do.

TABLE 97. DEATH RATES PER THOUSAND PATIENT VISITS TO THE VARIOUS EMERGENCY UNITS DURING THE MOST RECENT QUARTER[a]

Hospital Emergency Units (EU's) Involved		Number of Patients Per 1,000 Visits Who	
		Were "Dead on Arrival"[b]	Who Died While in the Emergency Unit[c]
ALL EU'S IN THE STUDY SAMPLE (N=23 Hospital EU's)	Mean:	2.59	0.78
	Range:	(0-11.5)	(0-4.59)
YOUR HOSPITAL'S EU			
EU' with:			
Low Patient Volume (n=8)		3.28	0.98
Medium Pat. Volume (n=8)		2.44	0.85
High Patient Volume (n=7)		1.98	0.44
EU's in:			
Church Operated Hospitals (n=7)		2.68	0.42
Osteopathic Hospitals (n=3)		2.10	0.48
All Other Hospitals (n=13)		2.66	1.09
EU's Located in:			
SMSA (urban) Areas (n=18)		2.57	0.90
Non-SMSA Areas (n=5)		2.68	0.41
EU's in Hospitals Having:			
Medical Teaching Affiliations (n=12)		2.81	0.90
No Medical Teaching Affiliations (n=11)		2.36	0.64
EU's in Hospitals Having:			
Emergency Personnel Training Programs (n=12)		2.49	0.58
No Training Programs (n=11)		2.70	0.99

Table 97 Continues

TABLE 97
(Continued)

---

[a] These findings are based on data from hospital records (RECS) supplied by the various institutions. Seven of the 30 institutions in the sample were unable to provide the necessary information and are therefore excluded.

[b] These rates were computed for the "most recent quarter," separately for each emergency unit, as follows: the total number of patients classified as "dead on arrival" was first divided by the total number of patient visits during the period, and then the resulting product was multiplied by 1,000. Subsequently, the obtained rates were averaged for the emergency units in each of the groupings shown.

[c] These rates were computed for the "most recent quarter," separately for each emergency unit, as follows: the total number of patients who died while in the emergency unit was divided by the total number of patient visits during the period, and then the resulting product was multiplied by 1,000. Subsequently, the obtained rates were averaged for the emergency units in each grouping shown.

The results in Table 97 also show the number of deaths per thousand patient visits considering only patients who died "while in the emergency unit" (who were not dead on arrival). This second death rate is much smaller than the first -- in fact only 30% the size of the first. Specifically, for the 23 EU's involved, the number of patients per thousand visits who died while in the emergency unit during the most recent quarter averages less than 1, or 0.78 exactly. Yet, the range across individual emergency units is considerable, from 0 to 4.59 deaths per thousand patient visits.

Based on the number of patients who died while in the emergency unit, the death rate is considerably greater on the average for EU's with a low, and also a medium patient volume, than for EU's with a high patient volume. Similarly, it is considerably greater for the EU's of the non-osteopathic hospitals which are not church operated than for the EU's of either the osteopathic or the church operated hospitals. Further, it is considerably greater for urban than for non-urban area EU's. And it is greater, but to a lesser extent, for the EU's of hospitals which have compared to those which do not have teaching affiliations, and for the EU's of hospitals which do not have emergency personnel training programs compared to those which do.

It is also interesting that the patterns of findings concerning the two death rate measures are basically the same when the following groupings of emergency units are compared: units with a high vs. a medium or low patient volume; the units of hospitals with vs. without medical teaching affiliation; and the units of hospitals with vs. without emergency personnel training programs. The patterns are not the same for the two death rates when emergency units are compared on the basis of location or on the basis of institutional control. The meaning of the differences and similarities found can not be determined at this stage of the research and must await more intensive analysis of the data. In the meantime, it is well to bear in mind that the patterns and differences found are based on data from only 23 of the EU's in the sample as well as on very small numbers of deaths. Even on the basis of such small numbers, on the other hand, the emergency units involved show considerable variability on both of the death rate measures discussed.

The Quality of Medical Management and Nursing Care for Patients with Certain Conditions

Because the composition of patient workload may vary from one emergency unit to another, significantly in some cases, in terms of such things as the proportion of patients who arrive in life-threatening condition or present complex medical requirements (see Chapter 1 for some relevant data), certain direct measures of the quality of medical and nursing care were needed with reference to specific categories of patients. Accordingly, the physicians (MDS) and the registered nurses (RNS) working in the various emergency units were asked, among other things, for their evaluations of (a) the quality of medical management, and (b) the quality of nursing care provided in their respective units for patients with the following selected conditions:

(1) Acute myocardial infarction, cardiac arrest, and ventricular fibrillation;

(2) Lacerations of the face or neck involving more than skin;

(3) Acute psychiatric illnesses -- suicide (depression), acute psychoses;

(4) Fractures or dislocations; and,

(5) Acute upper respiratory infections with stridor, epiglotitis, or asthmatic bronchitis.

Table 98 summarizes the physicians' (MDS) evaluations of the quality of medical management of cases in each of these categories. Considering all 30

EU's in the sample, the results show that, on the average, myocardial and related cases are the best managed from a medical standpoint. The overall mean score of the units for such cases is 1.82, indicating that these cases are managed slightly better than "very well." It is also interesting, however, that in some of the units the medical management of these cases is rated almost "excellent" on the average, while in other units it is rated only slightly better than just "good" (see the range of mean scores in Table 98).

At the other extreme, the quality of medical management of psychiatric cases in the 30 EU's is rated only slightly better than "good" (the overall mean score is 2.70) on the average. Moreover, inter-unit variability on this measure is extremely high. The range of unit mean scores is from 1.60 (indicating that the medical management of psychiatric cases is rated by the physicians midway between "excellent" and "very good") to 4.00 (indicating that it is rated only as "fair"). Obviously, myocardial infarction and similar other cardiac cases are managed significantly better than are acute psychiatric cases by the medical staffs of the emergency units studied.

The quality of medical management for the remaining three categories of patients -- lacerations..., fractures..., and upper respiratory infections... -- is rated equally favorably on the average. It is also rated more favorably (on the average) than is the management of acute psychiatric cases but somewhat less favorably than is the management of cardiac cases. The situation of individual emergency units, however, varies.

The results in Table 98 also show some differences among some of the groupings of emergency units. Briefly, the medical management of myocardial infarctions and similar cardiac cases is significantly better, on the average, in: the EU's of large compared to those of either medium-size or small hospitals (between the latter two groupings there is no difference); the EU's of

TABLE 98. THE QUALITY OF MEDICAL MANAGEMENT OF EMERGENCY UNIT PATIENTS IN SELECTED CONDITIONS, AS EVALUATED BY THE PHYSICIANS (MDS) WORKING IN THE UNITS[a]

Hospital Emergency Units (EU's) Involved		Quality of Medical Management for Patients With				
		Myocardial Infarction...	Facial Lacerations...	Psychiatric Illnesses...	Fractures or Dislocations	Respiratory Infections...
ALL EU'S IN THE STUDY SAMPLE (N= 30 Hospital EU's)	Mean:	1.82	1.92	2.70	1.91	1.91
	Range:	(1.20-2.67)	(1.33-2.57)	(1.60-4.00)	(1.11-3.00)	(1.33-2.67)
YOUR HOSPITAL'S EU						
EU's in:						
Small Hospitals (n=14)		1.97	2.01	2.78	2.07	2.05
Medium Hospitals (n=9)		1.82	1.88	2.63	1.80	1.77
Large Hospitals (n=7)		1.53	1.80	2.62	1.71	1.81
EU's in:						
Church Operated Hospitals (n=9)		1.85	2.04	2.47	2.09	2.02
Osteopathic Hospitals (n=3)		2.11	2.06	3.06	1.78	1.94
All Other Hospitals (n=18)		1.76	1.84	2.75	1.84	1.85
EU's Located in:						
SMSA (urban) Areas (n=21)		1.82	1.92	2.81	1.83	1.88
Non-SMSA Areas (n=9)		1.83	1.93	2.44	2.09	1.97
EU's in Hospitals Having:						
Medical Teaching Affiliations (n=17)		1.68	1.80	2.76	1.78	1.80
No Medical Teaching Affiliations (n=13)		2.00	2.08	2.61	2.08	2.06
EU's in Hospitals Having:						
Emergency Personnel Training Programs (n=15)		1.77	1.83	2.62	1.82	1.91
No Training Programs (n=15)		1.88	2.01	2.77	1.99	1.91

[a] These findings, reported here in the form of mean scores, are based on the responses of MDS from the various emergency units to the following multiple-part question: "Please consider the patients in the categories specified who visited this emergency unit over the past four-six weeks. On the average, how well were these patients managed from a medical standpoint?" The response alternatives were: (1) The medical management of (these) patients was excellent, (2) very good, (3) good, (4) fair, and (5) rather poor. For each category of patients specified, mean scores were first computed separately for each emergency unit and then averaged for the EU's in each grouping shown. The patient categories in question were as follows: "Acute myocardial infarction, cardiac arrest, and ventricular fibrillation cases"; "Lacerations of the face or neck involving more than skin"; "Acute psychiatric illnesses -- suicide (depression), acute psychoses"; "Fractures or dislocations"; and "Acute upper respiratory infections with stridor, epiglotitis, and asthmatic bronchitis cases."

the non-osteopathic hospitals which are not church operated compared to those of osteopathic hospitals; and the EU's of hospitals which have medical teaching affiliations compared to those which do not. Similarly, the management of fractures and dislocations is better in the EU's of large than in the EU's of small hospitals. And the management of acute psychiatric cases is better in: the EU's of church operated hospitals compared to those of hospitals which are not church operated, and in non-urban compared to urban area EU's. The data also show a general trend for all or nearly all of the five categories of patients to be slightly better managed, on the average, in the units of hospitals which have medical teaching affiliations, or emergency personnel training programs, compared to those which do not, and in urban compared to non-urban area units.

Registered nurses (RNS) also were asked to rate the quality of medical management for patients in the categories specified (data not shown). Overall, the evaluations provided by the nurses are very similar to those provided by the physicians, except that they are even less favorable concerning psychiatric cases and also somewhat less favorable concerning upper respiratory infection cases. Also, inter-unit variability is higher in the data from RNS than in the data from MDS (except with respect to psychiatric cases). Apart from these minor exceptions, agreement between the two groups of respondents is remarkably high.

The quality of nursing care. Corresponding evaluations by the registered nurses (RNS) at the various units of the quality of nursing care provided to patients in the five categories are summarized in Table 99. According to the overall mean scores of the 30 EU's on this measure, the quality of nursing care is best (on the average) for acute myocardial infarction and the other cardiac cases (the mean score is 1.57) and poorest for acute psychiatric cases (2.93), with

TABLE 99. THE QUALITY OF NURSING CARE PROVIDED TO EMERGENCY UNIT PATIENTS IN SELECTED CONDITIONS, AS EVALUATED BY THE REGISTERED NURSES (RNS) WORKING IN THE UNITS[a]

Hospital Emergency Units (EU's) Involved		Myocardial Infarction...	Facial Lacerations...	Psychiatric Illnesses...	Fractures or Dislocations	Respiratory Infections...
ALL EU'S IN THE STUDY SAMPLE (N=30 Hospital EU's)	Mean:	1.57	1.88	2.93	1.86	2.01
	Range:	(1.20-1.90)	(1.33-2.50)	(2.33-3.79)	(1.33-2.57)	(1.40-2.56)
YOUR HOSPITAL'S EU						
EU's in:						
Small Hospitals (n=14)		1.65	1.98	2.99	1.94	2.08
Medium Hospitals (n=9)		1.58	1.92	2.96	1.93	2.02
Large Hospitals (n=7)		1.41	1.65	2.75	1.60	1.87
EU's in:						
Church Operated Hospitals (n=9)		1.67	1.96	2.93	1.99	2.11
Osteopathic Hospitals (n=3)		1.55	1.90	3.12	1.78	2.05
All Other Hospitals (n=18)		1.53	1.84	2.89	1.81	1.95
EU's Located in:						
SMSA (urban) Areas (n=21)		1.56	1.85	2.90	1.81	1.95
Non-SMSA Areas (n=9)		1.61	1.96	2.99	1.97	2.16
EU's in Hospitals Having:						
Medical Teaching Affiliations (n=17)		1.51	1.84	2.91	1.76	2.02
No Medical Teaching Affiliations (n=13)		1.65	1.93	2.95	1.99	2.01
EU's in Hospitals Having:						
Emergency Personnel Training Programs (n=15)		1.56	1.81	2.85	1.83	1.96
No Training Programs (n=15)		1.58	1.95	3.00	1.89	2.06

[a] These findings, reported here in the form of mean scores, are based on the responses of RNS from the various emergency units to the following multiple-part question: "Please consider the patients in the categories specified who visited this emergency unit over the past four-six weeks. How would you evaluate the quality of nursing care that, on the average, patients in these categories received while in this emergency unit?" The response alternatives ranged from: "(1) The quality of nursing care for (these) patients was excellent,"... to "(5) it was rather poor." For each category of patients specified, mean scores were first computed separately for each emergency unit and then averaged for the EU's in each grouping shown. The patient categories in question were as follows: "Acute myocardial infarction, cardiac arrest, and ventricular fibrillation cases"; "Lacerations of the face or neck involving more than skin"; "Acute psychiatric illnesses -- suicide (depression), acute psychoses"; "Fractures or dislocations"; and "Acute upper respiratory infections with stridor, epiglotitis, and asthmatic bronchitis cases."

the other three categories of patients occupying intermediate positions in this respect. This pattern is identical to that concerning the medical management of the same cases as evaluated by MDS (Table 98). The data also indicate that the RNS evaluate the quality of nursing care slightly less favorably for upper respiratory infection cases than for lacerations or fractures and dislocations, while the MDS evaluated the medical management of patients in these categories equally favorably.

The findings concerning the quality of nursing care (Table 99) in the various groupings of emergency units, moreover, also parallel those on medical management very closely. There is a general trend, applying to all five categories of patients, for the quality of nursing care to be somewhat better (on the average) in: the EU's of large, compared to those of medium and small hospitals; the EU's of the non-osteopathic hospitals which are not church operated compared to those of the remaining hospitals; the urban compared to the non-urban area EU's; and the EU's of hospitals which have medical teaching affiliations, or emergency personnel training programs, compared to those which do not. In a few cases, moreover, the difference is significant (e.g., regarding laceration cases and fracture or dislocation cases in the EU's of large vs. other hospitals).

The data also show that the range of scores across individual emergency units concerning the quality of nursing care for patients in the five categories is smaller (for every category) than the corresponding range of scores concerning the quality of medical management (comparing Table 99 to Table 98). This suggests that the quality of nursing care, as rated by the RNS, is relatively more uniform across emergency units than is the quality of medical management, as rated by the MDS.

Finally, corresponding ratings of the quality of nursing care were also obtained from the physicians (MDS) working in the various emergency units (data not shown). The pattern of results from these data, as well as the trends concerning differences in the quality of nursing care among emergency unit groupings, are again very similar to those discussed above based on the data from the RNS. Inter-unit variability concerning the quality of nursing care for each category of patients (except fractures or dislocations) however, is greater based on the data from MDS than it is based on the data from RNS. (Based upon the evaluations provided by the physicians, therefore, the quality of nursing care for patients in the five categories is not more uniform than the quality of medical management across the emergency units studied.)

Considering all of the findings from all of the measures discussed in the present section as a set, it would appear that the clinical efficiency of the emergency units studied is moderately high, on the average, but not very high, except perhaps with regard to the treatment of myocardial infarction and similar other cardiac cases. With regard to the treatment of acute psychiatric cases, clinical efficiency is relatively low on the average.

The Quality of Overall Medical Care and Overall Nursing Care

Assessments of the quality of overall medical care, and also overall nursing care, provided in the various emergency units were obtained from qualified respondents <u>other than the "performers" themselves</u>. Specifically, the selected hospital physicians (HMDS) and the registered nurses (RNS) were asked to rate, on the basis of their own experience and information, the quality of overall <u>medical care</u> that patients generally receive in each unit. And, similarly, the selected hospital physicians (HMDS) and the physicians working in the emergency units (MDS) were asked to rate the overall quality of <u>nursing care</u>. The results based on these data are all presented in Table 100.

TABLE 100. THE QUALITY OF OVERALL MEDICAL CARE AND OVERALL NURSING CARE PROVIDED IN THE VARIOUS EMERGENCY UNITS, AS RATED BY CERTAIN NURSE AND PHYSICIAN RESPONDENTS (OTHER THAN THE PERFORMERS IN EACH CASE)

Hospital Emergency Units (EU's) Involved		The Quality of Medical Care, According to[a]		The Quality of Nursing Care, According to[b]	
		HMDS	RNS	HMDS	MDS
ALL EU'S IN THE STUDY SAMPLE (N=30 Hospital EU's)	Mean: Range:	2.08 (1.22-3.14)	2.71 (1.75-3.57)	1.81 (1.43-2.43)	2.36 (1.60-3.00)
YOUR HOSPITAL'S EU					
EU's in:					
Small Hospitals (n=14)		2.17	2.81	1.87	2.51
Medium Hospitals (n=9)		2.02	2.83	1.82	2.20
Large Hospitals (n=7)		1.97	2.37	1.69	2.27
EU's in:					
Church Operated Hospitals (n=9)		2.09	2.80	1.82	2.53
Osteopathic Hospitals (n=3)		2.05	2.62	1.86	2.62
All Other Hospitals (n=18)		2.08	2.69	1.80	2.23
EU's Located in:					
SMSA (urban) Areas (n=21)		2.01	2.59	1.76	2.39
Non-SMSA Areas (n=9)		2.23	3.00	1.95	2.28
EU's in Hospitals Having:					
Medical Teaching Affiliations (n=17)		2.01	2.65	1.78	2.23
No Medical Teaching Affiliations (n=13)		2.17	2.79	1.86	2.53
EU's in Hospitals Having:					
Emergency Personnel Training Programs (n=15)		1.92	2.63	1.70	2.33
No Training Programs (n=15)		2.24	2.79	1.93	2.39

Table 100 Continues

TABLE 100
(Continued)

---

^aThese findings, presented here in the form of mean scores, are based on the responses of selected hospital physicians (HMDS) from the various institutions who were not working in the emergency units, and on the responses of registered nurses (RNS) working in the emergency units, to the following question: "On the basis of your experience and information, how would you rate the quality of medical care that patients generally receive in this emergency unit?" In the case of HMDS, the response alternatives ranged from "(1) Excellent,"... to "(5) rather poor." In the case of RNS they ranged from "(1) Outstanding," followed by "(2) excellent,"... to "(6) rather poor" and "(7) poor." Using the data from each group of respondents, corresponding mean scores were first computed separately for each emergency unit and then averaged for the EU's in the particular categories shown. The lower the mean scores, the better the quality of care.

^bThese findings, presented here in the form of mean scores, are based on the responses of selected hospital physicians (HMDS), and on the responses of physicians (MDS) working in the various emergency units, to the following question: "On the basis of your experience and information, how would you rate the quality of nursing care that patients generally receive in this emergency unit?" The response alternatives in the case of HMDS formed a five-point scale, and those for MDS formed a seven-point scale, as in footnote "a." Mean scores were computed also as described in footnote "a." The lower the mean scores, the better the quality of care.

On the average, the quality of medical care in the 30 EU's studied is rated almost as "very good" by the selected physician respondents (HMDS). The overall mean score is 2.08 (on a five-point scale). Across individual emergency units, however, there is substantial variability. The unit mean scores range from 1.22 (signifying almost "excellent" medical care) to 3.14 (signifying slightly less than just "good" care). As rated by the registered nurses, the quality of medical care in the various units is slightly better than "very good" on the average. The overall mean score for the 30 EU's is 2.71 (on a seven-point scale). Inter-unit variability again is substantial; based on the data from RNS, unit mean scores range from 1.75 (signifying "excellent"-plus care) to 3.57 (signifying a level of care midway between "very good" and "good").

The evaluations by RNS and HMDS are in agreement that the quality of medical care is generally better, on the average, in: the EU's of large compared to those of medium-size and small hospitals; in urban compared to non-urban area EU's; and in the EU's of hospitals which have medical teaching affiliations, or emergency personnel training programs, compared to those which do not. These findings from the data provided by HMDS and RNS, moreover, are consistent with those in the preceding section concerning the medical management of patients in the five specific categories discussed there, as evaluated by the RNS and the MDS.

The quality of overall nursing care. Table 100 also presents the corresponding findings about nursing care. According to the selected hospital physicians (HMDS), the quality of nursing care that patients in the various units generally receive is slightly better than "very good" on the average (and also somewhat better than the quality of medical care). The overall mean score for the 30 EU's is 1.81 (on a five-point scale). Again, however, in some of the units the quality of nursing care is rated higher than in others, although inter-unit variability is not great. The mean scores of the units range from 1.43 (signifying a level of quality midway between "very good" and "excellent") to 2.43 (signifying a level midway between "good" and "very good").

The physicians working in the emergency unit (MDS) rate the quality of nursing care in the various units as almost "excellent" on the average. The overall mean score for the 30 EU's is 2.36 (on a seven-point scale). Across individual emergency units the quality of nursing care that on the average patients receive varies from midway between "excellent" and "outstanding" (1.60) to exactly "very good" (3.00). Some units are doing a better job than others. It is also interesting that, on the average, the MDS rate the quality of nursing care higher than the RNS rate the quality of medical care in the various units.

Other findings in Table 100 indicate that the quality of nursing care is generally higher in the EU's of hospitals which have medical teaching affiliations compared to those which do not (the difference is significant according to the data from MDS but not according to the data from HMDS). Similarly, it is higher in the EU's of non-osteopathic hospitals which are not church operated, compared to the EU's of osteopathic and church operated hospitals (the difference is significant based on the data from MDS only; the data from HMDS show no difference). With reference to hospital size, the quality of nursing care is lowest, on the average, in the EU's of the small hospitals. Nursing care also tends to be slightly (or directionally) better in the EU's of hospitals which have, compared to those which do not have, emergency personnel training programs. Finally, with reference to urban vs. non-urban location the results based on the data from the two groups of respondents are mixed. Overall, these findings are generally quite consistent with those in the preceding section concerning the quality of nursing care provided to patients in the five selected categories specified, as evaluated both by the RNS and the MDS.

The Quality of Medical Care and Nursing Care as Compared to the Quality of Care in the Emergency Units of Other Hospitals

The final table, Table 101, in this chapter shows how the physicians (MDS) and registered nurses (RNS) who are working in the emergency units studied evaluate the quality of medical and nursing care (respectively) provided in their units compared to the quality of care provided in the emergency units of other hospitals with which the respondents are familiar. In previous studies, a measure of this type has been found to discriminate very well between more and less efficient organizations and to yield valid and reliable assessments.

Considering first the data from MDS about medical care in the emergency units studied, the results show that the quality of medical care is judged to be somewhat higher than "generally better" (but not quite "much better"), on the average, than it is in the emergency units of other hospitals. The overall mean score on this measure for the 30 EU's in the sample is 2.62 (on the scale used, a score of 2.00 corresponds exactly to "much better" and a score of 3.00 corresponds exactly to "generally better"). Across individual emergency units, the relevant mean scores range from 1.60 (indicating a level midway between "outstanding" and "much better" care compared to the care provided in other hospital EU's) to 4.29 (indicating a quality of care almost "about the same" as in other hospital EU's, but in the direction of a "somewhat poorer"

TABLE 101. THE QUALITY OF MEDICAL CARE AND NURSING CARE IN THE VARIOUS EMERGENCY UNITS COMPARED TO THE QUALITY OF CARE IN THE UNITS OF OTHER HOSPITALS

Hospital Emergency Units (EU's) Involved		The Comparative Quality of	
		Medical Care, as Assessed by MDS[a]	Nursing Care, as Assessed by RNS[b]
ALL EU'S IN THE STUDY SAMPLE (N=30 Hospital EU's)	*Mean:* *Range:*	2.62 (1.60-4.29)	2.58 (1.50-3.43)
YOUR HOSPITAL'S EU			
EU's with:			
Low Patient Volume (n=10)		3.03	2.79
Medium Pat. Volume (n=10)		2.54	2.58
High Patient Volume (n=10)		2.29	2.37
EU's in:			
Church Operated Hospitals (n=9)		2.80	2.66
Osteopathic Hospitals (n=3)		2.76	2.32
All Other Hospitals (n=18)		2.51	2.59
EU's Located in:			
SMSA (urban) Areas (n=21)		2.61	2.51
Non-SMSA Areas (n=9)		2.65	2.75
EU's in Hospitals Having:			
Medical Teaching Affiliations (n=17)		2.33	2.39
No Medical Teaching Affiliations (n=13)		3.00	2.83
EU's in Hospitals Having:			
Emergency Personnel Training Programs (n=15)		2.60	2.36
No Training Programs (n=15)		2.64	2.81

Table 101 Continues

TABLE 101
(Continued)

---

^aThese findings, presented here in the form of mean scores, are based on the responses of physicians (MDS) working in the various emergency units to the following question: "Considering the emergency units of all other hospitals with which you are familiar, how would you estimate the quality of medical care provided in this particular emergency unit?" The response alternatives were: (1) The quality of medical care in this emergency unit is outstanding compared to most other emergency units, (2) it is much better than in most other emergency units, (3) it is generally better, (4) it is about the same as in most other emergency units, (5) it is somewhat poorer, (6) it is generally poorer, and (7) The quality of medical care in this unit is much poorer compared to most other emergency units. Of all the MDS who completed questionnaires for the study 93% were able to answer this question. Mean scores were first computed separately for each emergency unit and then averaged for the EU's in each grouping shown. The lower the scores, the more favorably the quality of medical care compares to the quality provided in other institutions.

^bThese findings, presented here in the form of mean scores, are based on the responses of registered nurses (RNS) working in the various emergency units to an identical question to that in footnote "a" but with reference to the quality of nursing care (instead of medical care). Of all the RNS who completed questionnaires for the study, 77% were able to answer the question. The obtained data in their case were treated in exactly the same manner as described in footnote "a." The lower the mean scores, the more favorably the quality of nursing care compares to the quality provided in other institutions.

level). Inter-unit variability is thus very high, suggesting much higher quality of medical care for some compared to other emergency units.

The results also show that the quality of medical care comparatively rated is, on the average, better in EU's with a high patient volume than EU's with a medium or low patient volume (particularly low volume). Similarly, it is better in the EU's of hospitals which are not church operated (excluding osteopathic hospitals) than the EU's of hospitals which are. And it is significantly better in the EU's of hospitals which have medical teaching affiliations than the EU's of hospitals which do not have such affiliations. The results show no difference on the present measure between urban and non-urban area EU's or between the EU's of hospitals having and not having emergency personnel training programs. Overall, these findings on the comparative quality of medical care are quite consistent with the non-comparative evaluations of medical care discussed in the preceding two sections (i.e., the ratings on the quality of medical care by qualified respondents other than the performers, and also the more specific ratings by performers and other respondents of the quality of medical management for patients in selected categories).

The quality of nursing care comparatively evaluated. The corresponding findings about the quality of nursing care, as evaluated by the registered nurses (RNS), are remarkably similar to the findings just discussed about medical care, as evaluated by the physicians (MDS), except that inter-unit variability is smaller concerning nursing care (though still considerable).

Considering first the data for the total sample, the results show that the quality of nursing care comparatively evaluated is midway between "generally better" and "much better," on the average, than it is in the emergency units of other hospitals with which the respondents are familiar. The overall mean score for the 30 EU's in the sample is 2.58. Across individual units the mean scores range from 1.50 (indicating a level exactly midway between "outstanding" and "much better" care) to 3.43 (indicating a level midway between "generally better" and "about the same" as in the units of other hospitals).

The results in Table 101 also show that the comparative quality of nursing care is significantly better (on the average) in: EU's with a high than with a low patient volume; the EU's of hospitals with than without medical teaching affiliations; and the EU's of hospitals with than without emergency personnel training programs. There is also a tendency for the quality of nursing care, when comparatively evaluated, to be somewhat (though not significantly) better in the EU's of hospitals which are not church operated than the EU's of those which are, and in urban than non-urban area EU's. Finally, once again, these findings are quite consistent with the corresponding findings in the preceding two sections concerning the quality of nursing care in the emergency units studied.

Summary

In this final chapter of the report the preliminary findings of the study about the clinical efficiency of the emergency units in the sample were presented and discussed in detail. Using data from several independent sources, and taking into account several legitimate perspectives (including those of the clinical staff of the units, of peers and associates in the rest of the hospital, and of patients), a wide variety of carefully constructed measures and indicators were considered. The results, which will be further examined in the forthcoming and more detailed analyses of the research, were here presented not as final conclusions but for the benefit and timely consideration of interested readers. It is, therefore, hoped that readers will exercise due caution in assessing the significance of the findings for their own institutions and that, in the process, they will also take into account the results presented in the other chapters of the report.

Concluding Comments

The main purpose of this special report of preliminary research findings was to provide the thirty hospitals and emergency units which participated in the research with useful information about the organization and effectiveness of the emergency units involved. Based on data from the medical and nursing staff of the units and other relevant respondents, including patients, and data from institutional records, descriptive and evaluative findings were presented on a number of important variables in the following major areas: the basic characteristics of emergency units; staff resources; current goal priorities, problems, and strengths; leadership and influence patterns; work relations and problem solving within the units; work relations with the parent hospitals; relations with the outside community; the reputation of emergency units and patient satisfaction; staff attitudes and satisfaction, or social efficiency; financial aspects and economic efficiency; and clinical efficiency in its various aspects.

For nearly all of the measures included in the more than 100 tables of the report, results were shown not only for the 30 hospital emergency units (EU's) in the study sample as a group, but also for certain groupings of units based on: hospital size or (alternatively) emergency unit patient volume, urban vs. non-urban location, institutional control (church operated vs. osteopathic vs. other hospitals), medical teaching affiliation, and the presence/absence of emergency personnel training programs. Additionally, in the copies of the report being sent to each participating institution, corresponding results based exclusively on the individual institution's data were shown. Furthermore, since most of the variables covered were measured with data from two or more groups of respondents, the findings were shown separately for each source of data involved.

As presented, therefore, the findings permit a variety of useful comparisons to be made -- across respondent groups, among particular groupings of hospitals or emergency units, between each of these groupings and all of the institutions in the study sample (viewed as a group), and between a hospital's own emergency unit and other such units. Thus, each table of results also provides useful "norms" against which the participating institutions may compare and evaluate their own organizational situation. In addition, of course, findings included in any particular chapter may be compared to relevant findings included in other chapters.

The range of emergency unit scores on the measures examined in most cases indicates substantial inter-unit differences (i.e., a good deal of variation from one unit to another) in the areas studied. The magnitude of this variation or inter-unit variability, however, depends on the specific area, on the specific measure, and to an extent also on the specific source of the data (sometimes, for example, the different groups of respondents involved did not evaluate a particular aspect of emergency unit functioning equally favorably).

Differences between emergency units, such as the above, are of great value to comparative research, because they make it possible to test ideas, to ascertain the relationships which may exist among particular variables of interest, and to arrive at conclusions which explain the observed differences that characterize the organizations under study. In short, they make possible many important analyses from which new knowledge and hypotheses can be generated. Technical analyses of this kind, in which the inter-unit differences found will be examined in detail, will be the main concern of the research for the duration of the project. The results from these analyses, along with the final conclusions of the research, will be made available in technical publications and in the final report of the project.

In many respects, however, the present report will probably be more useful to the hospitals and emergency units which took part in the study than will the forthcoming more technical publications. First, this special volume provides each participating institution with its own results, on the basis of which specific organizational strengths and weaknesses may be properly assessed. Second, it makes available to each emergency unit, on a relatively timely basis, important and heretofore unavailable information about many different aspects of its organizational situation, performance, and operations. Third, it makes it possible for a particular unit to compare itself to other units of interest (e.g., units having a similar patient volume or whose parent hospitals are of similar size, units in urban or non-urban areas, etc.) or to the "average" situation of all the emergency units studied.

In short, even though it contains only the preliminary findings of the study, the present report enables each emergency unit to find out how well it is doing, both comparatively and in an absolute sense, in each area of interest covered in the research.

To the participating institutions, it is hoped, this report offers a potential base for making "rational" decisions or needed improvements, in the light of the findings and in the context of the particular circumstances and constraints faced by each of them individually. The way and the extent to which the material is used depends on the individual emergency units and their parent hospitals. An institution is likely to benefit from it, however, in proportion to the time and effort that it is willing to invest to understand the findings and their implications. Proper utilization of the findings, in any event, would require a thorough review. The findings must be first studied and understood, as fully as possible, before they are put to use.

We could have written a shorter report, with considerably less effort and at substantially lower cost. We chose, instead, to prepare a relatively comprehensive report in the hope that all of the institutions which cooperated in the study, and their staffs and patients, may derive some benefit from the project.

Appendix

BACKGROUND INFORMATION ABOUT THE RESPONDENTS AND LOCAL POPULATIONS

This appendix presents some useful information about the characteristics of the individuals who provided data for the study. First, background data are presented about the several groups of respondents, including those working in the emergency unit (MDS, RNS, and LPNS) and in the parent hospital (HAS and HMDS) as well as the community respondents (CRS). Information is provided about the length of association with their respective institutions, their main fields of interest or professional specialization, and other factors which may have a bearing on their attitudes and outlook.

Second, the patients (PATS) who completed questionnaires for the study are described in terms of the number of years they have lived in their respective communities, their age and sex, and their education and family income. Third, certain information about the patients' reasons for going to the particular emergency units that they visited, as well as information about their usual sources of medical care, is also included.

Finally, some data from U.S. Census reports are presented regarding the local populations of the cities/towns in which the emergency units studied are located. These data show the percent of families with incomes below the "poverty level," the percent of the city's population classified as minority population, and the median school years completed by persons 25 years old or older. This information may provide yet another perspective about the type of community in which various hospital emergency units are located and the kind of service demands which may be placed on them.

In examining the data included in this appendix, the reader should note that the percentages and mean scores shown in the various tables (with the exception of Table 111) represent the percentage or average score for <u>individual respondents</u> rather than the mean or mean percentage score of <u>hospitals/emergency units</u>. The total number of respondents from <u>all</u> emergency units combined, in each case, is indicated near the top of the columns in each table. (The number of respondents for each of the various groupings of emergency units in Table 2, in the introduction to this report, may be greater than the corresponding number in the tables of the appendix because some individuals did not provide the relevant background information.)

Selected Characteristics of Particular Respondents

The first three tables show, for particular groups of respondents, their length of professional experience, length of association with their respective hospitals, and length of time that they have been working in their emergency units.

<u>Length of professional experience</u>. Table 102 focuses on the professional work experience of emergency unit physicians (MDS) and registered nurses (RNS), and of the selected physicians (HMDS) from the hospital outside the emergency unit who participated in the study. On the average, HMDS have been practicing medicine longer than the physicians (MDS) working in the emergency unit, the former having an average of 19.6 years of professional experience and the latter 12.3 years. The registered nurses (full- and part-time combined) of emergency units average 13.1 years of professional experience.

The MDS in emergency units with a medium patient volume have been practicing medicine for a shorter period of time than those in either low or high

TABLE 102. LENGTH OF PROFESSIONAL EXPERIENCE FOR SELECTED
GROUPS OF RESPONDENTS[a]

	Average Number of Years That		
Respondents Associated with	RNS Have Been Working in Nursing[b]	MDS Have Been Practicing Medicine[c]	HMDS Have Been Practicing Medicine[c]
ALL EMERGENCY UNITS (EU's) IN THE STUDY SAMPLE	13.1 (n=270)	12.3 (n=211)	19.6 (n=215)
EU's with:			
Low Patient Volume	14.1	12.7	16.8
Medium Pat. Volume	12.2	9.3	19.6
High Patient Volume	13.0	14.4	21.2
EU's in:			
Church Operated Hospitals	12.4	14.5	19.5
Osteopathic Hospitals	12.9	3.9	14.2
All Other Hospitals	13.4	12.1	20.6
EU's Located in:			
SMSA (urban) Areas	13.4	11.0	19.4
Non-SMSA Areas	12.1	15.5	20.1
EU's in Hospitals Having:			
Medical Teaching Affiliations	12.6	11.9	19.5
No Medical Teaching Affiliations	13.8	12.7	19.8
EU's in Hospitals Having:			
Emergency Personnel Training Programs	13.2	13.0	18.8
No Training Programs	13.0	11.5	20.5

[a] The results for each group are based on data about all of the individual respondents in the group from all institutions combined in each case. In other words, the numbers shown pertain to the membership of each group and are not institutional averages.

[b] Average number of years were computed from the responses of registered nurses (RNS) from the various emergency units to the following question: "How long have you been working as a nurse?"

[c] Average numbers of years were computed from the responses of emergency unit physicians (MDS), and selected hospital physicians (HMDS), to the following question: "How long have you been practicing medicine?"

patient volume EU's. The same is true, more markedly, of the MDS in osteopathic compared to other institutions. A similar pattern characterizes the HMDS. The latter, unlike the MDS, have been practicing medicine for a shorter period of time in hospitals whose emergency units have a low, compared to either a medium or a high patient volume. The RNS in the total sample, and also in most of the EU groupings, have been practicing nursing somewhat longer than the MDS have been practicing medicine. In three groupings, however, the reverse applies -- in EU's with a high patient volume, in church operated institutions, and in non-urban area EU's.

Length of association with present hospital. Information about the number of years that respondents have been associated with their present hospitals is provided in Table 103. The selected hospital physicians, averaging 13.7 years, generally have been associated with their present hospitals longer than have the hospital administrator respondents (12.0 years), the licensed practical nurses working full-time in the emergency unit (8.4 years), the registered nurses (7.8 years), or the emergency unit physicians (7.2 years). Exceptions to this pattern are the administrators in the non-urban area hospitals and in hospitals without medical teaching affiliations who, on the average, have been associated with their present institution slightly longer than have the selected physicians. It is rather interesting that, of all these groups, the emergency unit physicians and registered nurses have had the shortest association with their present hospitals.

The data also show that physicians working in low and high patient volume emergency units have been associated with their respective hospitals longer than have their colleagues in medium volume units. Further, they and the hospital administrators in non-urban areas have been associated with their

TABLE 103. LENGTH OF ASSOCIATION WITH THEIR RESPECTIVE INSTITUTIONS
FOR SELECTED GROUPS OF RESPONDENTS[a]

Respondents Associated With	Average Number of Years Associated with the Present Hospital for				
	HAS	HMDS	MDS	RNS	LPNS[b]
ALL EMERGENCY UNITS (EU'S) IN THE STUDY SAMPLE	12.0 (n=68)	13.7 (n=215)	7.2 (n=211)	7.8 (n=272)	8.4 (n=47)
EU's with:					
Low Patient Volume	10.9	11.6	8.3	7.3	3.7
Medium Pat. Volume	10.7	13.6	5.1	8.1	9.9
High Patient Volume	14.0	14.9	7.7	8.1	9.0
EU's in:					
Church Operated Hospitals	10.1	12.0	9.5	7.5	9.7
Osteopathic Hospitals	9.7	12.0	3.3	6.8	5.4
All Other Hospitals	13.3	14.5	6.3	8.2	8.7
EU's Located in:					
SMSA (urban) Areas	10.5	13.8	6.0	7.6	8.2
Non-SMSA Areas	16.3	13.4	10.3	8.5	9.4
EU's in Hospitals Having:					
Medical Teaching Affiliations	10.7	13.7	6.6	7.7	9.2
No Medical Teaching Affiliations	14.2	13.6	7.8	8.0	6.2
EU's in Hospitals Having:					
Emergency Personnel Training Programs	11.2	13.6	7.7	7.8	9.0
No Training Programs	13.0	13.8	6.7	7.8	7.9

[a] The results for each group are based on data about all of the individual respondents in the group from all institutions combined in each case. Accordingly, the numbers of years shown pertain to the membership of each group and are not institutional averages. Average numbers of years were computed from the responses of the members of each group to the following question: "How long have you been working in (associated with) this hospital?"

[b] Included in this group are only licensed practical nurses (LPNS) working full-time. However, not all of the emergency units had full-time LPNS.

present institutions longer than have their counterparts in urban area hospitals. Practical nurses who work full-time in emergency units with a low patient volume generally have been with their present hospitals considerably fewer years (only 3.7 years) than have those who work in emergency units with a medium or high patient volume (9.9 and 9.0 years, respectively). The length of association of registered nurses with their respective hospitals, which averages 7.8 years, does not vary significantly across the different groupings of emergency units.

Length of association with the emergency unit. Shown next, in Table 104, is the percentage of emergency unit physicians (MDS) and registered nurses (RNS) who have worked in their respective units for (a) less than one year and (b) four years or more. Overall, approximately 26% of the MDS, and also of the RNS, have worked in their present units for less than one year, but slightly more than 40% of them, in each case, have worked there for at least four years. Similarly (not shown in the table) 23% of the full-time practical nurses (LPNS) have worked in their respective EU's less than one year, while 43% have worked for four years or more. A number of differences across EU groupings with respect to these patterns may be also seen in Table 104.

Professional specialization. Emergency unit physicians and registered nurses were also asked to indicate their major field of interest or specialty (data are not presented in table form). Of the RNS, 51% mentioned "emergency nursing" or "emergency medicine" in response to this question. The balance indicated surgery and/or operating room specialties (11%), intensive care or cardiac care (9%), supervision or administrative nursing (7%), and various other fields which together account for about 21% of all the RNS. These patterns

TABLE 104. LENGTH OF ASSOCIATION WITH THEIR RESPECTIVE EMERGENCY UNITS
FOR THE PHYSICIANS (MDS) AND REGISTERED NURSES (RNS) WHO WORK THERE[a]

	Percent of Group Members Working in the Emergency Unit for			
	Less Than One Year		Four Years or More	
Respondents Associated With	MDS	RNS	MDS	RNS
ALL EMERGENCY UNITS (EU'S) IN THE STUDY SAMPLE	26.4% (n=208)	26.5% (n=268)	43.3% (n=208)	41.8% (n=268)
EU's with:				
Low Patient Volume	24.7	32.1	46.9	38.5
Medium Pat. Volume	29.5	25.3	32.8	42.7
High Patient Volume	25.8	23.5	48.5	43.5
EU's in:				
Church Operated Hospitals	23.3	32.0	52.1	38.7
Osteopathic Hospitals	29.4	21.4	29.4	32.1
All Other Hospitals	28.0	24.8	39.8	44.8
EU's Located in:				
SMSA (urban) Areas	26.0	26.5	40.0	40.3
Non-SMSA Areas	27.6	26.4	51.8	45.8
EU's in Hospitals Having:				
Medical Teaching Affiliations	25.2	22.9	46.8	40.1
No Medical Teaching Affiliations	27.8	31.5	39.2	44.1
EU's in Hospitals Having:				
Emergency Personnel Training Programs	23.1	24.3	45.2	43.9
No Training Programs	29.8	29.2	41.3	39.2

[a] The percentage figures shown for each group are based on data about all the individual respondents in the group from all institutions combined in each case. Accordingly, they pertain to the membership of each group and are not institutional averages. The percentages were computed from the responses of MDS and RNS to the following question: "How long have you been working in this emergency unit?"

differ somewhat across EU groupings. Most notably, a larger proportion of RNS in EU's with a high patient volume mention emergency nursing (59%) compared to the overall average of 51%, in contrast to their counterparts in EU's with a low patient volume (34%). Additionally, there is a larger percentage of supervisory/administrative and also surgery/operating room nurses, but a smaller percentage of nurses specializing in trauma, in church operated units than in not church operated (excluding osteopathic) units. Also, proportionately more of the emergency unit nurses are in supervision and administration in hospitals without medical teaching affiliations, and without emergency personnel training programs, than in hospitals with such affiliations or programs.

Compared to the large percentage of RNS who mentioned emergency nursing as their special field, a relatively small percentage of the physicians (MDS) working in the units specified "emergency medicine." Of a total of 212 responding physicians in this connection, only 12% indicated emergency medicine as their specialty. However, an additional 21% indicated surgery (including general surgery and "trauma medicine") or orthopedics as their field. It is also interesting to note, however, that 25% of all the MDS specified family practice or family medicine as their specialty -- the largest percentage of responses received by any single medical specialty/field. An additional 17% of the MDS mentioned internal medicine or cardiology. Of the remaining, 9% indicated "general practice," 6% pediatrics, 3% obstetrics/gynecology, and the balance (a total of 7%) indicated other fields.

The percentage of MDS specializing in emergency medicine varies greatly across emergency unit groupings. A much higher percentage of the MDS in osteopathic hospitals indicate emergency medicine (29%), for example, than of the MDS in other not church operated institutions (13%) or in church operated institutions (5%). Similarly, a higher percentage of the MDS in urban area units (14%) specialize in emergency medicine than in non-urban area units (5%). The same is true of MDS in hospitals with medical teaching affiliations (18%) than without such affiliations (4%), and in hospitals with emergency personnel training programs (16%) than without such programs (8%). Finally, the higher the patient volume of the units, the greater the percentage of MDS who specialize in emergency medicine.

Membership in certain professional associations. Emergency unit physicians and registered nurses also were asked whether they are currently members of the American College of Emergency Physicians (ACEP) or the Emergency Department Nurses Association (EDNA), respectively. About 22% of the RNS indicated that they are members of EDNA, and 25% of the MDS indicated that they are members of ACEP (data not shown in table form). A greater percentage of the MDS, and of the RNS, working in emergency units with a high, compared to low, patient volume report membership in these associations. RNS in osteopathic hospital units are less likely to belong to EDNA than are those working in the units of other hospitals; and MDS in church operated units are less likely to belong to ACEP than are those in not church operated units. Further, a much larger percentage of MDS in hospitals with medical teaching affiliations, and with emergency personnel training programs, belong to ACEP compared to MDS in hospitals without such affiliations or programs. A similar though weaker pattern characterizes the RNS with respect to membership in EDNA.

Demographic characteristics. Respondents working in the emergency units studied, as well as the hospital administrators, were asked to provide information about their age. In general, the administrators are the oldest group, followed by the emergency unit physicians, the registered nurses, and then the licensed practical nurses who work full-time in the units. (It should be recalled, however, that the administrators group includes the chief executive officer of each hospital, the next highest administrative officer, if any, who has responsibility for the emergency unit, and the hospital's director of nursing.) More specifically, 44% of the administrators, 20% of the physicians, 16% of the registered nurses, and 9% of the practical nurses are 50 years of age or older. Incidentally, 94% of the physicians working in the emergency units are male, while 98% of the registered nurses are female.

The Characteristics of Emergency Unit Patients Who Participated in the Study

The tables in this section provide background data about the patients (PATS) who completed questionnaires for the study, including demographic data and information about the patients' reasons for going to the particular units to which they went for care, and about the patients' usual sources of medical care. As noted in the introduction (p. 9) of this report, participating patients include those over 15 years of age who visited the emergency units at any time from 8:00 a.m. Friday until 12:00 p.m. Saturday of the week during which each particular hospital was scheduled for on-site data collection (excluding those who were unable to, or who preferred not to, consent). In reviewing the data in this section (particularly in Tables 106 and 107), therefore, the reader should keep in mind the group of patients involved.

The first table in the series, Table 105, concerns the length of time that patient respondents have lived in the communities in which they are currently living. Specifically, the table shows the percentage of PATS who have lived in their present communities for (a) two years or less and (b) more than ten years. Overall, more than half (57%) of the PATS have lived in their present communities for over ten years, and only about 20% of them

TABLE 105. THE LENGTH OF TIME PATIENT RESPONDENTS (PATS) HAVE LIVED IN THE COMMUNITIES IN WHICH THEY ARE CURRENTLY LIVING[a]

Respondents Associated With	The Percent of Patients Who Have Lived in Their Respective Communities for	
	Two Years or Less	More Than Ten Years
ALL EMERGENCY UNITS (EU'S) IN THE STUDY SAMPLE[b]	18.8% (n=388)	56.7% (n=388)
EU's with:		
Low Patient Volume	17.8	57.0
Medium Pat. Volume	20.5	55.4
High Patient Volume	18.3	57.4
EU's in:		
Church Operated Hospitals	15.1	54.7
Osteopathic Hospitals	20.0	51.1
All Other Hospitals	19.3	57.9
EU's Located in:		
SMSA (urban) Areas	20.7	53.9
Non-SMSA Areas	15.2	62.1
EU's in Hospitals Having:		
Medical Teaching Affiliations	19.6	54.2
No Medical Teaching Affiliations	17.6	60.8
EU's in Hospitals Having:		
Emergency Personnel Training Programs	18.6	56.4
No Training Programs	19.0	57.1

[a] The percentage figures shown are based on data about all of the individual patient respondents (PATS) from all institutions combined in each case. Accordingly they pertain to the collectivity of patients and are not institutional averages. The percentages were computed from the responses of PATS to the following question: "How long have you lived in the community in which you now live?"

[b] Two of the hospitals in the study sample did not allow patient participation, and their emergency unit patients are therefore not included.

have lived there less than two years. Moreover, there are no major differences across EU groupings with respect to the length of time that, on the average, patients have been living in their present communities. However, somewhat more of the patients in the urban area units, compared to other units, have lived in their respective communities for two years or less. And somewhat fewer of the patients in osteopathic hospitals, urban area hospitals, and hospitals with teaching affiliations (compared to the other institutions in each case) have lived in their present community longer than ten years.

Next, Table 106 shows the sex and age distributions of the patients (PATS) who completed questionnaires for the study. The same table also shows the sex distribution of the selected community respondents (CRS) who participated in the research. On the average, only 10% of the CRS are female, though the figure is somewhat higher for certain emergency unit groupings (including EU's with a medium patient volume, the EU's of osteopathic hospitals, and the EU's of hospitals without training programs). As would be expected, on the other hand, a much larger percentage of the patients, namely 52%, are female. The percentage of patients who are female is particularly high for EU's with a medium patient volume and EU's in osteopathic hospitals. Overall, 36.1% of the patient respondents are between 16 and 25 years of age, while 9.5% of them are 65 years old or older. Proportionately, more of the PATS in emergency units with a low, compared to either a medium or a high, patient volume are 16-25 years old. And more of the patients in EU's with a medium, compared to a low or high, patient volume are 65 years old or older.

Information about the formal education of patient respondents is summarized in Table 107. One-third of the patients have completed high school (but have not attended college), and an additional 25% of them have attended at least some college. The remaining patients have had less than a full high school

TABLE 106. PERCENT OF RESPONDENTS FROM EACH SPECIFIED GROUP WITH THE SEX AND AGE CHARACTERISTICS SHOWN[a]

Respondents Associated With	Percent of CRS, and Percent of PATS Who Are Female		Percent of PATS Who Are	
	CRS	PATS	16-25 Years Old	65 Years Old or Older
ALL EMERGENCY UNITS (EU'S) IN THE STUDY SAMPLE	10.0% (n=201)	52.1% (n=386)	36.1% (n=388)	9.5% (n=388)
EU's with:				
Low Patient Volume	11.4	38.5	44.3	7.6
Medium Pat. Volume	14.3	65.8	31.3	15.2
High Patient Volume	5.3	49.7	35.5	7.1
EU's in:				
Church Operated Hospitals	8.3	36.5	35.8	7.5
Osteopathic Hospitals	18.8	75.6	37.8	8.9
All Other Hospitals	9.6	51.2	35.9	10.0
EU's Located in:				
SMSA (urban) Areas	8.2	57.6	37.1	8.6
Non-SMSA Areas	13.4	41.2	34.1	11.4
EU's in Hospitals Having:				
Medical Teaching Affiliations	8.1	54.8	34.2	9.6
No Medical Teaching Affiliations	12.2	47.6	39.2	9.5
EU's in Hospitals Having:				
Emergency Personnel Training Programs	4.7	48.8	36.8	8.3
No Training Programs	15.8	55.7	35.3	10.9

[a] The percentage figures shown are based on information reported by the respondents themselves -- the patients (PATS), or the selected community respondents (CRS). They pertain to the collectivity of respondents from all institutions combined in each case, and are not institutional averages. (Two of the hospitals in the study sample did not allow patient participation, and their emergency unit patients are therefore not included. Furthermore, all patients who are included in the study, it should be recalled, were 16 years old or older.)

TABLE 107. PERCENT OF EMERGENCY UNIT PATIENTS (PATS) WITH
SPECIFIED LEVELS OF FORMAL EDUCATION[a]

	Percent of Patients Who Have	
Respondents Associated With	Had at Least Some College Education	Completed High School (but not attended college)
ALL EMERGENCY UNITS (EU'S) IN THE STUDY SAMPLE	25.5% (n=385)	33.0% (n=385)
EU's with:		
Low Patient Volume	25.4	35.4
Medium Pat. Volume	22.5	34.2
High Patient Volume	27.2	31.3
EU's in:		
Church Operated Hospitals	32.0	30.2
Osteopathic Hospitals	20.0	42.2
All Other Hospitals	25.1	32.1
EU's Located in:		
SMSA (urban) Areas	27.4	32.5
Non-SMSA Areas	21.6	33.8
EU's in Hospitals Having:		
Medical Teaching Affiliations	25.5	32.2
No Medical Teaching Affiliations	25.3	34.2
EU's in Hospitals Having:		
Emergency Personnel Training Programs	28.7	31.7
No Training Programs	21.9	34.4

[a]The percentage figures shown are based on the answers of patient respondents (PATS) to the following questionnaire item: "How much formal education have you had? (Check the highest completed)." The response alternatives were: (1) Grade school education only, (2) Some high school, (3) Completed high school, (4) Some college, (5) Completed college, (6) Completed more than four years of college, and (7) Other [Please write in:_____]. The percentages pertain to the collectivity of patient respondents from all institutions combined in each case, and are not institutional averages. (Two of the hospitals in the study did not allow patient participation, and their emergency unit patients are therefore not included. Furthermore, since all patients in the study are 16 years old or older, those in the younger age group obviously may have not yet completed their formal education.)

education. (It should be kept in mind that many of the patient respondents have not yet completed their formal education since a considerable number of them -- specifically 12% -- are between the ages of 16 and 18, and an even higher number -- 36% -- are between 16 and 25.) There are no significant differences across emergency unit groupings in the proportion of patients who have at least completed high school (around 59% on the average). However, the percent of patients who have had at least some college education is higher for church operated than for osteopathic emergency units. It is also somewhat higher for urban compared to non-urban area units, and for the units of hospitals which have, compared to those which do not have, emergency personnel training programs.

Table 108 provides data about the family income of patient respondents. It shows the percent of patients with family incomes (a) under $6,000 a year and (b) $20,000 a year or more. Overall, about 21% of the 351 patients who provided this information report a total family income of less than $6,000, and almost an equal proportion -- 22% -- report a family income of $20,000 or more. Proportionately, fewer of the patients in emergency units with a low, compared to either a medium or a high, patient volume report a low family income, and the same is true for patients in church operated compared to not church operated institutions. Conversely, a higher proportion of the patients in hospitals which are not church operated (excluding osteopathic institutions) report a high family income compared to patients in both osteopathic and church operated institutions. And, similarly, a larger proportion of the patients visiting urban, compared to non-urban, area EU's report a high family income.

TABLE 108. PERCENT OF PATIENT RESPONDENTS (PATS) REPORTING PARTICULAR LEVELS OF TOTAL FAMILY INCOME[a]

Respondents Associated With	Percent of Patients Reporting a Family Income of	
	Less than $6,000[b]	$20,000 or more
ALL EMERGENCY UNITS (EU'S) IN THE STUDY SAMPLE	21.1% (n=351)	22.2% (n=351)
EU's with:		
Low Patient Volume	12.3	23.3
Medium Pat. Volume	25.0	19.8
High Patient Volume	22.5	23.0
EU's in:		
Church Operated Hospitals	10.5	16.7
Osteopathic Hospitals	29.3	14.6
All Other Hospitals	21.7	24.4
EU's Located in:		
SMSA (urban) Areas	20.6	27.9
Non-SMSA Areas	22.1	11.0
EU's in Hospitals Having:		
Medical Teaching Affiliations	21.9	23.4
No Medical Teaching Affiliations	19.7	20.5
EU's in Hospitals Having:		
Emergency Personnel Training Programs	21.0	24.6
No Training Programs	21.3	19.4

[a] The percentage figures shown are based on the answers of patient respondents (PATS) to the following questionnaire item: "What was your total family income before taxes in 1976?" The response alternatives ranged from "(1) less than $2,000,"... to "(9) $30,000 or more." (Of all the patients in the study sample, 9.5% did not answer the question and are therefore excluded. Also excluded are patients from the two study hospitals which did not allow patient participation.) The percentages shown pertain to the collectivity of patient respondents from all institutions combined in each case and are not institutional averages.

Patients' Reasons for Going to the Particular Emergency Unit(s)

Each patient who participated in the study was asked the following question: "Why did you go to this particular emergency room instead of some other emergency room?" The question provided eleven different response alternatives, as shown in Table 109. Overall, the reason most frequently selected by the patients was: <u>This emergency room was the nearest one to go to</u> (selected by 31% of the PATS). The second and third most frequently selected reasons were: <u>I (or my family) had used this emergency room before</u> (25%), and <u>I knew that the hospital is a good one</u> (10%). These three reasons together account for the responses of two-thirds of all the patients who completed questionnaires for the study.

The data also show, however, that patient responses to the above question differ from the general pattern for some of the emergency unit groupings. For example, patients visiting EU's with a medium patient volume, and EU's in osteopathic hospitals, were much less likely than others to select "this emergency room was the nearest one to go to." Patients going to the units of osteopathic hospitals, and to medium patient volume units, were particularly likely to give as their reason "I (or my family) had used this emergency room before." This is also true of patients visiting emergency units in urban compared to non-urban areas, and units of hospitals with medical teaching affiliations compared to those without such affiliations.

After the third most frequently selected reason ("I knew that the hospital is a good one"), the reason chosen next most often was: <u>My doctor told me to go there</u> (8%). And the fifth most frequently given reason was: <u>This was the only available place to go for care</u> (selected by 6% of the patients). However, this last reason was given more often by patients who visited emergency units with a low patient volume (15%), units in non-urban areas (11%),

TABLE 109. PERCENT OF PATIENTS (PATS) GIVING PARTICULAR REASONS FOR HAVING "CHOSEN" TO GO TO THE EMERGENCY UNITS TO WHICH THEY WENT FOR CARE[a]

Hospital Emergency Units (EU's) Involved	Total Number of Patients	The Three Reasons Most Frequently Selected by Patients, and the Percent of Patients Selecting Them		
		First	Second	Third
ALL EU'S IN THE STUDY SAMPLE (N=28 Hospital EU's)	387	This EU was the nearest (31.5%)	Had used this EU before (25.1%)	The hospital is a good one (10.3%)
YOUR HOSPITAL'S EU				
EU's with:				
Low Patient Volume (n=9)	79	This EU was the nearest (38.0%)	Had used this EU before (20.3%)	It was the only available place (15.2%)
Medium Pat. Volume (n=10)	111	Had used this EU before (31.5%)	This EU was the nearest (15.3%)	The hospital is a good one (12.6%)
High Patient Volume (n=9)	197	This EU was the nearest (38.1%)	Had used this EU before (23.4%)	The hospital is a good one (10.2%)
EU's in:				
Church Operated Hospitals (n=8)	53	This EU was the nearest (37.7%)	Had used this EU before (17.0%)	My doctor told me to go to this EU (11.3%)
Osteopathic Hospitals (n=3)	45	Had used this EU before (46.7%)	My doctor told me to go to this EU (13.3%)	The hospital is a good one (8.9%)
All Other Hospitals (n=17)	289	This EU was the nearest (34.3%)	Had used this EU before (23.2%)	The hospital is a good one (11.1%)
EU's Located in:				
SMSA (urban) Areas (n=19)	256	This EU was the nearest (30.1%)	Had used this EU before (28.5%)	The hospital is a good one (11.3%)
Non-SMSA Areas (n=9)	131	This EU was the nearest (34.4%)	Had used this EU before (18.3%)	It was the only available place (11.5%)
EU's in Hospitals Having:				
Medical Teaching Affiliations (n=16)	239	Had used this EU before (28.9%)	This EU was the nearest (27.2%)	The hospital is a good one (13.4%)
No Medical Teaching Affiliations (n=12)	148	This EU was the nearest (38.5%)	Had used this EU before (18.9%)	It was the only available place (11.5%)
EU's in Hospitals Having:				
Emergency Personnel Training Programs (n=13)	204	This EU was the nearest (35.3%)	Had used this EU before (26.5%)	The hospital is a good one (11.3%)
No Training Programs (n=15)	183	This EU was the nearest (27.3%)	Had used this EU before (23.5%)	The hospital is a good one (9.3%)

[a] The results shown are based on the responses of recent patients (PATS) from the various emergency units to the following question: "Why did you go to this particular emergency room instead of some other emergency room? What would you say was the main reason?" The response alternatives were: (1) I (or my family) had used this emergency room before, (2) I thought this would be a good emergency room, (3) I knew that the hospital is a good one, (4) This emergency room was the nearest one to go to, (5) This was the only available place to go for care, (6) They just took me there, (7) My visit there was scheduled in advance, (8) My doctor told me to go there, (9) I wanted to see a particular doctor who worked there, (10) I was sent there from another emergency room or hospital, and (11) Some other reason. The percentages enclosed in parentheses after each reason in each row of the table are based on the corresponding "total number of patients" indicated. (Emergency unit patients from two of the study hospitals which did not allow patient participation are not included.)

and units in hospitals without medical teaching affiliations (11%). Other details may be seen in Table 109.

The Patients' Usual Source(s) of Medical Care

Patient respondents were also asked: "When you or a member of your family needs medical attention, where do you usually go for care?" Table 110 presents the findings, which are rather surprising. Overall, 76% of the patients report that they usually go to our regular family doctor for care. The second most frequently indicated source, but at a great distance, is a hospital emergency room (selected by 8% of the patients). The third and fourth most frequently chosen medical sources (with equal frequency) are: a private doctor's office but not a regular family doctor (6%), and a clinic which is not located in a hospital (also 6%).

Patients visiting emergency units with a high patient volume were more likely to report going to a hospital emergency room, and much less likely to report going to a clinic which is not located in a hospital than were patients visiting emergency units with a medium or low patient volume. Patients visiting the emergency units of urban area hospitals were less likely to report going to a hospital emergency room than were patients visiting non-urban area EU's. In contrast, the former were more likely to report going to a private doctor's office but not a regular family doctor than were the latter. Other details may be seen in Table 110.

Population Characteristics of the Cities in Which the Emergency Units are Located

The final table in this appendix and present report, Table 111, provides some background data from relevant U.S. Census reports published after the 1970 population census. These data indicate some of the population charac-

TABLE 110. PERCENT OF EMERGENCY UNIT PATIENTS (PATS) INDICATING PARTICULAR SOURCES AS THEIR "USUAL" SOURCES FOR MEDICAL CARE

Hospital Emergency Units (EU's) Involved	Total Number of Patients	The Three Sources Most Frequently Indicated by the Patients, and the Percent of Patients Selecting Them		
		First	Second	Third
ALL EU'S IN THE STUDY SAMPLE (N=28 Hospital EU's)	381	Our regular family doctor (76.1%)	A hospital emergency room (8.4%)	A doctor other than regular family doctor (6.3%); A clinic not in a hospital (6.3%)
YOUR HOSPITAL'S EU				
EU's with:				
Low Patient Volume (n=9)	79	Our regular family doctor (81.0%)	A clinic not in a hospital (8.9%)	A doctor other than regular family doctor (5.1%)
Medium Pat. Volume (n=10)	110	Our regular family doctor (70.0%)	A clinic not in a hospital (10.0%)	A doctor other than regular family doctor (7.3%)
High Patient Volume (n=9)	192	Our regular family doctor (77.6%)	A hospital emergency room (11.5%)	A doctor other than regular family doctor (6.3%)
EU's in:				
Church Operated Hospitals (n=8)	53	Our regular family doctor (73.6%)	A clinic not in a hospital (13.2%)	A doctor other than regular family doctor (5.7%); A hospital emergency room (5.7%)
Osteopathic Hospitals (n=3)	44	Our regular family doctor (84.1%)	A doctor other than regular family doctor (6.8%)	A clinic not in a hospital (4.5%)
All Other Hospitals (n=17)	284	Our regular family doctor (75.4%)	A hospital emergency room (9.9%)	A doctor other than regular family doctor (6.3%)
EU's Located in:				
SMSA (urban) Areas (n=19)	252	Our regular family doctor (75.0%)	A doctor other than regular family doctor (8.3%)	A hospital emergency room (6.7%); A clinic not in a hospital (6.7%)
Non-SMSA Areas (n=9)	129	Our regular family doctor (78.3%)	A hospital emergency room (11.6%)	A clinic not in a hospital (5.4%)
EU's in Hospitals Having:				
Medical Teaching Affiliations (n=16)	234	Our regular family doctor (72.2%)	A hospital emergency room (9.4%)	A doctor other than regular family doctor (7.7%)
No Medical Teaching Affiliations (n=12)	147	Our regular family doctor (82.3%)	A hospital emergency room (6.8%)	A clinic not in a hospital (4.8%)
EU's in Hospitals Having:				
Emergency Personnel Training Programs (n=13)	200	Our regular family doctor (78.5%)	A hospital emergency room (9.0%)	A doctor other than regular family doctor (7.0%)
No Training Programs (n=15)	181	Our regular family doctor (73.5%)	A clinic not in a hospital (8.3%)	A hospital emergency room (7.7%)

[a] The results shown are based on the responses of recent patients (PATS) from the various emergency units to the following question: "When you or a member of your family needs medical attention, where do you usually go for care?" The response alternatives were: (1) To our regular family doctor, (2) To a private doctor's office but not a regular family doctor, (3) To a clinic which is not located in a hospital, (4) To a hospital clinic (or outpatient department), (5) To a hospital emergency room, and (6) To some other care facility. The percentages enclosed in parentheses after each source of care in each row of the table are based on the corresponding "total number of patients" indicated. (Emergency unit patients from two of the study hospitals which did not allow patient participation are not included.)

TABLE 111. SELECTED CHARACTERISTICS OF THE POPULATION OF THE CITIES (TOWNS) IN WHICH THE STUDY HOSPITALS ARE LOCATED, BASED ON U.S. CENSUS DATA[a]

Cities/Towns Where the Hospital Emergency Units (EU's) Involved are Located		Median School Years Completed by Persons 25 Years Old or Older	Percent of Population Classified as Minority Population	Percent of Families With Income Below "Poverty Level"
ALL CITIES/TOWNS IN WHICH THE EU'S IN THE STUDY SAMPLE (N=30 Hospital EU's) ARE LOCATED	*Mean:*	12.1	6.8%	6.4%
	Range:	(10.5-14.5)	(0.1%-34.4%)	(1.2%-15.3%)
YOUR HOSPITAL'S CITY				
Cities Where Located, for EU's with:				
Low Patient Volume (n=10)		12.2	1.4	5.3
Medium Pat. Volume (n=10)		11.9	11.8	7.4
High Patient Volume (n=10)		12.2	7.2	6.5
Cities Where Located, for EU's in:				
Church Operated Hospitals (n=9)		11.9	7.3	6.5
Osteopathic Hospitals (n=3)		12.5	5.3	4.2
All Other Hospitals (n=18)		12.1	6.8	6.8
Cities Where Located, for EU's in:				
SMSA (urban) Areas (n=21)		12.2	8.8	5.8
Non-SMSA Areas (n=9)		11.8	2.2	7.9
Cities Where Located, for EU's in Hospitals With:				
Medical Teaching Affiliations (n=17)		12.2	8.6	6.6
No Medical Teaching Affiliations (n=13)		12.0	4.4	6.3
Cities Where Located, for EU's in Hospitals With:				
Emergency Personnel Training Programs (n=15)		12.2	4.9	6.0
No Training Programs (n=15)		12.0	8.7	6.9

[a] The background information presented in this table is in all cases based on data from relevant U.S. Census reports published after the last decennial U.S. Census (i.e., the 1970 Census).

teristics of the cities/towns in which the emergency units studied are located. The specific characteristics included are: median level of formal education; the proportion of the population classified as minority population; and the proportion of families with income below the "poverty level."

These population characteristics, of course, do not necessarily reflect the characteristics of the patients treated by the emergency units, or those of the patients who participated in the study, because hospitals serve patients from outside the cities as well. Furthermore, the data in Table 111 may differ from corresponding data provided by the patient respondents, since the latter information is more current, in addition to pertaining to the particular group of patients involved. Nevertheless, the data in Table 111 may be useful for comparing, at least in a gross way, the different community environments within which the various emergency units operate.

The first column in Table 111 shows, for the populations indicated, the median school years completed by persons 25 years old or older. For all the cities/towns combined (and properly averaged), the median number of school years completed is 12.1 years. However, the range across the individual cities/towns involved is substantial for this measure, from a median of only 10.5 school years (reflecting some high school education) to a median of 14.5 years (reflecting two and one-half years of college). On the other hand, the range of mean scores for cities in which particular groups of emergency units are located is very small (from 11.8 to 12.5 median school years), there being no significant differences among the EU groupings specified.

The cities in which the various emergency units are located also differ greatly from one another with respect to the percent of the population classified as minority population. Only 0.1% of the population of one of the cities, for example, is so classified, compared to 34.4% of the population of another one of the cities involved. The average figures for all the cities in which the EU's are located is 6.8%. There are also some differences among groups of cities in which particular groups of EU's are located. For example, the cities in which units with a medium patient volume are located have a higher percentage of minority population than do those in which units with a low patient volume are located. The percentage of the population classified as minority is also higher for cities/towns in urban (i.e., SMSA) areas than non-urban (i.e., non-SMSA) areas.

Finally, Table 111 shows the percent of families with incomes below the "poverty level" for the cities in which the emergency units are located. This ranges from a low of 1.2% to a high of 15.3%, depending upon the particular group of cities considered, and averages 6.4% for all of the cities/towns involved. The figure is relatively low for cities in which osteopathic hospital units, and also units with a low patient volume, are located.

The data in the present section of the appendix, it should be reiterated, do not necessarily depict the current situation of the cities/towns involved. Unlike all of the other data in the appendix, and in the report, they are considerably less recent and probably also less interesting. Nevertheless, they may be useful as supplementary information.

The study's special report to the participating institutions is now completed. It is hoped that all of them will find the report valuable. The research staff is profoundly grateful for the cooperation of every individual hospital, every individual emergency unit, and every individual respondent who provided data for the research.

PART III: THE RESEARCH INSTRUMENTS

PART III

THE RESEARCH INSTRUMENTS

The various instruments that were developed and used to collect the data for the study discussed in the present report are presented next. The sources of required data are also specified. The kinds of data needed for measuring the variables of concern to the study fall into five major categories: (a) data from the staff working in each emergency unit (EU) and from selected respondents in the rest of the hospital; (b) data from organizational records -- financial, personnel, patient census, and administrative records; (c) data from some of the patients treated in the EU; (d) data from selected individuals in the outside community with knowledge about each hospital EU; and (e) certain supplementary data from existing sources, such as U.S. Census reports and the AHA Guide to the Health Care Field. The instruments that were developed to obtain the relevant data in each case (except for the last category) are all included here.

The various instruments were designed to enable the research staff to collect the required data as economically as possible and without undue imposition on the hospitals or the individual respondents. Among other things, this meant that respondents from each relevant group were not asked to provide either surplus data or data on matters about which they had no personal knowledge. However, data about key variables had to be provided by respondents from two or more of the different groups in order to enable us to develop measures whose reliability and validity could be assessed. For these and other methodological reasons, therefore, the strategy was to maximize the independence of data sources relied upon for the measures.

Assessment of the criterion variables (e.g., clinical efficiency, economic efficiency, etc.) of the study required data from records, from staff and patients, and other sources. Assessment of certain control/moderator variables (e.g., organization size, location, etc.) required data mostly from organizational records and the sources in category (e) above. And assessment of most of the independent variables (and also some criterion and control variables) required data from individual respondents -- the doctors and nurses working in each EU, selected physicians in the rest of the hospital, key administrators, patients visiting the EU, and selected community respondents. To elicit the desired data, moreover, individual respondents had to be treated not only as "subjects" (to be asked information about themselves and their own work situation) but also as "observers" (to be asked to provide evaluative information about EU activities, performance, work relationships, etc.) having first-hand knowledge about specific aspects of the situation in the emergency unit.

Finally, some of the data could be obtained only by means of open-ended questions (e.g., data about EU strengths and weaknesses or needs, inter-institutional agreements, changes in the EU or the population being served), while other data required the construction of precisely formulated scale-type items (typically five-point scale items with ordinal, equal-appearing interval properties) or dictated construction of special lists, tables, and the like. Accordingly, and also for the purpose of maximizing respondent motivation and response rates, both personal interview and self-administered questionnaire forms had to be developed and used, along with an instrument to obtain data from different organizational records.

The particular instruments developed and corresponding data sources are:

	Instrument	Form Number	Length
1.	Administrators' Interview (personal interview)	Form 1, Part A	30 questions (about 45 minutes)
2.	Administrators' Questionnaire (self-administered)	Form 1, Part B	56 questions (about 30 min.)
3.	Emergency Unit Physicians' Interview	Form 2, Part A	23 questions (about 30 min.)
4.	Emergency Unit Physicians' Questionnaire	Form 2, Part B	65 questions (about 30 min.)
5.	Interview with Registered Nurses in Emergency Unit	Form 3, Part A	22 questions (about 30 min.)
6.	Questionnaire for Emergency Unit RN's	Form 3, Part B	84 questions (about 40 min.)
7.	Emergency Unit Supervising Nurse or Head Nurse "Supplement" (to #5 and #6)	Form 3, Part C	24 questions (about 45 min.)
8.	Interview for Selected Physicians in the Hospital (outside the emerg. unit)	Form 4	34 questions (about 45 min.)
9.	Interview for Selected Respondents from the Community	Form 5	27 questions (about 45 min.)
10.	Interview with Full-time Licensed Practical Nurses in Emergency Unit	Form 6	39 questions (about 45 min.)
11.	Special Instrument for Information from Various Institutional Records (structured format)	Form 7	26 questions (mostly multiple-part questions requiring a considerable number of work hours to complete)
12.	Emergency Unit Patient Questionnaire (mailed)	Form 8	54 questions (about 40 min.)

The several personal interview forms, for reasons already mentioned, incorporated a number of common questions, this number varying depending upon the particular groups of respondents that one might wish to compare. (In the case of emergency unit physicians and RN's, for example, there would be considerable overlap.) The same applies to the various questionnaire forms in relation to one another, although the patient questionnaire contains only a very few items in common with the other forms. The objective was to develop a well-coordinated set of instruments that would yield high-quality data with maximum possible efficiency concerning both the collection of information and the development of measures. The initial intention in developing the various instruments was to make use, where appropriate and available, of items or questions that had been used in previous relevant studies (either by project staff or by other researchers). Some such items were, therefore, incorporated in the various instruments, occasionally in their original format but most items in a suitably modified format to meet the requirements of the present study. However, it proved necessary to develop the large majority of the questions/items ourselves, so that most of the items in each and every instrument here presented are "new."

Instruments 1 and 2 in the above list were developed for the chief executive officer of each hospital and, with slight modification, for the next highest administrative official of the hospital (if any) directly responsible for the emergency service but not working in the emergency unit. Additionally, the modified version was intended for the hospital's director of nursing. Instrument 11 on the list was developed for completion by appropriate administrative staff (from personnel, records, fiscal section, etc.) as designated by the chief executive officer and under his supervision.

Instruments 3 and 4 were designed for all physicians, including the director, working in the emergency unit during the fieldwork period. Similarly, instruments 5 and 6 were designed for the registered nurses working in the emergency unit, whether full- or part-time, including the supervising nurse or head nurse. Instrument 7 was developed as a supplement to 5 and 6, to be completed only by the supervising nurse(s) of the emergency unit. And instrument 10 was designed for licensed practical nurses working in the emergency unit full-time.

Instrument 8 was developed for relevant key physicians in the hospital who had knowledge of, but were not working in, the emergency unit: the chief of the medical staff and the chairman of the medical executive committee; the chairman of the emergency department/room committee (if any); the chief pathologist and chief radiologist; the chairman of the trauma committee (if any); intensive care unit physician; the chairman of medical audit/records review committee; the director of medical education; and the heads of the four major services -- medicine, surgery, pediatrics, and obstetrics and gynecology.

Instrument 9 was designed for selected respondents from the community having contact with, or special knowledge about, each hospital's emergency unit. Eligible respondents in this group were: the local health department director or his designate; sheriff department, police department, and fire department representatives; the coroner or medical examiner; health systems agency (HSA) and emergency medical system (EMS) representatives, if any; ambulance company personnel (e.g., emergency medical technicians); and up to three additional individuals named by the chief executive officer of the hospital (when interviewed) as the "most knowledgeable individuals in the community outside the hospital concerning the emergency unit (of the hospital)."

Finally, instrument 12 was constructed for recent patients of the emergency unit. Eligible respondents from this group were all patients over 15 years of age visiting the emergency unit for care at any time from 8:00 AM Friday until

12:00 noon Saturday of the week during which each particular hospital was scheduled for on-site data collection. This arrangement was used in order not to omit "weekend patients," and to select patients able to complete a self-administered questionnaire (which would be mailed to them later). Further, the time interval was considered sufficient to yield, on the average, a total of 16 or more patients per emergency unit (the number committed to in the earlier grant application). Only patients who consented to participate in the study, of course, and who signed a written release making available their emergency visit record were eligible. (Eligible former patients of each study hospital were contacted by the research staff within three-four weeks after their emergency visit.)

Prior to data collection all of the instruments were properly pre-tested. Here, they are shown in their final form.

The University of Michigan
Institute for Social Research

Study 462312
Fall 1977

Hospital Administrators' Interview

HOSPITAL EMERGENCY SERVICES STUDY

FORM 1, PART A: ADMINISTRATORS' INTERVIEW

Interviewer: _____
Interview No.: _____
Date: _____

Study 462312   Fall 1977

FORM 1, PART A: ADMINISTRATORS' INTERVIEW

INTERVIEWER READ TO R:

> First, some general questions about the hospital and the emergency unit (i.e., the emergency room or department) here.

1. Within Hospital Administration at this institution, who is assigned principal administrative responsibility for the Emergency Unit?
IV:17

_____ _____
(NAME)   (TITLE/POSITION)

2. At the present time, does this hospital have an Emergency Room Committee or an
IV:18 Emergency Department Committee?

| 1. YES | 2. NO | 8. DON'T KNOW |

→ GO TO Q.3 (NEXT PAGE)

2a. Currently, who is chairing this committee?
IV:19

_____ _____
(NAME)   (TITLE/POSITION)

2b. How active, would you say, is this committee?
IV:20

Hospital Administrators' Interview

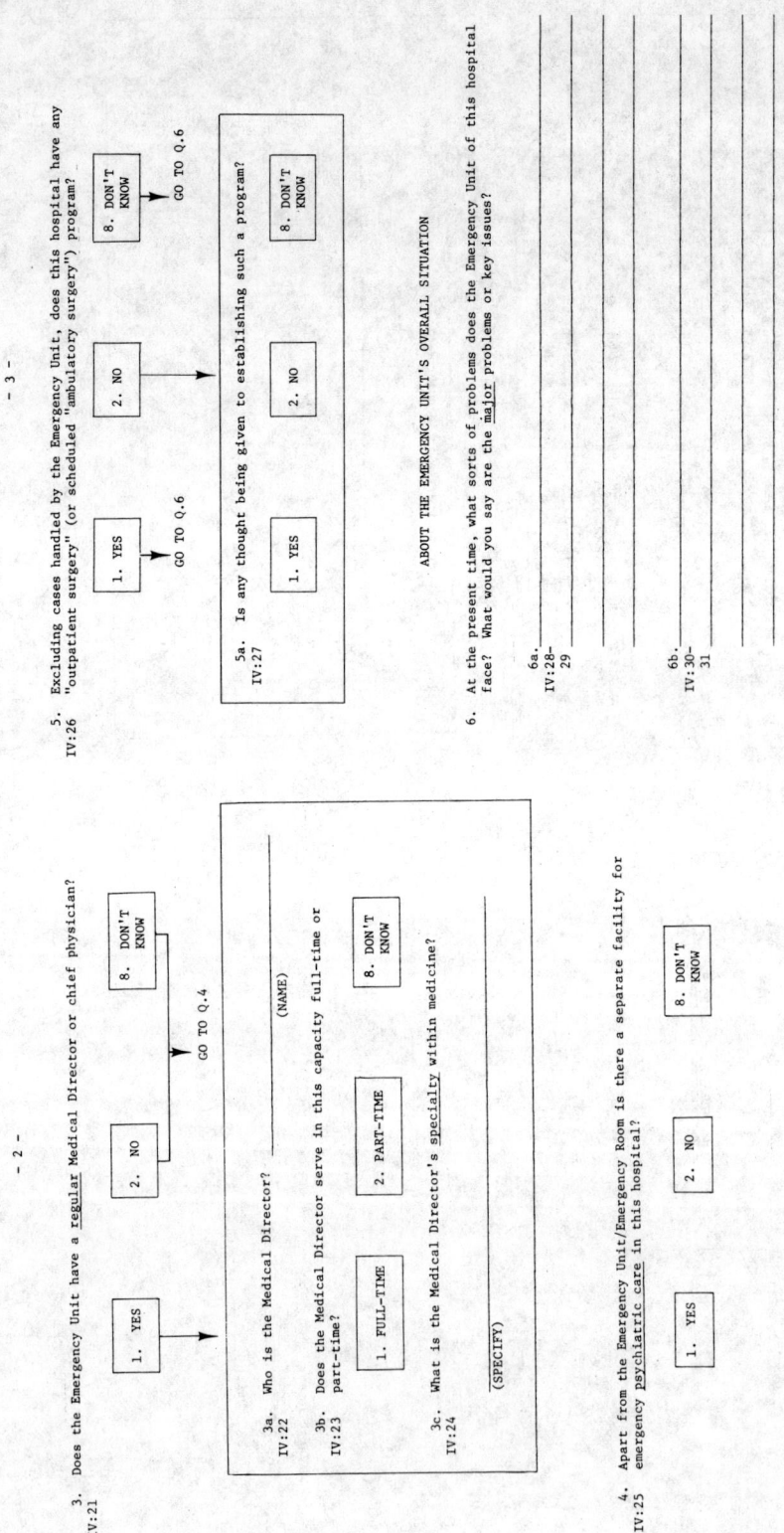

- 2 -

3. Does the Emergency Unit have a regular Medical Director or chief physician?
   IV:21

   1. YES → | 2. NO | 8. DON'T KNOW |
           GO TO Q.4

   3a. Who is the Medical Director?
   IV:22   (NAME)

   3b. Does the Medical Director serve in this capacity full-time or part-time?
   IV:23
   | 1. FULL-TIME | 2. PART-TIME | 8. DON'T KNOW |

   3c. What is the Medical Director's specialty within medicine?
   IV:24
   _____
   (SPECIFY)

4. Apart from the Emergency Unit/Emergency Room is there a separate facility for emergency psychiatric care in this hospital?
   IV:25
   | 1. YES | 2. NO | 8. DON'T KNOW |

- 3 -

5. Excluding cases handled by the Emergency Unit, does this hospital have any "outpatient surgery" (or scheduled "ambulatory surgery") program?
   IV:26
   | 1. YES | 2. NO | 8. DON'T KNOW |
   GO TO Q.6   GO TO Q.6

   5a. Is any thought being given to establishing such a program?
   IV:27
   | 1. YES | 2. NO | 8. DON'T KNOW |

ABOUT THE EMERGENCY UNIT'S OVERALL SITUATION

6. At the present time, what sorts of problems does the Emergency Unit of this hospital face? What would you say are the major problems or key issues?

6a. _____
IV:28- _____
29   _____

6b. _____
IV:30- _____
31   _____

6c. _____
IV:32- _____
33   _____

Hospital Administrators' Interview

- 4 -

7. What are the TWO or THREE most important areas, or respects, in which you consider this Emergency Unit to be particularly strong or especially outstanding?

7a.
IV:34-
35
_____
_____

7b.
IV:36-
37
_____
_____

7c.
IV:38-
39
_____
_____

8. And now, what are the TWO or THREE most important areas, or respects, in which you consider this Emergency Unit to be especially weak or to require the most improvement?

8a.
IV:40-
41
_____
_____

8b.
IV:42-
43
_____
_____

8c.
IV:44-
45
_____
_____

- 5 -

ABOUT PATIENT CARE ARRANGEMENTS AND THE PATIENTS

9. At the present time, does this Emergency Unit tend to concentrate on (or to specialize in) the treatment of any particular kinds of patients?
IV:46

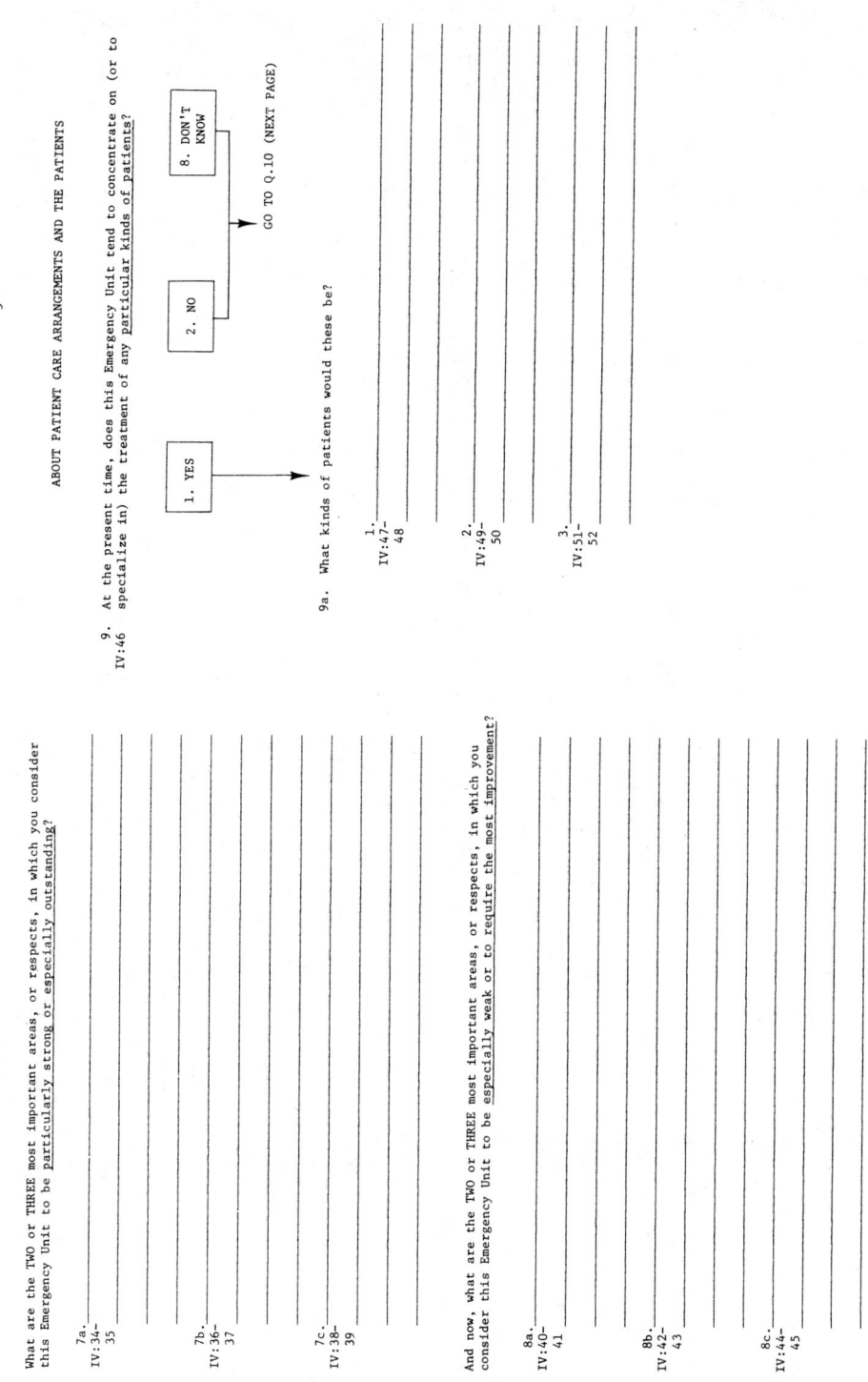

    1. YES   2. NO   8. DON'T KNOW
                        → GO TO Q.10 (NEXT PAGE)

9a. What kinds of patients would these be?

1.
IV:47-
48
_____
_____

2.
IV:49-
50
_____
_____

3.
IV:51-
52
_____
_____

Hospital Administrators' Interview

- 6 -

10. Are there any particular kinds of patients whose medical problems <u>cannot</u> be
IV:53 handled as adequately as they should be by this Emergency Unit?

    1. YES →
    2. NO → GO TO Q.11 (NEXT PAGE)
    8. DON'T KNOW →

    10a. Mainly, what kinds of patients would these be?

    1. _____
    IV:54-55
    2. _____
    IV:56-57
    3. _____
    IV:58-59

    10b. Why is it that these particular patients cannot be handled as adequately as they should?

    1. _____
    IV:60
    2. _____
    IV:61
    3. _____
    IV:62

- 7 -

11. What is your estimate of the average length of a patient visit to this Emergency
IV:63- Unit in a typical day? (I mean the average number of minutes from "time-in to
64   time-out" per patient visit.)

_____ (MINUTES)

12. Over the past four weeks, about what percent of the patients visiting this
IV:65- Emergency Unit, would you estimate, arrived in a "life-threatening" condition?
66

_____ (PERCENT)

13. And, about what percent of the patients visiting this Emergency Unit over the
IV:67- past four weeks, would you estimate, were "true emergencies"?
68

_____ (PERCENT)

Hospital Administrators' Interview

ABOUT RECENT CHANGES

14. In the past six months or so have any important changes or new ways of doing things
IV:69 been introduced in the Emergency Unit?

| 1. YES | 2. NO | 8. DON'T KNOW |

→ GO TO Q.15 (NEXT PAGE)

14a. What kinds of changes were these?

1.
IV:70-
   71 _____

2.
IV:72-
   73 _____

3.
IV:74-
   75 _____

14b. How well have they been working out?

1.
IV:76 _____

2.
IV:77 _____

3.
IV:78 _____

15. Currently, in this institution, are there any major changes being proposed for
V:17 the Emergency Unit?

| 1. YES | 2. NO | 8. DON'T KNOW |

→ GO TO Q.16 (NEXT PAGE)

15a. What kinds of changes would these be?

1.
V:18-
  19 _____

2.
V:20-
  21 _____

3.
V:22-
  23 _____

15b. How much support is there in the hospital for the proposed changes?

1.
V:24 _____

2.
V:25 _____

3.
V:26 _____

Hospital Administrators' Interview

- 10 -

16. Thinking now about the entire hospital, have there been any major changes in organization, services, or facilities in the past six months?
V:27

1. YES → 16a. What were these changes?
1. _____ V:28-29
2. _____ V:30-31
3. _____ V:32-33

16b. Did these changes have any significant impact—positive or negative—on the Emergency Unit?
1. _____ V:34
2. _____ V:35
3. _____ V:36

2. NO
8. DON'T KNOW
→ GO TO Q.17 (NEXT PAGE)

- 11 -

ABOUT CERTAIN ORGANIZATIONAL MATTERS

17. Some hospitals have formal mechanisms for monitoring the performance or the quality of work of their emergency unit. At the present time, does this institution have any such mechanisms?
V:37

1. YES → 17a. What would these mechanisms be?
1. _____ V:38-39
2. _____ V:40-41
3. _____ V:42-43

17b. How well have they been working out?
1. _____ V:44
2. _____ V:45
3. _____ V:46

2. NO
8. DON'T KNOW
→ GO TO Q.18 (NEXT PAGE)

Hospital Administrators' Interview

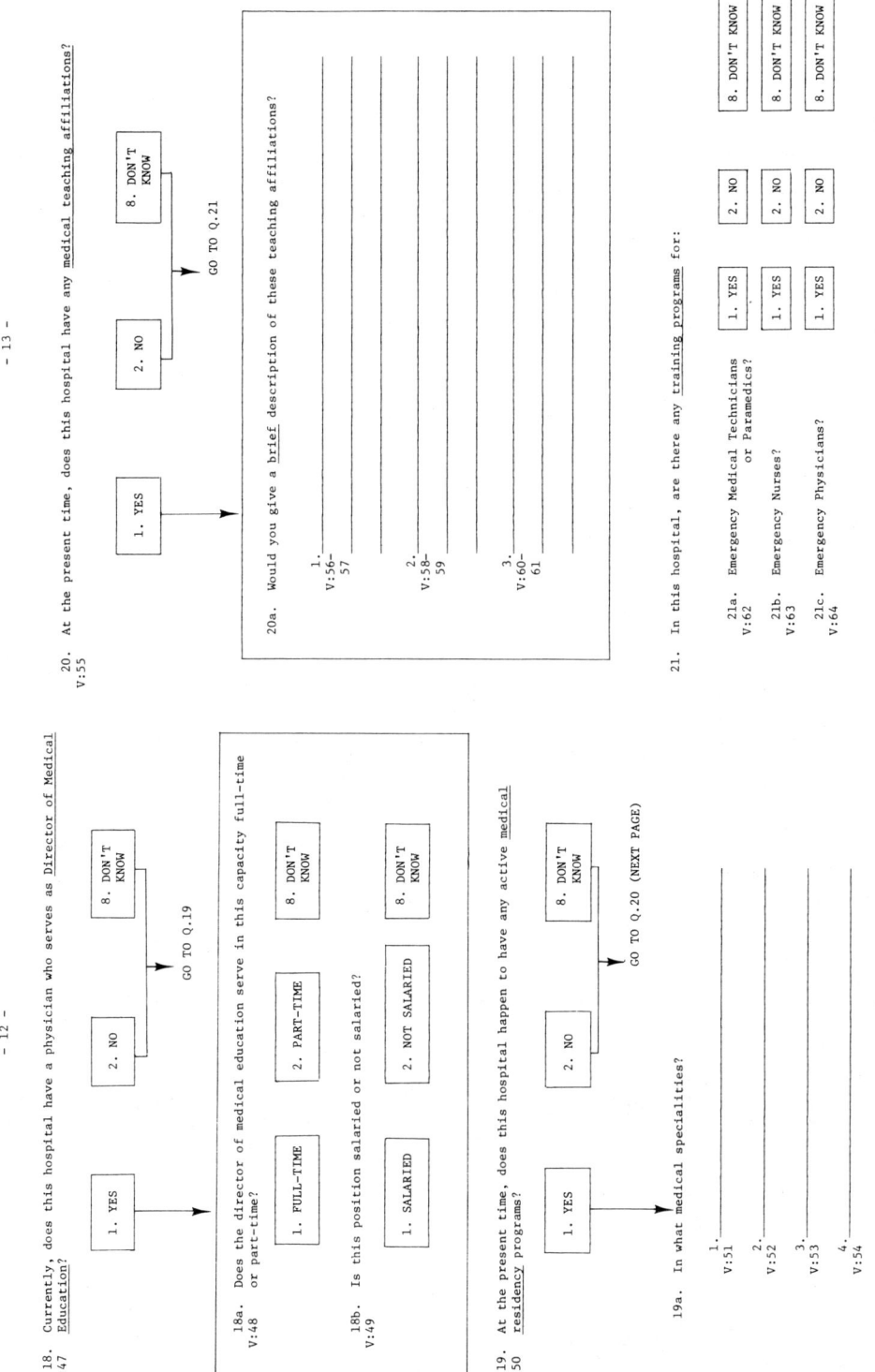

Hospital Administrators' Interview

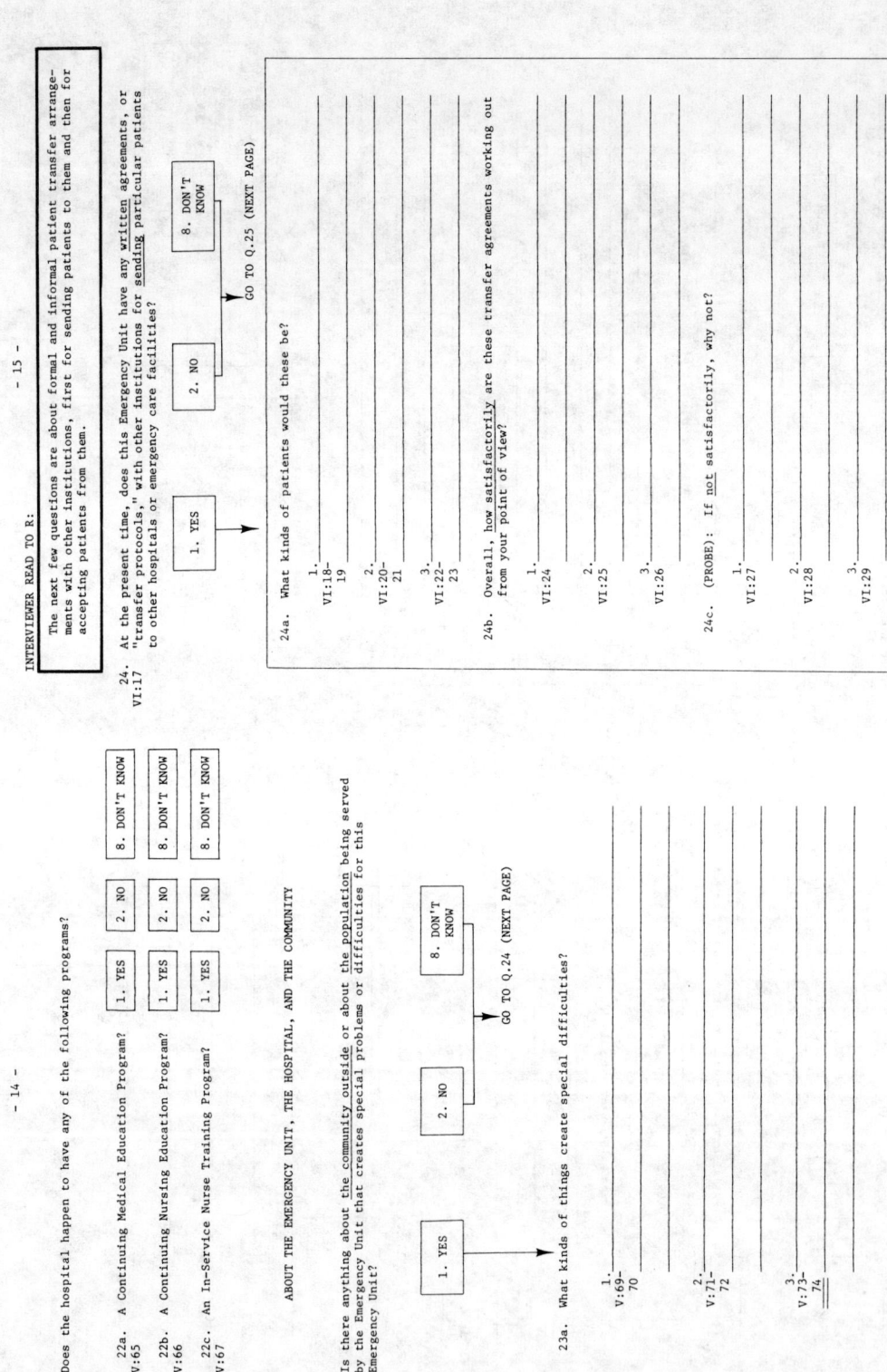

Hospital Administrators' Interview

25. What about informal transfer arrangements for sending particular patients to
VI:30 other facilities? Does the Emergency Unit have any?

[1. YES] →
[2. NO] → GO TO Q.26 (NEXT PAGE)
[8. DON'T KNOW] → GO TO Q.26 (NEXT PAGE)

25a. For what kinds of patients?

1. _____
VI:31-32

2. _____
VI:33-34

3. _____
VI:35-36

25b. Overall, how satisfactorily are these informal transfer arrangements working out from your point of view?

1. _____
VI:37

2. _____
VI:38

3. _____
VI:39

25c. (PROBE): If not satisfactorily, why not?

1. _____
VI:40

2. _____
VI:41

3. _____
VI:42

26. And what about accepting "transfer" patients? Does this Emergency Unit have any
VI:43 written agreements with other institutions for accepting transfer patients?

[1. YES] →
[2. NO] → GO TO Q.27 (NEXT PAGE)
[8. DON'T KNOW] → GO TO Q.27 (NEXT PAGE)

26a. What kinds of patients would these be?

1. _____
VI:44-45

2. _____
VI:46-47

3. _____
VI:48-49

26b. Overall, how satisfactorily are these transfer arrgements working out from your point of view?

1. _____
VI:50

2. _____
VI:51

3. _____
VI:52

26c. (PROBE): If not satisfactorily, why not?

1. _____
VI:53

2. _____
VI:54

3. _____
VI:55

Hospital Administrators' Interview

- 18 -

27. Finally, what about <u>informal</u> arrangements with other institutions for <u>accepting</u> transfer patients? Does this Emergency Unit have any?
VI:56

[1. YES] →

[2. NO] → GO TO Q.28

[8. DON'T KNOW] → GO TO Q.28 (NEXT PAGE)

27a. What kinds of patients would these be?

1. _____
VI:57-58

2. _____
VI:59-60

3. _____
VI:61-62

27b. Overall, how satisfactorily are these arrangements working out from your point of view?

1. _____
VI:63

2. _____
VI:64

3. _____
VI:65

27c. (PROBE): If <u>not</u> satisfactorily, why not?

1. _____
VI:66

2. _____
VI:67

3. _____
VI:68

- 19 -

28. Excluding patient transfer arrangements with other institutions, are there any emergency care facilities in the immediate area with which your Emergency Unit <u>collaborates</u> on some regular basis or in some significant way?
VI:69

[1. YES] →

[2. NO] → GO TO Q.29

[8. DON'T KNOW] → GO TO Q.29

28a. Would you briefly describe the nature of this collaboration:

1. _____
VI:70-71

2. _____
VI:72-73

29. At the present time, is there any BLS (Basic Life Support) or ALS (Advanced Life Support) "system" functioning in this community or the immediate area?
VI:74

[1. YES] →

[2. NO] → GO TO Q.30 (NEXT PAGE)

[8. DON'T KNOW] → GO TO Q.30 (NEXT PAGE)

29a. What kind of system would this be?
VI:75-76

Hospital Administrators' Interview

A FINAL QUESTION

30. All things considered, who would you say are the two or three most knowledgeable individuals in the community outside the hospital concerning this Emergency Unit?

PERSON'S NAME	POSITION (OCCUPATION, BUSINESS)	ORGANIZATION (OR PLACE OF WORK)
a.		
b.		
c.		

VI:77
VI:78
VI:79

INTERVIEWER READ TO R:

> Thank you very much. We are now finished with the first part of your interview. Next, we would like to have you complete the second part by filling out this more specific questionnaire.
>
> (INTERVIEWER: HAND THE RESPONDENT FORM 1, PART B, THE ADMINISTRATORS' QUESTIONNAIRE.)
>
> We greatly appreciate your cooperation.

Hospital Administrators' Questionnaire

The University of Michigan   Fall 1977

HOSPITAL EMERGENCY SERVICES STUDY

FORM 1, PART B: ADMINISTRATORS' QUESTIONNAIRE

Interviewer: _____
Interview No.: _____
Date: _____

HOSPITAL EMERGENCY SERVICES STUDY

FORM 1, PART B: ADMINISTRATORS' QUESTIONNAIRE

Institute for Social Research
The University of Michigan
Ann Arbor, Michigan

Study 462312
Fall 1977

Rights Reserved
The University of Michigan

INTRODUCTION

As you are answering the questions on the following pages, you will find that they are designed to supplement and extend the interview which you have completed. At the beginning, there are a few questions intended to provide some background information. Then, there are questions regarding hospital administration and the emergency unit, the emergency unit's priorities and goals, staffing and resources, patient care, work relations and problem solving, the overall operation of the emergency unit, the emergency unit and the community, and certain other aspects that were not covered in the interview. Most questions can be answered by checking (✓) one of the alternatives presented. If you do not find the exact alternative you desire, please check the one that comes closest or write your own answer. Thank you very much for your help; we appreciate your cooperation.

SOME BACKGROUND INFORMATION

1. How long have you been associated with this hospital? (Please enter number of years)
   I:17-18   _____ Years

2. How long have you been in your present position? (Please enter number of years)
   I:19-20   _____ Years

3. During the past five years, have you held the same or a similar position at any other health care institution? (Check one)
   I:21
   ____ (1) Yes
   ____ (2) No

4. What is your current title? (Please write in the correct title)
   I:22
   My current title is: _____

5. Professionally, what is your special interest within the broad field of administration? (Please write in)
   I:23
   My special interest is: _____

6. What is the highest professional or academic degree that you have earned? (Please write in)
   I:24
   Highest professional or academic degree: _____

7. What is your sex? (Check one)
   I:25
   ____ (1) Male
   ____ (2) Female

8. How old are you? (Check one)
   I:26
   ____ (1) 20 to 29 years
   ____ (2) 30 to 39 years
   ____ (3) 40 to 49 years
   ____ (4) 50 to 59 years
   ____ (5) 60 to 69 years
   ____ (6) 70 years or over

Hospital Administrators' Questionnaire

ABOUT HOSPITAL ADMINISTRATION AND THE EMERGENCY UNIT

9. From the point of view of being able to administer the emergency unit properly, on the whole how adequate is the information that Hospital Administration receives from the emergency unit? (Check one)
I:27
___ (1) Completely adequate
___ (2) Very adequate
___ (3) Fairly adequate
___ (4) Not so adequate
___ (5) Not adequate at all

10. Considering all the work-related contacts between Hospital Administration and the emergency unit, how satisfactory, would you say, are these contacts from the standpoint of administering the emergency unit properly? (Check one)
I:28
___ (1) Completely satisfactory
___ (2) Very satisfactory
___ (3) Fairly satisfactory
___ (4) Not so satisfactory
___ (5) Not satisfactory at all

11. In general, to what extent does the staff of the emergency unit understand and appreciate the constraints under which Hospital Administration operates? (Check one)
I:29
___ (1) They have an excellent understanding
___ (2) A very good understanding
___ (3) A good understanding
___ (4) A fair understanding
___ (5) They have a rather poor understanding

12. On the whole, to what extent does Hospital Administration understand and appreciate the work problems and needs of the emergency unit staff? (Check one)
I:30
___ (1) They have an excellent understanding
___ (2) A very good understanding
___ (3) A good understanding
___ (4) A fair understanding
___ (5) They have a rather poor understanding

13. From the standpoint of being able to provide the best emergency service possible, how much joint planning, would you say, is there between Hospital Administration and the emergency unit staff? (Check one)
I:31
___ (1) There is probably more than sufficient joint planning
___ (2) About the right amount of joint planning
___ (3) Somewhat less than is needed
___ (4) Much less than is needed
___ (5) There is no joint planning at all that I know of

14. How much difference, would you say, is there between the way the Hospital sees the job of doctors in the emergency unit and the way in which the doctors see their job? (Check one)
I:32
___ (1) A very small difference or no difference
___ (2) A small difference
___ (3) More than a small difference but not a considerable difference
___ (4) A considerable difference
___ (5) A very considerable difference

15. In this institution, to what extent does Hospital Administration do each of the following? (Check one for each line)

Extent to Which:

	To a very great extent (1)	To a great extent (2)	To a moderate extent (3)	To some extent (4)	Not at all (5)
Hospital Administration:					
I:33 Mediates differences between the emergency unit and other units in the hospital	☐	☐	☐	☐	☐
I:34 Determines policy for the emergency unit	☐	☐	☐	☐	☐
I:35 Determines the priorities and goals of the emergency unit	☐	☐	☐	☐	☐
I:36 Determines the relative allocation of hospital resources between the emergency unit and other hospital units	☐	☐	☐	☐	☐
I:37 Determines the operating budget of the emergency unit	☐	☐	☐	☐	☐
I:38 Evaluates the work of the emergency unit	☐	☐	☐	☐	☐
I:39 Mediates differences between the emergency unit and the community outside the hospital	☐	☐	☐	☐	☐

16. On the whole, how much influence would you say Hospital Administration has on each of the following? (Check one for each line)

Amount of Influence:

	Very considerable influence (1)	Considerable influence (2)	Moderate influence (3)	Little influence (4)	Very little or no influence (5)
Influence Regarding:					
I:40 The quality of care provided by this emergency unit	☐	☐	☐	☐	☐
I:41 The costs of emergency care	☐	☐	☐	☐	☐
I:42 How doctors and nurses in this emergency unit do their work	☐	☐	☐	☐	☐

Hospital Administrators' Questionnaire

17. At the present time, how is overall responsibility for each of the following kinds of decisions (or activities) divided between the emergency unit staff and other groups or individuals in the hospital. (Check one for each line)

Overall Responsibility:

Responsibility for:	Belongs exclusively to emergency unit staff (1)	Belongs mainly to emergency unit staff (2)	Is shared about equally between emergency unit staff and other hospital staff (3)	Belongs mainly to people outside the emergency unit (4)	Belongs exclusively to people outside the emergency unit (5)
I:43 Determining the priorities and goals of the emergency unit	☐	☐	☐	☐	☐
I:44 Establishing rules or procedures for patient care in the emergency unit	☐	☐	☐	☐	☐
I:45 Determining the emergency unit's operating budget	☐	☐	☐	☐	☐
I:46 Obtaining funds from outside the hospital for various emergency unit programs	☐	☐	☐	☐	☐
I:47 Evaluating the work of the emergency unit	☐	☐	☐	☐	☐
I:48 Deciding what tasks the different personnel in the emergency unit will perform or how their work roles are defined	☐	☐	☐	☐	☐

ABOUT EMERGENCY UNIT PRIORITIES AND GOALS

18. Hospital emergency units may emphasize different priorities and goals, some of which are listed below. Please rank these priorities in order of their importance to this hospital's Emergency Unit at the present time. (Place 1 in front of the one which is most important, 2 in front of the next most important, etc...., and 7 in front of the least important.)

Rank

- I:49 _____ Maintaining a good reputation in the community
- I:50 _____ Improving working conditions for the staff
- I:51 _____ Minimizing patient waiting time
- I:52 _____ Keeping the costs of the emergency service down
- I:53 _____ Maintaining high standards of patient care
- I:54 _____ Providing comprehensive emergency services
- I:55 _____ Maintaining a high level of patient satisfaction

19. Generally, how much influence does each of the following have over the priorities and goals of this emergency unit? (Check one for each group)

Amount of Influence:

Influence By:	Very considerable influence (1)	Considerable influence (2)	Moderate influence (3)	Little influence (4)	Very little or no influence (5)
I:56 The Board of Trustees or Governing Authority of the hospital	☐	☐	☐	☐	☐
I:57 Hospital Administration	☐	☐	☐	☐	☐
I:58 The doctors who work in the emergency unit	☐	☐	☐	☐	☐
I:59 The nurses who work in the emergency unit	☐	☐	☐	☐	☐
I:60 The Patients	☐	☐	☐	☐	☐
I:61 The Community Outside	☐	☐	☐	☐	☐

Hospital Administrators' Questionnaire

ABOUT STAFFING AND RESOURCES

20. At the present time, what is the basic medical staffing pattern for the emergency unit in this hospital? (Check one)
I:62
___ (1) Rotation of Attending Staff Physicians (without residents or interns)
___ (2) Combination of rotating Attending Staff With Residents or Interns
___ (3) Combination of non-rotating Attending Staff with Residents or Interns
___ (4) Physicians' Group on Contract (hospital-based group)
___ (5) Physicians' Group on Contract (not hospital-based)
___ (6) Medical Corporation on Contract
___ (7) Individual Physicians on Contract, full-time
___ (8) Part-time Individual Physicians on Contract
___ (9) Other than the above (please specify): _____

21. Of the following statements, which one would you say most accurately reflects the principles or policy governing medical staffing of the Emergency Unit at the present time? (Check one)
I:63
___ (1) The unit is staffed for "peak patient load"
___ (2) It is staffed for an "above average" patient volume but not for "peak load"
___ (3) The unit is staffed for an "average" level of patient volume

22. And, which of the following statements most accurately reflects the principles or policy governing the non-medical staffing (i.e., nursing personnel, etc.) of the emergency unit? (Check one)
I:64
___ (1) The unit is staffed for "peak patient load"
___ (2) It is staffed for an "above average" patient volume but not for "peak load"
___ (3) The unit is staffed for an "average" level of patient volume

23. How difficult is it for this hospital to recruit and maintain professional nursing staff for the Emergency Unit? (Check one)
I:65
___ (1) It is very easy
___ (2) Fairly easy
___ (3) Not as easy as it should be
___ (4) It is rather difficult
___ (5) It is very difficult

24. Considering what this emergency unit needs to provide high quality care to its patients at reasonable cost, how sufficient would you say is the quantity (amount) of each of the following resources? (Check one for each line)

The Quantity (Amount) Of These Resources Is:

Resources:	Completely sufficient (1)	Very sufficient (2)	Fairly sufficient (3)	Not so sufficient (4)	Not sufficient at all (5)
I:66 Medical staffing of the emergency unit	☐	☐	☐	☐	☐
I:67 RN staffing of the emergency unit	☐	☐	☐	☐	☐
I:68 Other staffing of the emergency unit	☐	☐	☐	☐	☐
I:69 The amount of total funds (total budget excluding capital funds) allocated to the emergency unit by the hospital	☐	☐	☐	☐	☐
I:70 The information received by emergency unit staff from other parts of the hospital	☐	☐	☐	☐	☐
I:71 The space (building space) controlled by the emergency unit	☐	☐	☐	☐	☐
I:72 All other physical facilities and equipment available to the emergency unit	☐	☐	☐	☐	☐

25. If, in the next two months, patient visits were to increase by 10%-15% but the quality of patient care were to remain at its current level, how well could the present staff of this emergency unit handle the increased patient volume? (Check one)
I:73
___ (1) The present staff could handle the increased volume without any difficulties
___ (2) It could handle it with some minor difficulties
___ (3) It could handle it with moderate difficulties
___ (4) It could handle it, but with great difficulties
___ (5) It could handle it, but with very great difficulties
___ (6) The present staff could not handle it at all

26. Considering the number of patients the staff now sees on an average day, what effect would a 10%-15% DECREASE in patient visits have on the quality of care provided by this emergency unit? (Check one)
I:74
___ (1) The quality of care would improve very considerably
___ (2) Quality would improve considerably
___ (3) Quality would improve moderately
___ (4) Quality would improve, but only a little
___ (5) Quality would improve very little
___ (6) The quality of care would not improve

Hospital Administrators' Questionnaire

---

27. Based on your knowledge and observations, how would you characterize the medical leadership of this emergency unit? (Check one)
I:75

___ (1) The medical leadership of the emergency unit is extremely effective
___ (2) Very effective
___ (3) Fairly effective
___ (4) Not so effective
___ (5) Not effective at all

28. Based on your knowledge and observations, how would you characterize the nursing leadership of the emergency unit? (Check one)
I:76

___ (1) The nursing leadership of the emergency unit is extremely effective
___ (2) Very effective
___ (3) Fairly effective
___ (4) Not so effective
___ (5) Not effective at all

29. In this hospital, is the emergency unit considered a separate "cost center" at the present time? (Check one)
I:77

___ (1) Yes
___ (2) No

ABOUT PATIENT CARE

30. Considering the emergency units of all other hospitals with which you are familiar, how would you estimate the overall quality of patient care provided in this particular emergency unit? (Check one)
II:17

___ (1) Overall, the quality of patient care in this emergency unit is outstanding compared to most other units
___ (2) It is much better than in most other emergency units
___ (3) It is generally better
___ (4) It is about the same as in most other units
___ (5) It is somewhat poorer
___ (6) It is generally poorer
___ (7) Overall, the quality of patient care in this emergency unit is much poorer compared to most other units
___ (8) I can't judge

31. Which of the following best describes this hospital's emergency unit (Emergency Room, Department) in terms of the services it provides? (Check one)
II:18

___ (1) The emergency unit here provides comprehensive emergency medical services
___ (2) It provides nearly comprehensive services
___ (3) It provides basic emergency services
___ (4) It provides more limited emergency medical services

32. For the purpose of answering this question, please assume that even in the very best of emergency units and under the most favorable circumstances, not every member of the MEDICAL STAFF is doing outstanding or excellent work consistently. With this assumption in mind, please indicate about how many of the doctors working in this emergency unit are doing outstanding or excellent work consistently. (Check one)
II:19

___ (1) More than 3 out of every 4 doctors are doing outstanding or excellent work consistently
___ (2) About 3 out of every 4 doctors
___ (3) About 2 out of every 3 doctors
___ (4) About 1 out of every 2 doctors
___ (5) About 1 out of every 3 doctors
___ (6) About 1 out of every 4 doctors
___ (7) Fewer than 1 out of every 4 doctors are doing outstanding or excellent work consistently

33. For the purpose of answering this question, please assume that even in the very best emergency units and under the most favorable circumstances, not every member of the PROFESSIONAL NURSING STAFF is doing outstanding or excellent work consistently. With this assumption in mind, please indicate about how many of the professional nurses in this emergency unit are doing outstanding or excellent work consistently. (Check one)
II:20

___ (1) More than 3 out of every 4 nurses are doing outstanding or excellent work consistently
___ (2) About 3 out of every 4 nurses
___ (3) About 2 out of every 3 nurses
___ (4) About 1 out of every 2 nurses
___ (5) About 1 out of every 3 nurses
___ (6) About 1 out of every 4 nurses
___ (7) Fewer than 1 out of every 4 nurses are doing outstanding or excellent work consistently

34. Considering the patient care practices and procedures used in the emergency unit at the present time, on the whole, how appropriate are they with respect to each of the following? (Check one for each line)

Care Practices and Procedures Are:

	Completely appropriate (1)	Very appropriate (2)	Fairly appropriate (3)	Not so appropriate (4)	Not appropriate at all (5)
With Respect to Enabling the Staff:					
II:21 To provide care of the highest quality possible	☐	☐	☐	☐	☐
II:22 To provide care at the lowest cost possible	☐	☐	☐	☐	☐
II:23 To provide care as promptly as it should be provided	☐	☐	☐	☐	☐

Hospital Administrators' Questionnaire

- 10 -

35. Considering the kind of service that this emergency unit provides to its patients,
II:24 how do you feel about what it charges the patients (or their insurance)? (Check one)

___ (1) Patient charges are too low considering the kind of service provided
___ (2) They are rather low
___ (3) They are about right
___ (4) They are rather high
___ (5) They are very high
___ (6) Patient charges are extremely high considering the kind of service provided
___ (8) I can't judge

ABOUT WORK RELATIONS AND PROBLEM SOLVING

36. Work problems in emergency units may be handled in a number of different ways, some of which may be more effective than others. Listed below are five different ways in which work problems might be handled. Please rank them from the one that is generally most effective in this hospital's emergency unit to the one that is least effective. (Place 1 in front of the way that is most effective, 2 in front of the next most effective way, etc...., and 5 in front of the least effective way.)

II:25 ___ Careful and precise timing and scheduling of tasks and work activities

II:26 ___ Correcting immediately any departures from the proper way of doing things

II:27 ___ Improving the staff's level of understanding of the work requirements of the unit so people can handle problems in a preventive way by anticipating them before they arise

II:28 ___ Trying to find better ways of doing things even when things operate smoothly and without problems

II:29 ___ Making sure that existing rules and regulations are followed by all concerned

37. Overall, how well do the different jobs and activities around the patient
II:30 fit together in the emergency unit? (Check one)

___ (1) They fit together extremely well
___ (2) Very well
___ (3) Fairly well
___ (4) Not so well
___ (5) Not well at all

38. In the emergency unit, to what extent do the different people
II:31 who have to work together take into account each other's work problems and needs as they go about doing their own activities? (Check one)

___ (1) To a very great extent
___ (2) A great extent
___ (3) A fair extent
___ (4) A small extent
___ (5) To a very small extent or not at all

- 11 -

39. All things considered, how much tension (friction, strain, or conflict) would you say is there between the groups specified in each of the following pairs? (Check one for each pair of groups)

Level of Tension:

Tension Between:	A high level of tension (1)	A moderate level of tension (2)	A low level of tension (3)	A very low level of tension (4)	No tension at all (5)
II:32 Emergency unit staff and Hospital Administration	☐	☐	☐	☐	☐
II:33 Doctors in the emergency unit and Hospital staff outside the emergency unit	☐	☐	☐	☐	☐
II:34 Nursing staff in the emergency unit and Hospital staff outside the emergency unit	☐	☐	☐	☐	☐
II:35 Doctors in the emergency unit and Nurses in the emergency unit	☐	☐	☐	☐	☐
II:36 Some nursing personnel in the emergency unit and Other nursing personnel in the emergency unit	☐	☐	☐	☐	☐
II:37 Some doctors in the emergency unit and Other doctors in the emergency unit	☐	☐	☐	☐	☐
II:38 Doctors in the emergency unit and Patients	☐	☐	☐	☐	☐
II:39 Nurses in the emergency unit and Patients	☐	☐	☐	☐	☐
II:40 Emergency unit staff and The community outside	☐	☐	☐	☐	☐

40. To what extent do the people in the emergency unit make an effort to
II:41 avoid creating problems or interferences with each other's duties and responsibilities? (Check one)

___ (1) To a very great extent
___ (2) A great extent
___ (3) A fair extent
___ (4) A small extent
___ (5) To a very small extent or not at all

41. To the best of your knowledge, how frequently are there unnecessary
II:42 work delays (avoidable delays) among the people whose work is related in the emergency unit? (Check one)

___ (1) Rarely or infrequently
___ (2) Not too frequently
___ (3) Fairly frequently
___ (4) Very frequently
___ (5) Extremely frequently

Hospital Administrators' Questionnaire

- 12 -

ABOUT THE OVERALL OPERATION OF THE EMERGENCY UNIT

42. Generally, how much influence does each of the following have on how this emergency unit operates? (Check one for each group)

Amount of Influence:

Influence By:	Very considerable influence (1)	Considerable influence (2)	Moderate influence (3)	Little influence (4)	Very little or no influence (5)
II:43 The Board of Trustees or Governing Authority of the hospital	☐	☐	☐	☐	☐
II:44 Hospital Administration	☐	☐	☐	☐	☐
II:45 The doctors who work in the emergency unit	☐	☐	☐	☐	☐
II:46 The nurses who work in the emergency unit	☐	☐	☐	☐	☐
II:47 The Patients	☐	☐	☐	☐	☐
II:48 The Community Outside	☐	☐	☐	☐	☐

43. Generally, how much influence should each of the following have on how this emergency unit operates? (Check one for each group)

Amount of Influence:

Influence By:	Very considerable influence (1)	Considerable influence (2)	Moderate influence (3)	Little influence (4)	Very little or no influence (5)
II:49 The Board of Trustees or Governing Authority of the hospital	☐	☐	☐	☐	☐
II:50 Hospital Administration	☐	☐	☐	☐	☐
II:51 The doctors who work in the emergency unit	☐	☐	☐	☐	☐
II:52 The nurses who work in the emergency unit	☐	☐	☐	☐	☐
II:53 The Patients	☐	☐	☐	☐	☐
II:54 The Community Outside	☐	☐	☐	☐	☐

- 13 -

ABOUT THE EMERGENCY UNIT AND THE COMMUNITY

44. At the present time, what kind of reputation does this emergency unit have in
II:55 the community outside? (Check one)

___ (1) This emergency unit has an excellent reputation in the community
___ (2) A very good reputation
___ (3) A good reputation
___ (4) A fair reputation
___ (5) This emergency unit has a rather poor reputation in the community

45. Do the people in the community seem to
II:56 have adequate information about the services which this emergency unit can and cannot provide? (Check one)

Most people seem to have:

___ (1) Completely adequate information
___ (2) Very adequate information
___ (3) Fairly adequate information
___ (4) Not so adequate information
___ (5) Inadequate information

46. Some communities are quite active in
II:57 applying pressures on hospitals for better, less costly, or more extensive services from hospital emergency units. On the whole, how much pressure of this type is currently being applied to this hospital and/or its emergency unit? (Check one)

___ (1) A very great amount of community pressure
___ (2) A great amount
___ (3) A fair amount
___ (4) A small amount
___ (5) A very small amount or none at all

47. The emergency health care needs of
II:58 communities change from time to time. How well has the emergency unit of your hospital been able to keep up and respond to such changes? (Check one)

___ (1) Extremely well
___ (2) Very well
___ (3) Fairly well
___ (4) Not too well
___ (5) Not well at all

48. On the whole, how adequately would
II:59 you say is this emergency unit meeting current community expectations regarding the services it provides? (Check one)

___ (1) Extremely adequately
___ (2) Very adequately
___ (3) Fairly adequately
___ (4) Not so adequately
___ (5) Not adequately at all

49. All things considered, how realistic
II:60 would you say are the community's expectations regarding the services provided by this emergency unit? (Check one)

___ (1) Extremely realistic
___ (2) Very realistic
___ (3) Fairly realistic
___ (4) Not so realistic
___ (5) Not realistic at all

Hospital Administrators' Questionnaire

50. To what extent is Hospital Administration able to get sufficient information
II:61   about the emergency care needs of the community when desired? (Check one)

    ___ (1) To a very great extent
    ___ (2) To a great extent
    ___ (3) To a fair extent
    ___ (4) To a small extent
    ___ (5) To a very small extent or not at all

51. At the present time, to what extent is this hospital or emergency unit collaborating
    with other hospitals, emergency units, or relevant service agencies for the following
    purposes? (Check one for each line)

    It Is Collaborating:

Purpose:	To a very great extent (1)	To a great extent (2)	To a fair extent (3)	To a small extent (4)	To a very small extent or not at all (5)
II:62 To provide better or less costly emergency medical services to the community	☐	☐	☐	☐	☐
II:63 To facilitate or improve the work of this emergency unit	☐	☐	☐	☐	☐
II:64 To share useful information about the emergency medical needs of the community	☐	☐	☐	☐	☐
II:65 To establish or maintain special emergency care facilities or a regional system	☐	☐	☐	☐	☐
II:66 To train emergency medical technicians or other emergency service personnel	☐	☐	☐	☐	☐

52. Considering all of the work-related contacts that the staff of the emergency unit
    have with each of the following, how satisfactory would you say are their contacts
    from the standpoint of accomplishing the work of this emergency unit? (Check one
    for each line)

    These Contacts Are:

Emergency Unit Staff Contacts With:	Completely satisfactory (1)	Very satisfactory (2)	Fairly satisfactory (3)	Not so satisfactory (4)	Not satisfactory at all (5)	They have no contacts with this personnel (0)
II:67 Sheriff's department personnel	☐	☐	☐	☐	☐	___
II:68 Police department personnel	☐	☐	☐	☐	☐	___
II:69 Fire department personnel	☐	☐	☐	☐	☐	___
II:70 Private ambulance services personnel	☐	☐	☐	☐	☐	___
II:71 Public safety department personnel	☐	☐	☐	☐	☐	___
II:72 Local health department personnel	☐	☐	☐	☐	☐	___
II:73 Coroner or medical examiner(s)	☐	☐	☐	☐	☐	___
II:74 Health Systems Agency (HSA) personnel	☐	☐	☐	☐	☐	___

53. With approximately how many of the personnel from these outside groups would you
II:75   say the work-related contacts of the emergency unit staff are tense or strained
    at the present time? (Check one)

    ___ (1) Contacts with very few or none of these personnel are tense/strained
    ___ (2) Contacts with a few of these personnel are tense/strained
    ___ (3) Contacts with some of these personnel are tense/strained
    ___ (4) Contacts with many of these personnel are tense/strained
    ___ (5) Emergency unit staff contacts with all or nearly all of these personnel
            are tense/strained
    ___ (8) I don't know

Hospital Administrators' Questionnaire

- 16 -

54. On the whole, how much influence would you say outside agencies and regulatory bodies (like state and local health agencies, HSA's, PSRO's, etc.) have on each of the following? (Check one for each line)

Amount of Influence:

Influence Regarding:	Very considerable influence (1)	Considerable influence (2)	Moderate influence (3)	Little influence (4)	Very little or no influence (5)
III:17 The priorities and goals of this emergency unit	☐	☐	☐	☐	☐
III:18 How this emergency unit operates	☐	☐	☐	☐	☐
III:19 The quality of care provided by this emergency unit	☐	☐	☐	☐	☐
III:20 How the doctors and nurses in this emergency unit do their work	☐	☐	☐	☐	☐
III:21 The costs of emergency care	☐	☐	☐	☐	☐

55. On the whole, how much influence SHOULD these outside agencies and regulatory bodies (like state and community health agencies, HSA's, PSRO's, etc.) have on each of the following? (Check one for each line)

Amount of Influence:

Influence Regarding:	Very considerable influence (1)	Considerable influence (2)	Moderate influence (3)	Little influence (4)	Very little or no influence (5)
III:22 The priorities and goals of this emergency unit	☐	☐	☐	☐	☐
III:23 How this emergency unit operates	☐	☐	☐	☐	☐
III:24 The quality of care provided by this emergency unit	☐	☐	☐	☐	☐
III:25 How the doctors and nurses in this emergency unit do their work	☐	☐	☐	☐	☐
III:26 The costs of emergency care	☐	☐	☐	☐	☐

- 17 -

56. From the point of view of being able to administer the emergency unit properly, on the whole, how adequate is the information that Hospital Administration has about the requirements and working of these outside health agencies and regulatory bodies? (Check one)

III:27

___ (1) Completely adequate
___ (2) Very adequate
___ (3) Fairly adequate
___ (4) Not so adequate
___ (5) Not adequate at all

THANK YOU VERY MUCH. WE APPRECIATE YOUR COOPERATION.

The University of Michigan
Institute for Social Research

Study 462312
Fall 1977

HOSPITAL EMERGENCY SERVICES STUDY

FORM 2, PART A: EMERGENCY UNIT PHYSICIANS' INTERVIEW

Interviewer: _____
Interview No.: _____
Date: _____

EU Physicians' Interview

Study 462312   Fall 1977

FORM 2, PART A: EMERGENCY UNIT PHYSICIANS' INTERVIEW

First, some general questions about the emergency unit (i.e., the emergency room or department) here.

1. Does this Emergency Unit tend to concentrate on (or to specialize in) the treatment
IV:17 of any particular kinds of patients?

┌─────────┐   ┌───────┐   ┌──────────┐
│ 1. YES │   │ 2. NO │   │ 8. DON'T │
│   │   │   │   │   KNOW │
└────┬────┘   └───┬───┘   └─────┬────┘
     │   │   │
     ▼   └──────────────┴─── GO TO Q.2 (NEXT PAGE)

1a. What kinds of patients would these be?

1. _____
IV:18-
19   _____

2. _____
IV:20-
21   _____

3. _____
IV:22-
23   _____

EU Physicians' Interview

- 2 -

2. At the present time, what sorts of problems does the Emergency Unit of this hospital face? What would you say are the <u>major</u> problems or key issues?

a. _____
IV:24- _____
   25   _____

b. _____
IV:26- _____
   27   _____

c. _____
IV:28- _____
   29   _____

3. What are the TWO or THREE most important areas, or respects, in which you consider this Emergency Unit to be particularly strong or especially outstanding?

a. _____
IV:30- _____
   31

b. _____
IV:32- _____
   33

c. _____
IV:34- _____
   35   _____

- 3 -

4. And now, what are the TWO or THREE most important areas, or respects, in which you consider this emergency unit to be especially weak or to require the most improvement?

a. _____
IV:36- _____
   37   _____

b. _____
IV:38- _____
   39

c. _____
IV:40- _____
   41

EU Physicians' Interview

- 4 -

INTERVIEWER READ TO R:

The next few questions are about patient transfer arrangements with other institutions, first for sending patients to them, and then for accepting patients from them.

5. Currently, does this Emergency Unit have any written agreements ("transfer protocols") or informal arrangements with other institutions for sending particular patients to other hospitals or emergency care facilities?
IV:42

[1. YES] → [2. NO] [8. DON'T KNOW]
                    → GO TO Q.6 (NEXT PAGE)

5a. What kinds of patients would these be?

1.
IV:43-44
2.
IV:45-46
3.
IV:47-48

5b. Overall, how satisfactorily are these transfer arrangements working out from your point of view?

1.
IV:49
2.
IV:50
3.
IV:51

5c. (PROBE): If not satisfactorily, why not?

1.
IV:52
2.
IV:53
3.
IV:54

- 5 -

6. And what about accepting "transfer" patients? Does this Emergency Unit have any written agreements or informal arrangements with other institutions for accepting transfer patients?
IV:55

[1. YES] → [2. NO] [8. DON'T KNOW]
                    → GO TO Q.7 (NEXT PAGE)

6a. For what kinds of patients?

1.
IV:56-57
2.
IV:58-59
3.
IV:60-61

6b. Overall, how satisfactorily are these transfer arrangements working out from your point of view?

1.
IV:62
2.
IV:63
3.
IV:64

6c. (PROBE): If not satisfactorily, why not?

1.
IV:65
2.
IV:66
3.
IV:67

EU Physicians' Interview

- 6 -

ABOUT THE PATIENTS VISITING THE EMERGENCY UNIT

7. Are there any particular kinds of patients whose medical problems cannot be handled as adequately as they should be by this Emergency Unit?
IV:68

☐ 1. YES →

☐ 2. NO

☐ 8. DON'T KNOW → GO TO Q.8

7a. Mainly, what kinds of patients would these be?

1.
IV:69-70 _____

2.
IV:71-72 _____

3.
IV:73-74 _____

7b. Why is it that these particular patients cannot be handled as adequately as they should?

1.
IV:75 _____

2.
IV:76 _____

3.
IV:77 _____

8. In your opinion, about what percent of the patients visiting this Emergency Unit over the past four weeks were seriously ill or seriously injured?
V:17-18

_____ (PERCENT)

- 7 -

9. And, about what percent of the patients visiting this emergency unit over the past four weeks would you estimate should have gone to a private physician or had a problem that could have been handled in a doctor's office instead of the Emergency Unit?
V:19-20

_____ (PERCENT)

10. Of all the patients visiting the Emergency Unit in the past four weeks, about what percent do you estimate were seen by a doctor within the first 15 minutes after arriving here?
V:21-22

_____ (PERCENT)

11. Could you please also give me your estimate of the average length of a patient visit to this Emergency Unit in a typical day? (I mean average number of minutes from "time-in to time-out" per patient visit.)
V:23-24

_____ (NUMBER OF MINUTES)

EU Physicians' Interview

- 8 -

12. Some hospitals have formal mechanisms for monitoring the performance or the quality of work of their emergency unit. At the present time, does this institution have any such mechanisms?

V:25

| 1. YES | 2. NO | 8. DON'T KNOW |

→ GO TO Q.13 (NEXT PAGE)

12a. What would these mechanisms be?

1. _____
V:26-
27   _____

2. _____
V:28-
29   _____

3. _____
V:30-
31   _____

12b. How well have they been working out?

1. _____
V:32   _____

2. _____
V:33   _____

3. _____
V:34   _____

- 9 -

ABOUT THE EMERGENCY UNIT AND THE COMMUNITY

13. At the present time, what kind of reputation does this Emergency Unit have in the community outside? Would you say it has an excellent reputation, a very good reputation, a good reputation, a fair reputation, or a rather poor reputation?

V:35-36

| 1. AN EXCELLENT REPUTATION | 2. A VERY GOOD REPUTATION | 3. A GOOD REPUTATION | 4. A FAIR REPUTATION | 5. A RATHER POOR REPUTATION |

14. Is there anything about the community outside or about the population being served by the Emergency Unit that creates special problems or difficulties for this Emergency Unit?

V:37

| 1. YES | 2. NO | 8. DON'T KNOW |

→ GO TO Q.15 (NEXT PAGE)

14a. What kinds of things create special difficulties?

1. _____
V:38-
39   _____

2. _____
V:40-
41   _____

3. _____
V:42-
43   _____

EU Physicians' Interview

- 10 -

15. The emergency health care needs of communities change from time to time. How well has the Emergency Unit of this hospital been able to keep up and respond to
V:44- such changes? Would you say it has kept up extremely well, very well, fairly
45 well, not so well, or not well at all?

| 1. EXTREMELY WELL | 2. VERY WELL | 3. FAIRLY WELL | 4. NOT SO WELL | 5. NOT WELL AT ALL |

16. Please think about the work-related contacts that emergency unit staff have with
V:46- outside groups like the police, fire department, sheriff's department, local
47 health department, medical examiners, and ambulance service personnel.

On the whole, how satisfactory do you consider these contacts from the standpoint of accomplishing the work of the Emergency Unit? In general, are they completely satisfactory, very satisfactory, fairly satisfactory, not so satisfactory, or not satisfactory at all?

| 1. COMPLETELY SATISFACTORY | 2. VERY SATISFACTORY | 3. FAIRLY SATISFACTORY | 4. NOT SO SATISFACTORY | 5. NOT SATISFACTORY AT ALL |

ABOUT THE WORK SITUATION AND WORK RELATIONS IN THE EMERGENCY UNIT

17. On the whole, what do you think of this Emergency Unit as a place to work?
V:48- Would you say it is an excellent place, a very good place, a good place, a fair
49 place, or a rather poor place to work?

| 1. IT IS AN EXCELLENT PLACE TO WORK | 2. A VERY GOOD PLACE | 3. A GOOD PLACE | 4. A FAIR PLACE | 5. A RATHER POOR PLACE |

- 11 -

18. Overall, how well do the different jobs and activities around the patient fit together in this Emergency Unit? (I mean the activities of the different people
V:50- who are working in the Emergency Unit.) Do they fit together extremely well, very
51 well, fairly well, not so well, or not well at all?

| 1. EXTREMELY WELL | 2. VERY WELL | 3. FAIRLY WELL | 4. NOT SO WELL | 5. NOT WELL AT ALL |

19. Generally, to what extent do the nurses in this Emergency Unit make adjustments in their work activities in order to facilitate the work of the medical staff?
V:52- Would you say they make adjustments to a very great extent, a great extent, a
53 fair extent, a small extent, or to a very small extent or not at all?

| 1. TO A VERY GREAT EXTENT | 2. A GREAT EXTENT | 3. A FAIR EXTENT | 4. A SMALL EXTENT | 5. TO A VERY SMALL EXTENT OR NOT AT ALL |

20. All things considered, how adequate for your work needs is the information that you generally receive from others working in the Emergency Unit? Would you say
V:54- it is completely adequate, very adequate, fairly adequate, not so adequate, or not
55 adequate at all?

| 1. COMPLETELY ADEQUATE | 2. VERY ADEQUATE | 3. FAIRLY ADEQUATE | 4. NOT SO ADEQUATE | 5. NOT AT ALL ADEQUATE |

EU Physicians' Interview

- 12 -

21. And, what about the information that you generally receive from people in other parts or departments of the hospital outside the Emergency Unit? Is it completely adequate, very adequate, fairly adequate, not so adequate, or not adequate at all for your needs?

V:56-57

| 1. COMPLETELY ADEQUATE | 2. VERY ADEQUATE | 3. FAIRLY ADEQUATE | 4. NOT SO ADEQUATE | 5. NOT ADEQUATE AT ALL |

22. When you request services or support from others in the hospital outside the Emergency Unit (for example, ancillary services, administrative support, cooperation from other medical units), on the whole, how satisfactorily are your requests met? Are most of these requests met completely satisfactorily, very satisfactorily, fairly satisfactorily, not so satisfactorily, or not satisfactorily at all?

V:58-59

| 1. COMPLETELY SATISFACTORILY | 2. VERY SATISFACTORILY | 3. FAIRLY SATISFACTORILY |

| 4. NOT SO SATISFACTORILY | 5. NOT SATISFACTORILY AT ALL |

- 13 -

A FINAL QUESTION

23. At the present time, who would you say are the TWO or THREE most influential individuals in this hospital concerning the Emergency Unit's situation and operation?

    NAME   POSITION OR TITLE

a. _____
V:60

b. _____
V:61

c. _____
V:62

INTERVIEWER READ TO R:

```
Thank you very much. We are now finished with the first part of your
interview. Next, we would like to have you complete the second part
by filling out this more specific questionnaire.

INTERVIEWER: HAND THE RESPONDENT FORM 2, PART B - EMERGENCY UNIT
PHYSICIANS' QUESTIONNAIRE.

We greatly appreciate your cooperation.
```

EU Physicians' Questionnaire

The University of Michigan   Fall 1977

HOSPITAL EMERGENCY SERVICES STUDY

FORM 2, PART B: EMERGENCY UNIT PHYSICIANS' QUESTIONNAIRE

Institute for Social Research
The University of Michigan
Ann Arbor, Michigan

Study 462312
Fall 1977

Rights Reserved
The University of Michigan

I N T R O D U C T I O N

As you are answering the questions on the following pages, you will find that they are designed to supplement and extend the interview which you have completed. At the beginning, there are a few questions intended to provide some background information. Then, there are questions regarding the emergency unit and the community, the priorities and operation of the emergency unit, resources and workload, patient care, work relations, work procedures, your work, and certain other aspects that were not covered in the interview. Most questions can be answered by checking (✓) one of the alternatives presented. If you do not find the exact alternative you desire, please check the one that comes closest or write your own answer. Thank you very much for your help; we appreciate your cooperation.

SOME BACKGROUND INFORMATION

1. How long have you been practicing medicine? (Please enter number of years)
I:17-18
_____ Years

2. How long have you been associated with this hospital? (Please enter number of years)
I:19-20
_____ Years

3. How long have you been working in this Emergency Unit? (Check one)
I:21
____ (1) Less than one year
____ (2) One year or more but less than two years
____ (3) Two years or more but less than four years
____ (4) Four years or more but less than ten years
____ (5) Ten years or more

4. At the present time, are you working in this Emergency Unit on a regular basis? (Check one)
I:22
____ (1) Yes
____ (2) No

5. Ordinarily, about how many hours a week do you work in this Emergency Unit? (Write in number of hours)
I:23-24
_____ Hours per week

Form 2, Part B: Emergency Unit Physicians' Questionnaire

Hospital Emergency Services Study

The University of Michigan

Interviewer: _____
Interview No.: _____
Date: _____

EU Physicians' Questionnaire

- 2 -

6. Professionally, what is your major field of interest or specialty within medicine? (Please write in)
I:25

Major field (specialty): _____

7. At the present time are you board-certified or board-eligible in any medical specialty? (Check one)
I:26
___ (1) Yes
___ (2) No

8. Are you currently a member of the American College of Emergency Physicians? (Check one)
I:27
___ (1) Yes
___ (2) No

9. Are you on the staff of any other hospital(s) at the present time? (Check one)
I:28
___ (1) Yes
___ (2) No

10. What is your sex? (Check one)
I:29
___ (1) Male
___ (2) Female

11. How old are you? (Check one)
I:30
___ (1) 20 to 29 years
___ (2) 30 to 39 years
___ (3) 40 to 49 years
___ (4) 50 to 59 years
___ (5) 60 to 69 years
___ (6) 70 years or over

ABOUT THE EMERGENCY UNIT AND THE COMMUNITY

12. On the whole, how adequately would you say is this emergency unit meeting current community expectations regarding the services it provides? (Check one)
I:31
___ (1) Extremely adequately
___ (2) Very adequately
___ (3) Fairly adequately
___ (4) Not so adequately
___ (5) Not adequately at all

13. All things considered, how realistic would you say are the community's expectations regarding the services provided by this emergency unit? (Check one)
I:32
___ (1) Extremely realistic
___ (2) Very realistic
___ (3) Fairly realistic
___ (4) Not so realistic
___ (5) Not realistic at all

14. Some communities are quite active in applying pressure on hospitals for better, less costly, or more extensive services to be provided by hospital emergency units. On the whole, how much pressure of this type is currently being applied to this hospital and/or its emergency unit? (Check one)
I:33
___ (1) A very great amount of community pressure is being applied
___ (2) A great amount
___ (3) A fair amount
___ (4) A small amount
___ (5) A very small amount or none at all

- 3 -

15. Considering the kind of service that this emergency unit provides to its patients, how do you feel about what it charges the patients (or their insurance) for their care? (Check one)
I:34
___ (1) Patient charges are too low considering the kind of service provided
___ (2) They are rather low
___ (3) They are about right
___ (4) They are rather high
___ (5) They are very high
___ (6) Patient charges are extremely high considering the kind of service provided
___ (8) I can't judge

16. On the whole, how much influence would you say outside agencies and regulatory bodies (like state and local health agencies, HSA's, PSRO's, etc.) have on each of the following? (Check one for each line)

Amount of Influence:

Influence on:	Very considerable influence (1)	Considerable influence (2)	Moderate influence (3)	Little influence (4)	Very little or no influence (5)
I:35 The quality of care provided by this emergency unit	☐	☐	☐	☐	☐
I:36 How the doctors and nurses in this emergency unit do their work	☐	☐	☐	☐	☐
I:37 The costs of emergency care here	☐	☐	☐	☐	☐

17. From the point of view of being able to do your work properly, on the whole, how adequate is the information that you have about the requirements and workings of these outside health agencies and regulatory bodies? (Check one)
I:38
___ (1) Completely adequate
___ (2) Very adequate
___ (3) Fairly adequate
___ (4) Not so adequate
___ (5) Not adequate at all

EU Physicians' Questionnaire

18. Please think of all the patients who were brought to this emergency unit by
I:39- ambulance over the past four weeks. For what percent of these patients,
40   would you say, did the ambulance personnel do their job "right"?
    (Write in %)

    _____ %

19. At the present time, how much medical control would you say is there over the
I:41 activities performed by emergency medical technicians and ambulance personnel
    who bring patients to this emergency unit? (Check one)

    ____ (1) There is very considerable medical control over the
             activities performed by these personnel
    ____ (2) There is considerable medical control
    ____ (3) There is moderate medical control
    ____ (4) There is some, but little medical control
    ____ (5) There is very little or no medical control over
             the activities performed by these personnel

ABOUT THE PRIORITIES AND OPERATION OF THE EMERGENCY UNIT

20. Hospital emergency units may emphasize different priorities and goals, some of
    which are listed below. Please rank these priorities in order of their impor-
    tance to this emergency unit. (Place 1 in front of the one which is the most
    important, 2 in front of the next most important, etc...., and 7 in front of
    the one which is the least important.)
    Rank

    I:42 _____ Maintaining a good reputation in the community
    I:43 _____ Improving working conditions for the staff
    I:44 _____ Minimizing patient waiting time
    I:45 _____ Keeping the costs of the emergency service down
    I:46 _____ Maintaining high standards of patient care
    I:47 _____ Providing comprehensive emergency services
    I:48 _____ Maintaining a high level of patient satisfaction

21. In emergency units like this, work problems may be handled in a number of
    different ways, some of which may be more effective than others. Listed
    below are some ways that are perhaps being used here. Please rank them from
    the one that is generally most effective to the one that is least effective
    in this emergency unit. (Place 1 in front of the way that is most effective,
    2 in front of the next most effective way, etc...., and 5 in front of the
    least effective way.)
    Rank

    I:49 _____ Careful and precise timing and scheduling of tasks and work
                activities
    I:50 _____ Correcting immediately any departures from the proper way of
                doing things
    I:51 _____ Improving the staff's level of understanding of the work
                requirements of the unit so people can handle problems in
                a preventive way by anticipating them before they arise
    I:52 _____ Trying to find better ways of doing things even when things
                operate smoothly and without problems
    I:53 _____ Making sure that existing rules and regulations are followed
                by all concerned

22. Generally, how much influence does each of the following have on how this
    emergency unit operates? (Check one for each group)

    Amount of Influence:

Influence By:	Very consid-erable influence (1)	Consider-able influence (2)	Moderate influence (3)	Little influence (4)	Very little or no influence (5)
I:54 The Board of Trustees or Governing Authority of this hospital	☐	☐	☐	☐	☐
I:55 Hospital Administration	☐	☐	☐	☐	☐
I:56 The doctors who work in the emergency unit	☐	☐	☐	☐	☐
I:57 The nurses who work in the emergency unit	☐	☐	☐	☐	☐
I:58 The patients	☐	☐	☐	☐	☐
I:59 The community outside	☐	☐	☐	☐	☐

EU Physicians' Questionnaire

23. Generally, how much influence should each of the following have on how this emergency unit operates? (Check one for each group)

Amount of Influence:

Influence By:	Very considerable influence (1)	Considerable influence (2)	Moderate influence (3)	Little influence (4)	Very little or no influence (5)
I:60 The Board of Trustees or Governing Authority of this hospital	☐	☐	☐	☐	☐
I:61 Hospital Administration	☐	☐	☐	☐	☐
I:62 The doctors who work in the emergency unit	☐	☐	☐	☐	☐
I:63 The nurses who work in the emergency unit	☐	☐	☐	☐	☐
I:64 The patients	☐	☐	☐	☐	☐
I:65 The community outside	☐	☐	☐	☐	☐

Appropriateness of Procedures

24. Please think of the various medical treatment and nursing care procedures used
I:66 in this emergency unit. On the whole, are most of them appropriate from the standpoint of enabling the staff to provide care of the highest quality possible? (Check one)

_____ (1) All or almost all of the medical and nursing procedures used in this unit are very appropriate
_____ (2) The large majority of them are
_____ (3) The majority of them are
_____ (4) About half of them are
_____ (5) Fewer than half of them are very appropriate

25. Again, thinking of the same proce-
I:67 dures, are most of them appropriate from the standpoint of enabling the staff to provide care at the lowest cost possible? (Check one)

_____ (1) All or almost all of them are very appropriate
_____ (2) The large majority of them are
_____ (3) The majority of them are
_____ (4) About half of them are
_____ (5) Fewer than half of them are very appropriate

26. Lastly, are most of these same
I:68 procedures appropriate from the standpoint of enabling the staff to provide care as promptly as it should be provided? (Check one)

_____ (1) All or almost all of them are very appropriate
_____ (2) The large majority of them are
_____ (3) The majority of them are
_____ (4) About half of them are
_____ (5) Fewer than half of them are very appropriate

ABOUT RESOURCES AND WORKLOAD

27. Considering what this emergency unit needs to provide high quality care to its patients at reasonable cost, how sufficient would you say is the quantity (amount) of each of the following resources? (Check one for each resource)

The Quantity (Amount) of These Resources is:

Resources:	Completely sufficient (1)	Very sufficient (2)	Fairly sufficient (3)	Not so sufficient (4)	Not sufficient at all (5)
I:69 Medical staffing of the emergency unit	☐	☐	☐	☐	☐
I:70 RN staffing of the emergency unit	☐	☐	☐	☐	☐
I:71 Other staffing of the emergency unit	☐	☐	☐	☐	☐
I:72 The amount of total funds (total budget excluding capital funds) allocated to the emergency unit by the hospital	☐	☐	☐	☐	☐
I:73 The information received by emergency unit staff from other parts of the hospital	☐	☐	☐	☐	☐
I:74 The space (building space) and physical facilities belonging to the emergency unit	☐	☐	☐	☐	☐

EU Physicians' Questionnaire

28. If, in the next two months, patient visits were to increase by 10%-15% but the quality of patient care were to remain at its current level, how well could the present staff of this emergency unit handle the increased patient volume? (Check one)
I:75

    ___ (1) The present staff could handle the increased volume without any difficulties
    ___ (2) It could handle it with some minor difficulties
    ___ (3) It could handle it with moderate difficulties
    ___ (4) It could handle it, but with great difficulties
    ___ (5) It could handle it, but with very great difficulties
    ___ (6) The present staff could not handle it at all

29. Considering the number of patients the staff now sees on an average day, what effect would a 10%-15% DECREASE in patient visits have on the quality of care provided by this emergency unit? (Check one)
I:76

    ___ (1) The quality of care would improve very considerably
    ___ (2) It would improve considerably
    ___ (3) It would improve moderately
    ___ (4) It would improve a little
    ___ (5) It would improve very little
    ___ (6) The quality of care would not improve

30. Please think about the 5% of the patients visiting this emergency unit over the past four weeks who presented the most complicated problems in terms of their medical care requirements. Overall, how well prepared would you say was this emergency unit to handle these complicated cases? (Check one)
I:77

    ___ (1) Extremely well prepared
    ___ (2) Very well prepared
    ___ (3) Fairly well prepared
    ___ (4) Not so well prepared
    ___ (5) Not well prepared at all

31. Considering all patient visits to this emergency unit over the past four-six weeks, approximately how many patients do you estimate were there in each of the categories specified? (Check one for each category)

The Number of Emergency Patients Was:

Category:	Considerable (1)	Moderate (2)	Small (3)	Very small (4)	Zero (There were no such patients) (5)
II:17 Acute Myocardial Infarction, Cardiac Arrest, and Ventricular Fibrillation cases	☐	☐	☐	☐	☐
II:18 Lacerations of the Face or Neck involving more than skin	☐	☐	☐	☐	☐
II:19 Acute Psychiatric Illnesses — suicide(depression), acute psychoses	☐	☐	☐	☐	☐
II:20 Fractures or Dislocations	☐	☐	☐	☐	☐
II:21 Acute Upper Respiratory Infections with Stridor, Epiglotitis, and Asthmatic Bronchitis cases	☐	☐	☐	☐	☐
II:22 Rape Cases	☐	☐	☐	☐	☐
II:23 Infants with Blood Disorders, Dehydration, Congenital Anomalies, or Respiratory Distress Syndrome	☐	☐	☐	☐	☐
II:24 Spinal Injuries or Closed Head Injuries with subdural hematomas or neurologic deficit	☐	☐	☐	☐	☐
II:25 Drug Abuse cases	☐	☐	☐	☐	☐
II:26 Burns of the face, ears, hands, feet, or perineum, and Burns involving 10% or more of total body surface area with 2% or more third degree	☐	☐	☐	☐	☐

EU Physicians' Questionnaire

32. Over the past four weeks, about what percent of the patients visiting this emergency unit arrived in what you would judge to be a "life-threatening" condition? (Please write in %) _____ %
II:27-28

33. Thinking of the patients who visited this emergency unit over the past four weeks, about how many of them would you say presented rather unusual problems or unique medical requirements? (Write in %) _____ %
II:29-30

34. About what percent of the patients visiting this emergency unit over the past four weeks, would you estimate had reached an "advanced state" in terms of the pathological progression of the illness or injury involved? (Write in %) _____ %
II:31-32

35. About what percent of the patients coming to this emergency unit over the past four weeks do you estimate arrived by ambulance or other emergency vehicle? (Write in %) _____ %
II:33-34

ABOUT PATIENT CARE

36. On the basis of your experience and information, how would you rate the quality of nursing care that patients generally receive in this emergency unit? (Check one)
II:35

____ (1) Nursing care in this emergency unit is outstanding
____ (2) Excellent
____ (3) Very good
____ (4) Good
____ (5) Fair
____ (6) Rather poor
____ (7) Nursing care in this emergency unit is poor

37. Considering the emergency units of all other hospitals with which you are familiar, how would you estimate the quality of medical care provided in this particular emergency unit? (Check one)
II:36

____ (1) The quality of medical care in this emergency unit is outstanding compared to most other emergency units
____ (2) It is much better than in most other emergency units
____ (3) It is generally better
____ (4) It is about the same as in most other emergency units
____ (5) It is somewhat poorer
____ (6) It is generally poorer
____ (7) The quality of medical care in this emergency unit is much poorer compared to most other emergency units
____ (8) I can't judge

38. For the purpose of answering this question, please assume that even in the very best emergency units and under the most favorable circumstances, not every member of the PROFESSIONAL NURSING STAFF is doing outstanding or excellent work consistently. With this assumption in mind, please indicate about how many of the professional nurses in this emergency unit are doing outstanding or excellent work consistently. (Check one)
II:37

____ (1) More than 3 out of every 4 nurses are doing outstanding or excellent work consistently
____ (2) About 3 out of every 4 nurses
____ (3) About 2 out of every 3 nurses
____ (4) About 1 out of every 2 nurses
____ (5) About 1 out of every 3 nurses
____ (6) About 1 out of every 4 nurses
____ (7) Fewer than 1 out of every 4 nurses are doing outstanding or excellent work consistently

39. For the purpose of answering this question, please assume that even in the very best emergency units and under the most favorable circumstances, not every member of the MEDICAL STAFF is doing outstanding or excellent work consistently. With this assumption in mind, please indicate about how many of the doctors working in this emergency unit are doing outstanding or excellent work consistently. (Check one)
II:38

____ (1) More than 3 out of every 4 doctors are doing outstanding or excellent work consistently
____ (2) About 3 out of every 4 doctors
____ (3) About 2 out of every 3 doctors
____ (4) About 1 out of every 2 doctors
____ (5) About 1 out of every 3 doctors
____ (6) About 1 out of every 4 doctors
____ (7) Fewer than 1 out of every 4 doctors are doing outstanding or excellent work consistently

EU Physicians' Questionnaire

40. Please consider the patients in the categories specified who visited this emergency unit over the past four-six weeks. On the average, how well were these patients managed from a medical standpoint? (Check one for each category)

The Medical Management of Emergency Patients in This Category Was:

Category:	Excellent (1)	Very good (2)	Good (3)	Fair (4)	Rather poor (5)	There were no such patients (0)
II:39 Acute Myocardial Infarction, Cardiac Arrest, and Ventricular Fibrillation cases	☐	☐	☐	☐	☐	
II:40 Lacerations of the Face or Neck involving more than skin	☐	☐	☐	☐	☐	
II:41 Acute Psychiatric Illnesses—suicide(depression), acute psychoses	☐	☐	☐	☐	☐	
II:42 Fractures or Dislocations	☐	☐	☐	☐	☐	
II:43 Acute Upper Respiratory Infections with Stridor, Epiglottitis, and Asthmatic Bronchitis cases	☐	☐	☐	☐	☐	
II:44 Rape cases	☐	☐	☐	☐	☐	
II:45 Infants with Blood Disorders, Dehydration, Congenital Anomalies, or Respiratory Distress Syndrome	☐	☐	☐	☐	☐	
II:46 Spinal Injuries or Closed Head Injuries with subdural hematomas or neurologic deficit	☐	☐	☐	☐	☐	
II:47 Drug Abuse cases	☐	☐	☐	☐	☐	
II:48 Burns of the face, ears, hands, feet, or perineum, and Burns involving 10% or more of total body surface area with 2% or more third degree	☐	☐	☐	☐	☐	

41. Please consider the patients in the categories specified who visited this emergency unit over the past four-six weeks. How would you evaluate the quality of nursing care that, on the average, patients in these particular categories received while in this emergency unit? (Check one for each category)

The Quality of Nursing Care for Patients in this Category Was:

Category:	Excellent (1)	Very good (2)	Good (3)	Fair (4)	Rather poor (5)	There were no such patients (0)
II:49 Acute Myocardial Infarction, Cardiac Arrest, and Ventricular Fibrillation cases	☐	☐	☐	☐	☐	
II:50 Lacerations of the Face or Neck involving more than skin	☐	☐	☐	☐	☐	
II:51 Acute Psychiatric Illnesses—suicide(depression), acute psychoses	☐	☐	☐	☐	☐	
II:52 Fractures or Dislocations	☐	☐	☐	☐	☐	
II:53 Acute Upper Respiratory Infections with Stridor, Epiglottitis, and Asthmatic Bronchitis cases	☐	☐	☐	☐	☐	
II:54 Rape cases	☐	☐	☐	☐	☐	
II:55 Infants with Blood Disorders, Dehydration, Congenital Anomalies, or Respiratory Distress Syndrome	☐	☐	☐	☐	☐	
II:56 Spinal Injuries or Closed Head Injuries with subdural hematomas or neurologic deficit	☐	☐	☐	☐	☐	
II:57 Drug Abuse cases	☐	☐	☐	☐	☐	
II:58 Burns of the face, ears, hands, feet, or perineum, and Burns involving 10% or more of total body surface area with 2% or more third degree	☐	☐	☐	☐	☐	

EU Physicians' Questionnaire

ABOUT WORK RELATIONS IN EMERGENCY UNIT

42. On the whole, to what extent does the nursing staff understand and appreciate the work problems and needs of the medical staff in this emergency unit? (Check one)
II:59

____ (1) They have an excellent understanding
____ (2) A very good understanding
____ (3) A good understanding
____ (4) A fair understanding
____ (5) They have a rather poor understanding

43. On the whole, to what extent does the medical staff understand and appreciate the work problems and needs of the nursing staff in this emergency unit? (Check one)
II:60

____ (1) They have an excellent understanding
____ (2) A very good understanding
____ (3) A good understanding
____ (4) A fair understanding
____ (5) They have a rather poor understanding

44. Here in the emergency unit, to what extent do the different people who have to work together take into account each other's work problems and needs as they go about doing their own activities? (Check one)
II:61

____ (1) To a very great extent
____ (2) A great extent
____ (3) A fair extent
____ (4) A small extent
____ (5) To a very small extent or not at all

45. On the whole, how successful are the people in this emergency unit in coming up with better ways of fitting together their related work efforts and activities? (Check one)
II:62

____ (1) Extremely successful
____ (2) Very successful
____ (3) Moderately successful
____ (4) Not so successful
____ (5) Not successful at all

46. To what extent are the various interrelated tasks and activities well-timed in the everyday work of this emergency unit? (Check one)
II:63

____ (1) All related tasks and activities are extremely well-timed
____ (2) They are very well-timed
____ (3) They are fairly well-timed
____ (4) They are not so well-timed
____ (5) They are not well-timed at all

47. In this emergency unit, to what extent do you feel that you can rely on others whose work is related to yours (or affects your work) to do their jobs right? (Check one)
II:64

____ (1) To a very great extent
____ (2) A great extent
____ (3) A fair extent
____ (4) A small extent
____ (5) To a very small extent or not at all

48. How frequently do the people in this emergency unit do their jobs in a way which ensures that their joint efforts and activities will fit together smoothly? (Check one)
II:65

____ (1) Always or nearly always
____ (2) Very frequently
____ (3) Fairly frequently
____ (4) Not so frequently
____ (5) Infrequently

49. All things considered, how much tension (friction, strain, or conflict) would you say is there between the groups specified in each of the following pairs? (Check one for each pair)

Level of Tension:

Tension Between:	A high level of tension (1)	A moderate level of tension (2)	A low level of tension (3)	A very low level of tension (4)	No tension at all (5)
II:66 Emergency unit staff and Hospital Administration	☐	☐	☐	☐	☐
II:67 Doctors in the emergency unit and Hospital staff outside the emergency unit	☐	☐	☐	☐	☐
II:68 Doctors in the emergency unit and Nurses in the emergency unit	☐	☐	☐	☐	☐
II:69 Some doctors in the emergency unit and Other doctors in the emergency unit	☐	☐	☐	☐	☐
II:70 Doctors in the emergency unit and Patients	☐	☐	☐	☐	☐
II:71 Emergency unit staff and The community outside	☐	☐	☐	☐	☐

50. To what extent do the people in this emergency unit make an effort to avoid creating problems or interferences with each other's duties and responsibilities? (Check one)
II:72

____ (1) To a very great extent
____ (2) A great extent
____ (3) A fair extent
____ (4) A small extent
____ (5) To a very small extent or not at all

51. After problems arise in the work activities of people who have to work together, corrections often are tried or steps taken to handle the problem. Generally, how effective are such corrective efforts in this emergency unit? (Check one)
II:73

____ (1) Completely effective
____ (2) Very effective
____ (3) Fairly effective
____ (4) Not so effective
____ (5) Not effective at all

EU Physicians' Questionnaire

52. On the whole, to what extent does Hospital Administration understand and appre-
II:74 ciate the work problems and needs of the emergency unit staff? (Check one)

    ___ (1) They have an excellent understanding
    ___ (2) A very good understanding
    ___ (3) A good understanding
    ___ (4) A fair understanding
    ___ (5) They have a rather poor understanding

ABOUT WORK PROCEDURES

53. From the standpoint of enabling the medical and nursing staff in this emergency unit to provide patients with emergency care of the highest quality possible at reasonable cost, how appropriate would you say are each of the following procedures? (Check one for each kind of procedure)

On the Whole, These Procedures Are:

Procedures:	Completely appropriate (1)	Very appropriate (2)	Fairly appropriate (3)	Not so appropriate (4)	Not appropriate at all (5)	There are no such procedures in this unit (0)
II:75 Receiving and registering patients who visit this emergency unit	☐	☐	☐	☐	☐	___
II:76 The initial screening (triage) of patients	☐	☐	☐	☐	☐	___
II:77 The examination and testing of patients	☐	☐	☐	☐	☐	___
II:78 Preparing patients for their discharge (including patient teaching and instruction for follow-up care)	☐	☐	☐	☐	☐	___
II:79 The procedures for patient disposition	☐	☐	☐	☐	☐	___

54. Emergency unit personnel often rely on different arrangements or bases to ensure that everyone contributes properly to the work and operation of the unit. Generally, to what degree do the personnel of this unit rely on—or count on—each of the following for this particular purpose? (Check one for each item)

Degree to Which They Rely:

Rely On:	To a very high degree (1)	To a high degree (2)	To a fair degree (3)	To a small degree (4)	To a very small degree (5)
III:17 The current policies of this institution	☐	☐	☐	☐	☐
III:18 The existing standards of clinical practice and clinical decision making	☐	☐	☐	☐	☐
III:19 Regularly scheduled meetings or conferences, written reports, and the like	☐	☐	☐	☐	☐
III:20 The autonomy and discretion of the professional staff	☐	☐	☐	☐	☐

55. When work procedures or the procedures
III:21 of the unit are neither clear-cut nor well-established, how well do the work activities of the different staff fit together? (Check one)

    ___ (1) Their activities fit together extremely well
    ___ (2) Very well
    ___ (3) Fairly well
    ___ (4) Not so well
    ___ (5) Their activities do not fit together well at all

56. In general, how well-planned are
III:22 the work assignments of the different people who have to work together in this emergency unit? (Check one)

    ___ (1) Extremely well-planned
    ___ (2) Very well-planned
    ___ (3) Fairly well-planned
    ___ (4) Not so well-planned
    ___ (5) Not well-planned at all

EU Physicians' Questionnaire

ABOUT YOUR WORK HERE

57. People who work together often are able to anticipate each other's work problems
III:23 and needs spontaneously or automatically. To what extent are most of the people
you work with in this emergency unit able to anticipate your work problems and
needs? (Check one)

___ (1) To a very great extent
___ (2) A great extent
___ (3) A fair extent
___ (4) A small extent
___ (5) To a very small extent
        or not at all

58. While working in this emergency unit,
III:24 to what extent do you generally find
yourself unable to do your work properly and on time UNTIL others who
work with you have first completed
what they were supposed to do?
(Check one)

___ (1) To a very considerable
        extent
___ (2) To a considerable extent
___ (3) To a moderate extent
___ (4) To a small extent
___ (5) To a very small extent or
        not at all

59. While working in this emergency
III:25 unit, to what extent do you
generally find yourself unable
to do your work properly or on
time UNLESS others who are working
with you also are doing their work
properly and on time? (Check one)

___ (1) To a very considerable
        extent
___ (2) To a considerable extent
___ (3) To a moderate extent
___ (4) To a small extent
___ (5) To a very small extent
        or not at all

60. When working in the emergency unit, do you feel any pressure for better perfor-
III:26 mance over and above what you think is reasonable? (Check one)

___ (1) I feel no pressure at all over and above what is reasonable
___ (2) A very small amount of pressure
___ (3) A small amount of pressure
___ (4) A moderate amount of pressure
___ (5) A great amount of pressure

61. If you feel any pressure over and above what is reasonable, what is the main
III:27 source of this pressure? (Check one)

___ (0) I feel no pressure over and above what is reasonable
___ (1) The main source of the pressure is my colleagues or peers
___ (2) The medical director
___ (3) Hospital Administration
___ (4) The Nursing staff
___ (5) Myself
___ (6) Poor or inadequate performance by others
___ (7) The work load
___ (8) Things outside the hospital
___ (9) Something else, other than the above

62. Personally, how strongly identified with or how strongly committed do you feel
III:28 you are to this emergency unit? (Check one)

___ (1) Extremely strongly
___ (2) Very strongly
___ (3) Moderately strongly
___ (4) Fairly strongly
___ (5) Not strongly

63. Considering your work efforts and   64. Considering your work efforts and
III:29 contributions here, how satisfied   III:30 contributions, how satisfied are
are you with the financial or   you with all of the non-financial
monetary rewards that you derive   rewards that you derive from working
from your work? (Check one)   in this emergency unit? (Check one)

___ (1) Completely satisfied   ___ (1) Completely satisfied
___ (2) Very satisfied   ___ (2) Very satisfied
___ (3) Fairly satisfied   ___ (3) Fairly satisfied
___ (4) Not so satisfied   ___ (4) Not so satisfied
___ (5) Not satisfied at all   ___ (5) Not satisfied at all

65. IF YOU CARE TO MAKE ANY ADDITIONAL COMMENTS, PLEASE USE THE SPACE BELOW OR THE
REVERSE SIDE.

III:31-32 a. _____
           _____

III:33-34 b. _____
           _____

THANK YOU VERY MUCH. WE APPRECIATE YOUR COOPERATION.

EU Registered Nurses' Interview

- 426 -

The University of Michigan
Institute for Social Research

Study 462312
Fall 1977

HOSPITAL EMERGENCY SERVICES STUDY

FORM 3, PART A: <u>INTERVIEW WITH REGISTERED NURSES (RN's) IN THE EMERGENCY UNIT</u>

Interviewer: _____
Interview No.: _____
Date: _____

Study 462312   Fall 1977

<u>FORM 3, PART A</u>: INTERVIEW WITH REGISTERED NURSES (RN's) IN THE EMERGENCY UNIT

First, some questions about the emergency unit (i.e., the emergency room or department) here.

1. On the whole, what do you think of this Emergency Unit as a place to work? Would
IV:17- you say it is an excellent place, a very good place, a good place, a fair place,
18   or a rather poor place to work?

| 1. IT IS AN EXCELLENT PLACE TO WORK | 2. A VERY GOOD PLACE | 3. A GOOD PLACE | 4. A FAIR PLACE | 5. A RATHER POOR PLACE |

2. At the present time, what sorts of problems does the Emergency Unit of this hospital face? What would you say are the <u>major</u> problems or key issues?

a. _____
IV:19-
20 _____

b. _____
IV:21-
22 _____

c. _____
IV:23-
24 _____

EU Registered Nurses' Interview

3. What are the TWO or THREE most important areas, or respects, in which you consider this Emergency Unit to be particularly strong or especially outstanding?

a.
IV:25-26 _____
_____
_____

b.
IV:27-28 _____
_____
_____

c.
IV:29-30 _____
_____
_____

4. And now, what are the TWO or THREE most important areas, or respects, in which you consider this Emergency Unit to be especially weak or to require the most improvement?

a.
IV:31-32 _____
_____
_____

b.
IV:33-34 _____
_____
_____

c.
IV:35-36 _____
_____
_____

5. In the past six months or so, have any important changes or new ways of doing things been introduced in the Emergency Unit?
IV:37

   1. YES   2. NO   8. DON'T KNOW
                 ↓   ↓
              GO TO Q.6 (NEXT PAGE)

   5a. What kinds of changes were these?

   1.
   IV:38-39 _____
   _____

   2.
   IV:40-41 _____
   _____

   3.
   IV:42-43 _____
   _____

   5b. How well have they been working out?

   1.
   IV:44 _____
   _____

   2.
   IV:45 _____
   _____

   3.
   IV:46 _____
   _____

EU Registered Nurses' Interview

ABOUT THE EMERGENCY UNIT AND THE COMMUNITY

6. Is there anything about the community outside or about the population being served by the Emergency Unit that creates special problems or difficulties for this Emergency Unit?

IV:47

| 1. YES | 2. NO | 8. DON'T KNOW |

2. NO and 8. DON'T KNOW → GO TO Q.7

6a. What kinds of things create special difficulties?

1. _____
IV:48-49

2. _____
IV:50-51

3. _____
IV:52-53

7. At the present time, what kind of reputation does this Emergency Unit have in the community outside? Would you say it has an excellent reputation, a very good reputation, a good reputation, a fair reputation, or a rather poor reputation?

IV:54-55

| 1. AN EXCELLENT REPUTATION | 2. A VERY GOOD REPUTATION | 3. A GOOD REPUTATION | 4. A FAIR REPUTATION | 5. A RATHER POOR REPUTATION |

8. The emergency health care needs of communities change from time to time. How well has the Emergency Unit of this hospital been able to keep up with and respond to these changes? Would you say it has responded extremely well, very well, fairly well, not so well, or not well at all?

IV:56-57

| 1. EXTREMELY WELL | 2. VERY WELL | 3. FAIRLY WELL | 4. NOT SO WELL | 5. NOT WELL AT ALL |

ABOUT THE PATIENTS IN THE EMERGENCY UNIT

9. In this hospital, are there any specific procedures for sending Emergency Unit patients to the rest of the hospital? (I mean for admitting patients or transferring patients from the Emergency Unit to some other part of this hospital?)

IV:58

| 1. YES | 2. NO | 8. DON'T KNOW |

2. NO and 8. DON'T KNOW → GO TO Q.10 (NEXT PAGE)

9a. Would you briefly describe the nature of these procedures?
IV:59-60

9b. On the whole, how well would you say are these procedures working out from your point of view?
IV:61

EU Registered Nurses' Interview

10. Does this Emergency Unit tend to concentrate on (or to specialize in) the
IV:62 treatment of any particular kinds of patients?

    1. YES   2. NO   8. DON'T KNOW

                    GO TO Q.11 (NEXT PAGE)

10a. What kinds of patients would these be?

    1. _____
    IV:63-
      64

    2. _____
    IV:65-
      66

    3. _____
    IV:67-
      68

11. Are there any particular kinds of patients whose medical problems cannot be
IV:69 handled as adequately as they should be by this Emergency Unit?

    1. YES   2. NO   8. DON'T KNOW

                    GO TO Q.12 (NEXT PAGE)

11a. Mainly, what kinds of patients would these be?

    1. _____
    IV:70-
      71

    2. _____
    IV:72-
      73

    3. _____
    IV:74-
      75

11b. Why is it that these particular patients cannot be handled as adequately
     as they should?

    1. _____
    IV:76

    2. _____
    IV:77

    3. _____
    IV:78

EU Registered Nurses' Interview

- 8 -

12. Of all the patients visiting the Emergency Unit over the past four weeks, about
V:17- what percent, would you estimate, arrived by ambulance or other emergency
18   vehicle?

_____ (PERCENT)

13. Of all the patients visiting the Emergency Unit in the past four weeks, about
V:19- what percent do you estimate were seen by a doctor within the first 15 minutes
20   after arriving here?

_____ (PERCENT)

14. Could you please also give me your estimate of the average length of a patient
V:21- visit to this Emergency Unit in a typical day? (I mean average number of minutes
22   "from time-in to time-out" per patient visit.)

_____ (NUMBER OF MINUTES)

15. In your judgment, about what percent of the patients visiting this Emergency
V:23- Unit over the past four weeks were "true emergencies"?
24

_____ (PERCENT)

- 9 -

ABOUT WORK RELATIONS IN THE EMERGENCY UNIT

16. Overall, how well do the different jobs and activities around the patient fit
    together in this Emergency Unit? (I mean the activities of the different people
V:25- who are working in the Emergency Unit.) Do they fit together extremely well, very
26   well, fairly well, not so well, or not well at all?

| 1. EXTREMELY WELL | 2. VERY WELL | 3. FAIRLY WELL | 4. NOT SO WELL | 5. NOT WELL AT ALL |

17. Generally, to what extent do the doctors who work in this Emergency Unit make
    adjustments in their work activities in order to facilitate the work in the
V:27- Emergency Unit? Would you say -- to a very great extent, to a great extent,
28   to a fair extent, to a small extent, or not at all?

| 1. TO A VERY GREAT EXTENT | 2. A GREAT EXTENT | 3. A FAIR EXTENT | 4. A SMALL EXTENT | 5. TO A VERY SMALL EXTENT OR NOT AT ALL |

18. When you need help or advice from the doctors here in deciding what to do for
V:29- emergency patients, how do you feel about the help or advice that you can get
30   from them?

_____
_____
_____
_____
_____
_____
_____
_____

EU Registered Nurses' Interview

19. Considering the training and professional experience that you have had, how do you feel about the amount of discretion or judgment that the doctors in the Emergency Unit allow you to use at work? On the whole, do they allow you -- about the right amount of discretion, more than enough discretion, somewhat less discretion than they should, or much less discretion than they should?
V:31-32

| 1. MORE THAN ENOUGH DISCRETION | 2. ABOUT THE RIGHT AMOUNT OF DISCRETION | 3. SOMEWHAT LESS DISCRETION THAN THEY SHOULD | 4. MUCH LESS DISCRETION THAN THEY SHOULD |

1. INTERVIEWER CHECKPOINT

   ☐ R IS A HEAD NURSE OR NURSING SUPERVISOR ⟶ GO TO CLOSING STATEMENT (NEXT PAGE). INTERVIEW COMPLETED.

   ☐ R IS NOT A HEAD NURSE OR NURSING SUPERVISOR ⟶ GO TO Q.20 (BELOW)

20. And how about the discretion that the supervising nurse or supervising nurses in the Emergency Unit allow you? Is it about the right amount of discretion, more than enough, somewhat less than it should be, or much less than it should be?
V:33-34

| 1. MORE THAN ENOUGH DISCRETION | 2. ABOUT THE RIGHT AMOUNT OF DISCRETION | 3. SOMEWHAT LESS DISCRETION THAN IT SHOULD BE | 4. MUCH LESS DISCRETION THAN IT SHOULD BE |

21. When you need help or advice at work from the supervising nurse, or supervising nurses, in the Emergency Unit, how do you feel about the help or advice that you can get?
V:35-36

_____
_____
_____
_____
_____
_____
_____

22. Finally, how frequently does the supervising nurse who is your immediate superior in the Emergency Unit let you know how well you are doing your job and whether or not you are doing it properly? Would you say (she/he) lets you know about as frequently as she should, more frequently than she should, somewhat less frequently than she should, or much less frequently than she should?
V:37-38

| 1. MORE FREQUENTLY THAN SHE SHOULD | 2. ABOUT AS FREQUENTLY AS SHE SHOULD | 3. SOMEWHAT LESS FREQUENTLY THAN SHE SHOULD | 4. MUCH LESS FREQUENTLY THAN SHE SHOULD |

INTERVIEWER READ TO R:

Thank you very much. We are now finished with the first part of your interview. Next, we would like to have you complete the second part by filling out this more specific questionnaire.

INTERVIEWER: HAND THE RESPONDENT FORM 3, PART B - QUESTIONNAIRE FOR EMERGENCY UNIT RN's.

We greatly appreciate your cooperation.

EU Registered Nurses' Questionnaire

The University of Michigan   Fall 1977

HOSPITAL EMERGENCY SERVICES STUDY

FORM 3, PART B: QUESTIONNAIRE FOR EMERGENCY UNIT RN's

Institute for Social Research
The University of Michigan
Ann Arbor, Michigan

Study 462312   Rights Reserved
Fall 1977   The University of Michigan

I N T R O D U C T I O N

As you are answering the questions on the following pages, you will find that they are designed to supplement and extend the interview which you have completed. At the beginning, there are a few questions intended to provide some background information. Then, there are questions regarding the emergency unit and the community, the priorities and operation of the emergency unit, resources and workload, patient care, work relations in the emergency unit, work procedures, your work here, and certain other aspects that were not covered in the interview. Most questions can be answered by checking (✓) one of the alternatives presented. If you do not find the exact alternative you desire, please check the one that comes closest or write your own answer. Thank you very much for your help; we appreciate your cooperation.

SOME BACKGROUND INFORMATION

1. How long have you been working as a nurse? (Please enter number of years)
I:17-18
_____ Years

2. How long have you been working in this hospital? (Please enter number of years)
I:19-20
_____ Years

3. How long have you been working in this Emergency Unit? (Check one)
I:21
___ (1) Less than one year
___ (2) One year or more but less than two years
___ (3) Two years or more but less than four years
___ (4) Four years or more but less than ten years
___ (5) Ten years or more

4. At the present time, are you working in the Emergency Unit on a regular basis? (Check one)
I:22
___ (1) Yes
___ (2) No

5. Ordinarily, about how many hours a week do you work in this Emergency Unit?
I:23-24 (Write in number of hours)
_____ Hours per week

Interviewer: _____
Interview No.: _____
Date: _____

HOSPITAL EMERGENCY SERVICES STUDY

FORM 3, PART B: QUESTIONNAIRE FOR EMERGENCY UNIT RN's

EU Registered Nurses' Questionnaire

6. What shift are you working on at the present time? (Check one)
I:25
___ (1) Day Shift
___ (2) Afternoon (Evening) Shift
___ (3) Night Shift
___ (4) I rotate

7. Professionally, what is your main field of interest (or speciality) within nursing? (Please write in)
I:26
Main field: _____

8. Have you had any special training in emergency nursing? (Check one)
I:27
___ (1) Yes
___ (2) No

9. What nursing degree do you hold? (Check your highest degree)
I:28
___ (1) A Diploma
___ (2) An Associate Degree
___ (3) A Baccalaureate (B.S., B.S.N.)
___ (4) A Master's Degree
___ (5) Other

10. What is your sex? (Check one)
I:29
___ (1) Female
___ (2) Male

11. How old are you? (Check one)
I:30
___ (1) Under 25 years
___ (2) 25 to 29 years
___ (3) 30 to 34 years
___ (4) 35 to 39 years
___ (5) 40 to 49 years
___ (6) 50 to 59 years
___ (7) 60 years or over

12. What is your present marital status? (Check one)
I:31
___ (1) Married
___ (2) Not married

13. At the present time, are you a member of the Emergency Department Nurses' Association (EDNA)? (Check one)
I:32
___ (1) Yes
___ (2) No

ABOUT THE EMERGENCY UNIT AND THE COMMUNITY

14. On the whole, how adequately would you say is this emergency unit meeting current community expectations regarding the services it provides? (Check one)
I:33
___ (1) Extremely adequately
___ (2) Very adequately
___ (3) Fairly adequately
___ (4) Not so adequately
___ (5) Not adequately at all

15. All things considered, how realistic would you say are the community's expectations regarding the services provided by this emergency unit? (Check one)
I:34
___ (1) Extremely realistic
___ (2) Very realistic
___ (3) Fairly realistic
___ (4) Not so realistic
___ (5) Not realistic at all

16. Do the people in the community seem to have adequate information about the services which this emergency unit can and cannot provide? (Check one)
I:35
Most people seem to have:
___ (1) Completely adequate information
___ (2) Very adequate information
___ (3) Fairly adequate information
___ (4) Not so adequate information
___ (5) Inadequate information

17. Considering the kind of service that this emergency unit provides to its patients, how do you feel about what it charges the patients (or their insurance) for their care? (Check one)
I:36
___ (1) Patient charges are too low considering the kind of service provided
___ (2) They are rather low
___ (3) They are about right
___ (4) They are rather high
___ (5) They are very high
___ (6) Patient charges are extremely high considering the kind of service provided
___ (8) I can't judge

18. On the basis of your experience and information while working here, about how many of the patients speak very well of this emergency unit? (Check one)
I:37
___ (1) All patients without exception speak very well of this emergency unit
___ (2) Nearly all of the patients speak very well of it
___ (3) The large majority of the patients speak very well of it
___ (4) A little over half of the patients speak very well of it
___ (5) About half of the patients speak very well of it
___ (6) Less than half of the patients speak very well of it
___ (7) Only a few of the patients speak very well of this emergency unit

19. Please think about all the ambulance personnel that the staff of this emergency unit have dealt with over the past four weeks. About how many of these personnel, would you say, provided the staff with adequate information about the incoming patients? (Check one)
I:38
___ (1) All ambulance personnel, without exception, provided the staff with adequate information
___ (2) Nearly all of them did
___ (3) The large majority of them did
___ (4) A little over half of them did
___ (5) About half of them did
___ (6) Fewer than half of them did
___ (7) Only a few of them provided the staff with adequate information

EU Registered Nurses' Questionnaire

- 4 -

20. Please think about the work-related contacts that emergency unit staff have with outside groups like the police, fire department, sheriff's department, local health department, medical examiners, and ambulance service personnel. With approximately how many of the personnel from these outside groups would you say the work-related contacts of the emergency unit staff are tense or strained at the present time? (Check one)

I:39
    (8) ___ I don't know
    (1) ___ Contacts with very few or none of these personnel are tense/strained
    (2) ___ Contacts with a few of these personnel are tense/strained
    (3) ___ Contacts with some of these personnel are tense/strained
    (4) ___ Contacts with many of these personnel are tense/strained
    (5) ___ Emergency unit staff contacts with all or nearly all of these personnel are tense/strained

ABOUT THE PRIORITIES AND OPERATION OF THE EMERGENCY UNIT

21. Hospital emergency units may emphasize different priorities and goals, some of which are listed below. Please rank these priorities in order of their importance to this emergency unit. (Place 1 in front of the one which is the most important, 2 in front of the next most important, etc....., and 7 in front of the one which is the least important.

Rank

I:40 ___ Maintaining a good reputation in the community
I:41 ___ Improving working conditions for the staff
I:42 ___ Minimizing patient waiting time
I:43 ___ Keeping the costs of the emergency service down
I:44 ___ Maintaining high standards of patient care
I:45 ___ Providing comprehensive emergency services
I:46 ___ Maintaining a high level of patient satisfaction

22. In emergency units like this, work problems may be handled in a number of different ways, some of which may be used more than others. Listed below are some ways that are perhaps being used here. Please rank them from the one that is generally used the most to the one that is used the least in this emergency unit. (Place 1 in front of the way which is most used, 2 in front of the next most used way, etc....., and 5 in front of the least used way.)

Rank

I:47 ___ Letting the people involved in the problem or affected by the problem make whatever adjustments are needed to deal with the problem
I:48 ___ Allocating sufficient authority, along with proper accountability, to the various personnel according to their jobs
I:49 ___ Allowing people sufficient discretion and flexibility to do their work
I:50 ___ Having clear and detailed job definitions for all involved
I:51 ___ Calling attention to relevant rules, procedures, and information and then letting people decide what to do next or how to proceed

- 5 -

23. Generally, how much influence does each of the following have over the priorities and goals of the emergency unit? (Check one for each group)

Amount of Influence:

Influence By:	Very considerable influence (1)	Considerable Influence (2)	Moderate Influence (3)	Little Influence (4)	Very little or no influence (5)
I:52 The Board of Trustees or Governing Authority of the hospital	☐	☐	☐	☐	☐
I:53 Hospital Administration	☐	☐	☐	☐	☐
I:54 Doctors who work in the emergency unit	☐	☐	☐	☐	☐
I:55 Nurses who work in the emergency unit	☐	☐	☐	☐	☐
I:56 The Patients	☐	☐	☐	☐	☐
I:57 Health Agencies and Regulatory Bodies (e.g., HSA, PSRO, etc.)	☐	☐	☐	☐	☐
I:58 The Community outside	☐	☐	☐	☐	☐

EU Registered Nurses' Questionnaire

Medical and Nursing Procedures

24. On the whole, in this emergency unit, how well performed (or how well carried
I:59 out) are the medical treatment and nursing care procedures from the standpoint
of providing patient care of the highest quality possible? (Check one)

The large majority of these procedures are:

___ (1) Extremely well performed
___ (2) Very well performed
___ (3) Fairly well performed
___ (4) Not so well performed
___ (5) Not performed well at all

25. On the whole, in this emergency unit, how well performed (or how well carried
I:60 out) are the medical treatment and nursing care procedures from the standpoint
of providing patient care at the lowest cost possible? (Check one)

The large majority of these procedures are:

___ (1) Extremely well performed
___ (2) Very well performed
___ (3) Fairly well performed
___ (4) Not so well performed
___ (5) Not performed well at all

26. On the whole, in this emergency unit, how well performed (or how well carried
I:61 out) are the medical treatment and nursing care procedures from the standpoint
of providing patient care as promptly as it should be provided? (Check one)

The large majority of these procedures are:

___ (1) Extremely well performed
___ (2) Very well performed
___ (3) Fairly well performed
___ (4) Not so well performed
___ (5) Not performed well at all

ABOUT RESOURCES AND WORKLOAD

27. Considering this emergency unit's requests to the hospital for resources of each
of the following kinds, on the whole, how successful is the emergency unit in
obtaining the requested resources? (Check one for each resource)

Usually, This Unit Obtains:

Requested Resources:	All or nearly all of what it requests (1)	Most of what it requests (2)	About half of what it requests (3)	Less than half of what it requests (4)	I don't know (8)
I:62 Medical staff to work in the emergency unit	☐	☐	☐	☐	
I:63 Medical specialists on-call to the emergency unit	☐	☐	☐	☐	
I:64 RN's to work in the emergency unit	☐	☐	☐	☐	
I:65 Other personnel to work in the emergency unit	☐	☐	☐	☐	
I:66 Funds (total budget excluding capital funds)	☐	☐	☐	☐	
I:67 Information needed by emergency unit staff from other parts of the hospital	☐	☐	☐	☐	
I:68 Space for the emergency unit	☐	☐	☐	☐	
I:69 All other physical facilities and equipment	☐	☐	☐	☐	

EU Registered Nurses' Questionnaire

- 8 -

28. Considering what this emergency unit needs to provide high quality care to its patients at reasonable cost, how adequate would you say is the quality of each of the following resources? (Check one for each resource)

The Quality of These Resources Is:

Resources:	Completely adequate (1)	Very adequate (2)	Fairly adequate (3)	Not so adequate (4)	Not adequate at all (5)
I:70 Medical staffing of the emergency unit	☐	☐	☐	☐	☐
I:71 RN staffing of the emergency unit	☐	☐	☐	☐	☐
I:72 Other emergency unit staffing	☐	☐	☐	☐	☐
I:73 The information received by emergency unit staff from other parts of the hospital	☐	☐	☐	☐	☐
I:74 The layout of the emergency unit facility	☐	☐	☐	☐	☐
I:75 The physical facilities and equipment available to the emergency unit	☐	☐	☐	☐	☐

29. If, in the next two months, patient visits were to increase by 10%-15% but the
I:76 quality of patient care were to remain at its current level, how well could the present staff of this emergency unit handle the increased patient volume? (Check one)

___ (1) The present staff could handle the increased volume without any difficulties
___ (2) It could handle it with some minor difficulties
___ (3) It could handle it with moderate difficulties
___ (4) It could handle it, but with great difficulties
___ (5) It could handle it, but with very great difficulties
___ (6) The present staff could not handle it at all

30. Considering the number of patients the staff now sees on an average day, what
I:77 effect would a 10%-15% DECREASE in patient visits have on the quality of care provided by this emergency unit? (Check one)

___ (1) The quality of care would improve very considerably
___ (2) It would improve considerably
___ (3) It would improve moderately
___ (4) It would improve a little
___ (5) It would improve very little
___ (6) The quality of care would not improve

- 9 -

31. When you request the services, assistance, or support of others in the hospital (outside the emergency unit), on the whole, how satisfactorily are your requests met by each of the following? (Check one for each item)

Usually, Most of These Requests Are Met:

Requests For:	Completely satisfactorily (1)	Very satisfactorily (2)	Fairly satisfactorily (3)	Not so satisfactorily (4)	Not satisfactorily at all (5)
II:17 The services of medical specialists from the hospital who are "on-call"	☐	☐	☐	☐	☐
II:18 Ancillary services from various units in the hospital (outside the emergency unit)	☐	☐	☐	☐	☐
II:19 The cooperation or assistance of the inpatient medical services or departments in the hospital	☐	☐	☐	☐	☐
II:20 The cooperation or assistance of the non-emergency outpatient clinics (if any) of the hospital	☐	☐	☐	☐	☐
II:21 Administrative service or support from the hospital	☐	☐	☐	☐	☐

32. Please think about the 5% of the patients visiting this emergency unit over the
II:22 past four weeks who presented the most complicated problems in terms of their nursing care requirements. Overall, how well prepared would you say was this emergency unit to handle these complicated cases? (Check one)

___ (1) Extremely well prepared
___ (2) Very well prepared
___ (3) Fairly well prepared
___ (4) Not so well prepared
___ (5) Not well prepared at all

- 437 -

EU Registered Nurses' Questionnaire

33. Considering all patient visits to this emergency unit over the past four-six weeks, approximately how many patients do you estimate were there in each of the categories specified? (Check one for each category)

The Number of Emergency Patients Was:

Category:	Consid-erable (1)	Moder-ate (2)	Small (3)	Very small (4)	Zero (There were no such patients) (5)
II:23 Acute Myocardial Infarction, Cardiac Arrest, and Ventricular Fibrillation cases	☐	☐	☐	☐	☐
II:24 Lacerations of the Face or Neck involving more than skin	☐	☐	☐	☐	☐
II:25 Acute Psychiatric Illnesses—suicide (depression), acute psychoses	☐	☐	☐	☐	☐
II:26 Fractures or Dislocations	☐	☐	☐	☐	☐
II:27 Acute Upper Respiratory Infections with Stridor, Epiglottis, and Asthmatic Bronchitis cases	☐	☐	☐	☐	☐
II:28 Rape Cases	☐	☐	☐	☐	☐
II:29 Infants with Blood Disorders, Dehydration, Congenital Anomalies, or Respiratory Distress Syndrome	☐	☐	☐	☐	☐
II:30 Spinal Injuries or Closed Head Injuries with subdural hematomas or neurologic deficit	☐	☐	☐	☐	☐
II:31 Drug Abuse cases	☐	☐	☐	☐	☐
II:32 Burns of the face, ears, hands, feet, or perineum, and Burns involving 10% or more of total body surface area with 2% or more third degree	☐	☐	☐	☐	☐

34. What is your estimate of the average length of a patient visit to this Emergency
II:33- Unit in a typical day? (Write in estimated number of minutes)
34

The average length of patient visits
to this Emergency Unit is about _____ minutes.

35. Over the past four weeks, about what percent of the patients visiting this
II:35- emergency unit arrived in what you would judge to be a "life threatening"
36 condition? (Write in %)

_____ %

36. In your opinion, about what percent of the patients visiting this emergency unit
II:37- over the past four weeks were seriously ill or seriously injured? (Write in %)
38

_____ %

ABOUT PATIENT CARE

37. On the basis of your experience and information, how would you rate the quality
II:39 of medical care that patients generally receive in this emergency unit?
(Check one)

_____ (1) Medical care in this
          emergency unit is
          outstanding
_____ (2) Excellent
_____ (3) Very good
_____ (4) Good
_____ (5) Fair
_____ (6) Rather poor
_____ (7) Medical care in this
          emergency unit is poor

EU Registered Nurses' Questionnaire

38. Considering the emergency units of all other hospitals with which you are familiar, how would you estimate the quality of nursing care provided in this particular emergency unit? (Check one)

II:40

___ (1) The quality of nursing care in this emergency unit is outstanding compared to most other units
___ (2) It is much better than in most other emergency units
___ (3) It is generally better
___ (4) It is about the same as in most other units
___ (5) It is somewhat poorer
___ (6) It is generally poorer
___ (7) The quality of nursing care in this emergency unit is much poorer compared to most other units
___ (8) I can't judge

39. For the purpose of answering this question, please assume that even in the very best emergency units and under the most favorable circumstances, not every member of the MEDICAL STAFF is doing outstanding or excellent work consistently. With this assumption in mind, please indicate about how many of the doctors working in this emergency unit are doing outstanding or excellent work consistently. (Check one)

II:41

___ (1) More than 3 out of every 4 doctors are doing outstanding or excellent work consistently
___ (2) About 3 out of every 4 doctors
___ (3) About 2 out of every 3 doctors
___ (4) About 1 out of every 2 doctors
___ (5) About 1 out of every 3 doctors
___ (6) About 1 out of every 4 doctors
___ (7) Fewer than 1 out of every 4 doctors are doing outstanding or excellent work consistently

40. For the purpose of answering this question, please assume that even in the very best emergency units and under the most favorable circumstances, not every member of the PROFESSIONAL NURSING STAFF is doing outstanding or excellent work consistently. With this assumption in mind, please indicate about how many of the professional nurses in this emergency unit are doing outstanding or excellent work consistently. (Check one)

II:42

___ (1) More than 3 out of every 4 nurses are doing outstanding or excellent work consistently
___ (2) About 3 out of every 4 nurses
___ (3) About 2 out of every 3 nurses
___ (4) About 1 out of every 2 nurses
___ (5) About 1 out of every 3 nurses
___ (6) About 1 out of every 4 nurses
___ (7) Fewer than 1 out of every 4 nurses are doing outstanding or excellent work consistently

41. Please consider the patients in the categories specified who visited this emergency unit over the past four-six weeks. How would you evaluate the quality of nursing care that, on the average, patients in these categories received while in this emergency unit? (Check one for each category)

The Quality of Nursing Care for Patients in this Category Was:

Category:	Excellent (1)	Very good (2)	Good (3)	Fair (4)	Rather poor (5)	There were no such patients (0)
II:43 Acute Myocardial Infarction, Cardiac Arrest, and Ventricular Fibrillation cases	☐	☐	☐	☐	☐	☐
II:44 Lacerations of the Face and Neck involving more than skin	☐	☐	☐	☐	☐	☐
II:45 Acute Psychiatric Illnesses—suicide(depression), acute psychoses	☐	☐	☐	☐	☐	☐
II:46 Fractures or Dislocations	☐	☐	☐	☐	☐	☐
II:47 Acute Upper Respiratory Infections with Stridor, Epiglotitis, and Asthmatic Bronchitis cases	☐	☐	☐	☐	☐	☐
II:48 Rape cases	☐	☐	☐	☐	☐	☐
II:49 Infants with Blood Disorders, Dehydration, Congenital Anomalies, or Respiratory Distress Syndrome	☐	☐	☐	☐	☐	☐
II:50 Spinal Injuries or Closed Head Injuries with subdural hematomas or neurologic deficit	☐	☐	☐	☐	☐	☐
II:51 Drug Abuse cases	☐	☐	☐	☐	☐	☐
II:52 Burns of the face, ears, hands, feet, or perineum, and Burns involving 10% or more of total body surface area with 2% or more third degree	☐	☐	☐	☐	☐	☐

EU Registered Nurses' Questionnaire

42. Please consider the patients in the categories specified who visited this emergency unit over the past four-six weeks. On the average, how well were these patients managed from a medical standpoint? (Check one for each category)

The Medical Management of Emergency Patients in this Category Was:

Category:	Excellent (1)	Very good (2)	Good (3)	Fair (4)	Rather poor (5)	There were no such patients (0)
II:53 Acute Myocardial Infarction, Cardiac Arrest, and Ventricular Fibrillation cases	☐	☐	☐	☐	☐	
II:54 Lacerations of the Face or Neck involving more than skin	☐	☐	☐	☐	☐	
II:55 Acute Psychiatric Illnesses--suicide(depression), acute psychoses	☐	☐	☐	☐	☐	
II:56 Fractures or Dislocations	☐	☐	☐	☐	☐	
II:57 Acute Upper Respiratory Infections with Stridor, Epiglotitis, and Asthmatic Bronchitis cases	☐	☐	☐	☐	☐	
II:58 Rape cases	☐	☐	☐	☐	☐	
II:59 Infants with Blood Disorders, Dehydration, Congenital Anomalies, or Respiratory Distress Syndrome	☐	☐	☐	☐	☐	
II:60 Spinal Injuries or Closed Head Injuries with subdural hematomas or neurologic deficit	☐	☐	☐	☐	☐	
II:61 Drug Abuse cases	☐	☐	☐	☐	☐	
II:62 Burns of the face, ears, hands, feet, or perineum, and Burns involving 10% or more of total body surface area with 2% or more third degree	☐	☐	☐	☐	☐	

ABOUT WORK RELATIONS IN THE EMERGENCY UNIT

43. On the whole, to what extent does the medical staff understand and appreciate the work problems and needs of the nursing staff in this emergency unit? (Check one)
II:63
___ (1) They have an excellent understanding
___ (2) A very good understanding
___ (3) A good understanding
___ (4) A fair understanding
___ (5) They have a rather poor understanding

44. On the whole, to what extent does the nursing staff understand and appreciate the work problems and needs of the medical staff in this emergency unit? (Check one)
II:64
___ (1) They have an excellent understanding
___ (2) A very good understanding
___ (3) A good understanding
___ (4) A fair understanding
___ (5) They have a rather poor understanding

45. Here in the emergency unit, to what extent do the different people who have to work together take into account each other's work problems and needs as they go about doing their own activities? (Check one)
II:65
___ (1) To a very great extent
___ (2) A great extent
___ (3) A fair extent
___ (4) A small extent
___ (5) To a very small extent or not at all

46. On the whole, how successful are the people in this emergency unit in coming up with better ways of fitting together their related work efforts and activities? (Check one)
II:66
___ (1) Extremely successful
___ (2) Very successful
___ (3) Moderately successful
___ (4) Not successful
___ (5) Not successful at all

47. To what extent are the various inter-related tasks and activities well-timed in the everyday work of this emergency unit? (Check one)
II:67
___ (1) All related tasks and activities are extremely well-timed
___ (2) They are very well-timed
___ (3) They are fairly well-timed
___ (4) They are not so well-timed
___ (5) They are not well-timed at all

48. In this emergency unit, to what extent do you feel that you can rely on others whose work is related to yours (or affects your work) to do their job right? (Check one)
II:68
___ (1) To a very great extent
___ (2) A great extent
___ (3) A fair extent
___ (4) A small extent
___ (5) To a very small extent or not at all

49. How frequently do the people in this emergency unit do their jobs in a way which ensures that their joint efforts and activities will fit together smoothly? (Check one)
II:69
___ (1) Always or nearly always
___ (2) Very frequently
___ (3) Fairly frequently
___ (4) Not so frequently
___ (5) Infrequently

50. In your experience while working in this emergency unit, how frequently are there unnecessary or avoidable work delays among the people whose work is related? (Check one)
II:70
___ (1) Rarely or infrequently
___ (2) Not too frequently
___ (3) Fairly frequently
___ (4) Very frequently
___ (5) Extremely frequently

EU Registered Nurses' Questionnaire

51. From the standpoint of being able to provide patients with care of the highest quality possible, how much joint planning, would you say, is there between the doctors and nurses in this emergency unit? (Check one)
III:71

    ____ (1) There is probably more than sufficient joint planning
    ____ (2) About the right amount of joint planning
    ____ (3) Somewhat less joint planning than is needed
    ____ (4) Much less than is needed
    ____ (5) There is no joint planning at all that I know of

52. All things considered, how much tension (friction, strain, or conflict) would you say is there between the groups specified in each of the following pairs? (Check one for each pair)

Tension Between:	A high level of tension (1)	A moderate level of tension (2)	A low level of tension (3)	A very low level of tension (4)	No tension at all (5)
III:17 Emergency unit staff and Hospital Administration	☐	☐	☐	☐	☐
III:18 Doctors in the emergency unit and Hospital staff outside the emergency unit	☐	☐	☐	☐	☐
III:19 Nursing staff in the emergency unit and Hospital staff outside the emergency unit	☐	☐	☐	☐	☐
III:20 Doctors in the emergency unit and Nurses in the emergency unit	☐	☐	☐	☐	☐
III:21 Some nursing personnel in the emergency unit and Other nursing personnel in the emergency unit	☐	☐	☐	☐	☐
III:22 Some doctors in the emergency unit and Other doctors in the emergency unit	☐	☐	☐	☐	☐
III:23 Doctors in the emergency unit and Patients	☐	☐	☐	☐	☐
III:24 Nurses in the emergency unit and Patients	☐	☐	☐	☐	☐
III:25 Emergency unit staff and The community outside	☐	☐	☐	☐	☐

53. In general, how adequately do the doctors here explain things to nursing personnel about the condition and needs of patients? (Check one)
III:26

    ____ (1) Extremely adequately
    ____ (2) Very adequately
    ____ (3) Fairly adequately
    ____ (4) Not so adequately
    ____ (5) Not adequately at all

54. To what extent do the people in this emergency unit make an effort to avoid creating problems or interferences with each other's duties and responsibilities? (Check one)
III:27

    ____ (1) To a very great extent
    ____ (2) A great extent
    ____ (3) A fair extent
    ____ (4) A small extent
    ____ (5) To a very small extent or not at all

55. After problems arise in the work activities of people who have to work together, corrections often are tried or steps are taken to handle the problems. Generally, how effective are such corrective efforts in this emergency unit? (Check one)
III:28

    ____ (1) Completely effective
    ____ (2) Very effective
    ____ (3) Fairly effective
    ____ (4) Not so effective
    ____ (5) Not effective at all

56. Generally, to what degree do the different people who have to work together in this emergency unit see the other person's viewpoint in their working relationships? (Check one)
III:29

    ____ (1) To a very high degree
    ____ (2) To a high degree
    ____ (3) To a fair degree
    ____ (4) To a low degree
    ____ (5) To a very low degree

57. Judging from their attitudes and behaviors here at work, to what degree do the doctors in this emergency unit show genuine acceptance of the interrelatedness between medical and nursing activities? (Check one)
III:30

    ____ (1) To a very high degree
    ____ (2) To a high degree
    ____ (3) To a fair degree
    ____ (4) To a small degree
    ____ (5) To a very small degree or not at all

58. Aside from their work with patients, how much interest do the doctors here take in this emergency unit? (Check one)
III:31

    ____ (1) Aside from their work with patients, most doctors are extremely interested in this emergency unit
    ____ (2) Most doctors are very interested
    ____ (3) Most doctors are fairly interested
    ____ (4) Most doctors are not so interested
    ____ (5) Aside from their work with patients, most doctors take no interest in this emergency unit

59. In general, to what extent do your work contacts with people from other units or departments in the hospital (i.e., people whose work is related to yours) facilitate your work in the emergency unit? (Check one)
III:32

    ____ (1) To a very great extent
    ____ (2) A great extent
    ____ (3) A moderate extent
    ____ (4) A small extent
    ____ (5) To a very small extent or not at all

EU Registered Nurses' Questionnaire

ABOUT WORK PROCEDURES

60. In this emergency unit, who usually performs each of the following activities? (Check one for each activity)

Activities:	Only by a doctor (1)	Only by a professional person (2)	Either by a doctor or by a professional nurse (3)	By a clerk or a secretary (4)	By some one other than the preceding (5)	No one performs this activity (0)
III:33 Admitting the patients into the emergency unit	☐	☐	☐	☐	☐	
III:34 The initial screening (or triage) of patients	☐	☐	☐	☐	☐	
III:35 Preparing patients for their discharge and instructing them for follow-up care	☐	☐	☐	☐	☐	
III:36 Making arrangements for follow-up care in the case of patients who require such care	☐	☐	☐	☐	☐	
III:37 Checking to see that decisions concerning the disposition of patients are actually carried out	☐	☐	☐	☐	☐	

61. Generally, how well performed (or how well carried out) are each of the following activities in this emergency unit?

Activities:	Extremely well performed (1)	Very well performed (2)	Fairly well performed (3)	Not so well performed (4)	Not well performed (5)
III:38 Receiving and registering patients who visit this emergency unit	☐	☐	☐	☐	☐
III:39 The initial screening (triage) of patients	☐	☐	☐	☐	☐
III:40 The examination and testing of patients	☐	☐	☐	☐	☐
III:41 Preparing patients for their discharge (including patient teaching and instruction for follow-up care)	☐	☐	☐	☐	☐
III:42 The procedures for patient disposition and discharge	☐	☐	☐	☐	☐

62. Emergency unit personnel often rely on different arrangements or bases to ensure that everyone contributes properly to the work and operation of the unit. Generally, to what degree do the personnel of this unit rely on -- or count on -- each of the following for this particular purpose? (Check one for each item)

Rely On:

	To a very high degree (1)	To a high degree (2)	To a fair degree (3)	To a small degree (4)	To a very small degree (5)
III:43 The existing standards for clinical practice and clinical decision making	☐	☐	☐	☐	☐
III:44 Unwritten rules, standards, or understandings about what should be done or how things should be done here	☐	☐	☐	☐	☐
III:45 The authority arrangements and power structure of the hospital	☐	☐	☐	☐	☐
III:46 Written organizational rules, regulations and procedures, and existing job descriptions	☐	☐	☐	☐	☐
III:47 Informal communication structure -- unscheduled ways of exchanging ideas and sharing relevant information about the work or the unit	☐	☐	☐	☐	☐

63. When work procedures or the procedures of the unit are neither clear-cut nor III:48 well-established, how well do the work activities of the different staff fit together? (Check one)

___ (1) Their activities fit together extremely well
___ (2) Very well
___ (3) Fairly well
___ (4) Not so well
___ (5) Their activities do not fit together well at all

- 442 -

EU Registered Nurses' Questionnaire

- 20 -

ABOUT YOUR WORK HERE

64. Generally, how much variety would you say is there in the activities which you perform on the job in this emergency unit? (Check one)
III:49

____ (1) Very considerable variety
____ (2) Considerable variety
____ (3) Moderate variety
____ (4) Some variety
____ (5) Little or very little variety

65. Considering what you think you should be doing in your work here, how well is your working time divided among the various tasks and activities that make up your job? (Check one)
III:50

____ (1) My working time is divided exactly the way it should be divided
____ (2) It is divided almost the way it should be divided
____ (3) It should be divided somewhat differently
____ (4) It should be divided differently
____ (5) My working time should be divided much differently than it is

66. People who work together often are able to anticipate each other's work problems and needs spontaneously or automatically. To what extent are most of the people you work with in this emergency unit able to anticipate your work problems and needs? (Check one)
III:51

____ (1) To a very great extent
____ (2) A great extent
____ (3) A fair extent
____ (4) A small extent
____ (5) To a very small extent or not at all

67. In general, how clearly defined are the various rules and regulations which affect your work in the emergency unit? (Check one)
III:52

____ (1) Generally, they are defined as clearly as they should be defined
____ (2) They are defined almost as clearly as they should be defined
____ (3) They should be defined somewhat more clearly
____ (4) They should be defined more clearly
____ (5) Generally, they should be defined much more clearly

68. How much difference, would you say, is there between the way the hospital sees the job of the nurses in the emergency unit and the way in which the nurses see their job? (Check one)
III:53

____ (1) A very small difference or no difference
____ (2) A small difference
____ (3) More than a small difference, but not a considerable difference
____ (4) A considerable difference
____ (5) A very considerable difference

69. To what extent are you able to use your judgment and discretion in carrying out your work activities here in the emergency unit? (Check one)
III:54

____ (1) To a very great extent
____ (2) A great extent
____ (3) A fair extent
____ (4) A small extent
____ (5) To a very small extent or not at all

- 21 -

70. To what extent do you find that you have to do things on your job that you feel should be the responsibility of other people in the emergency unit? (Check one)
III:55

____ (1) To a very great extent
____ (2) A great extent
____ (3) A fair extent
____ (4) A small extent
____ (5) To a very small extent or not at all

71. While working in this emergency unit, to what extent do you generally find yourself unable to do your work properly and on time UNLESS others who are working with you also are doing their work properly and on time? (Check one)
III:56

____ (1) To a very considerable extent
____ (2) To a considerable extent
____ (3) To a moderate extent
____ (4) To a small extent
____ (5) To a very small extent or not at all

72. While working in this emergency unit, to what extent do you generally find yourself unable to do your work properly and on time UNTIL others who work with you have first completed what they were supposed to do? (Check one)
III:57

____ (1) To a very considerable extent
____ (2) To a considerable extent
____ (3) To a moderate extent
____ (4) To a small extent
____ (5) To a very small extent or not at all

73. To what extent do you generally find that others who work here with you are unable to do their work properly or on-time UNTIL you yourself have completed first what you were supposed to do? (Check one)
III:58

____ (1) To a very considerable extent
____ (2) To a considerable extent
____ (3) To a moderate extent
____ (4) To a small extent
____ (5) To a very small extent or not at all

74. Ordinarily, to what extent does your own work in the emergency unit depend on direct contacts with personnel from other parts of the hospital outside the emergency unit? (Check one)
III:59

____ (1) To a very great extent
____ (2) To a great extent
____ (3) To a fair extent
____ (4) To a small extent
____ (5) To a very small extent or not at all

EU Registered Nurses' Questionnaire

75. On the whole, about how many of the tasks or activities that you currently per-
III:60- form here on the job are actually planned or specified ahead of time? (Write in %)
61
_____ %

76. About how many of these same tasks or activities, in your opinion, reasonably
III:62- could be planned or specified ahead of time? (Write in %)
63
_____ %

77. At work in the emergency unit, do you feel any pressure for better performance
III:64 over and above what you think is reasonable? (Check one)

_____ (1) I feel no pressure at all over
          and above what is reasonable
_____ (2) A very small amount of pressure
_____ (3) A small amount of pressure
_____ (4) A moderate amount of pressure
_____ (5) A great amount of pressure
_____ (6) I feel a very great amount of
          pressure over and above what is
          reasonable

78. If you feel any pressure over and above what is reasonable, what is the
III:65 main source of this pressure? (Check one)

_____ (0) I feel no pressure over and above
          what is reasonable
_____ (1) The main source of the pressure is my
          superiors
_____ (2) My colleagues or peers
_____ (3) The medical staff
_____ (4) The work load
_____ (5) Myself
_____ (6) Poor or inadequate performance by others
_____ (7) The patients or their relatives
_____ (8) Things outside the hospital
_____ (9) Something else, other than the above

79. In your daily work here, do you usually perform a great many tasks for relatively
III:66 few patients or a relatively few tasks for a great many patients? (Check one)

_____ (1) I usually perform a great many tasks
          for relatively few patients
_____ (2) Many tasks for relatively few patients
_____ (3) A fair number of tasks for a fair number
          of patients
_____ (4) Relatively few tasks for many patients
_____ (5) I usually perform very few tasks for a
          great many patients

80. On the whole, how adequate for your work needs is the information that you
    normally receive from each of the following? (Check one for each group)

The Information I Receive Is:

Information From:	Completely adequate (1)	Very adequate (2)	Fairly adequate (3)	Not so adequate (4)	Not adequate at all (5)
III:67 The physicians in this emergency unit	☐	☐	☐	☐	☐
III:68 Other nurses in this emergency unit	☐	☐	☐	☐	☐
III:69 Other personnel in the emergency unit	☐	☐	☐	☐	☐
III:70 The emergency unit patients	☐	☐	☐	☐	☐
III:71 Personnel from other parts of the hospital outside the emergency unit	☐	☐	☐	☐	☐

EU Registered Nurses' Questionnaire

- 24 -

81. How strongly identified with or how strongly committed do you feel you are to each of the following? (Check one for each line)

I Feel Identified:

	Extremely strongly (1)	Very strongly (2)	Moderately strongly (3)	Fairly strongly (4)	Not strongly (5)
With:					
III:72 This hospital	☐	☐	☐	☐	☐
III:73 This emergency unit	☐	☐	☐	☐	☐
III:74 Your profession	☐	☐	☐	☐	☐
III:75 The community served by this hospital	☐	☐	☐	☐	☐

82. On the whole, how much opportunity does your job in this emergency unit offer
III:76 for using your own skills and knowledge? (Check one)

___ (1) A very great opportunity
___ (2) A great opportunity
___ (3) A moderate opportunity
___ (4) Some opportunity
___ (5) Little or no opportunity

83. Considering your work efforts and contributions here, how satisfied
III:77 are you with the financial or monetary rewards that you derive from your work in this emergency unit? (Check one)

___ (1) Completely satisfied
___ (2) Very satisfied
___ (3) Fairly satisfied
___ (4) Not so satisfied
___ (5) Not satisfied at all

84. Considering your work efforts and contributions here, how satisfied
III:78 are you with all of the non-financial rewards that you derive from working in this emergency unit? (Check one)

___ (1) Completely satisfied
___ (2) Very satisfied
___ (3) Fairly satisfied
___ (4) Not so satisfied
___ (5) Not satisfied at all

THANK YOU VERY MUCH. WE APPRECIATE YOUR COOPERATION.

- 445 -

EU Supervisory/Head Nurses' Questionnaire

The University of Michigan   Fall 1977

HOSPITAL EMERGENCY SERVICES STUDY

FORM 3, PART C: SRN/HN SUPPLEMENT

(To be completed only by the Supervising Nurse and/or Head Nurse of the Emergency Unit. If the Emergency Unit has both a Nursing Supervisor and a Head Nurse, each of them is requested to complete this supplement independently.)

Interviewer: _____
Interview No.: _____
Date: _____

HOSPITAL EMERGENCY SERVICES STUDY

FORM 3, PART C: SRN/HN SUPPLEMENT

Institute for Social Research
The University of Michigan
Ann Arbor, Michigan

Study 462312
Fall 1977

Rights Reserved
The University of Michigan

I N T R O D U C T I O N

This is a special supplementary form to be completed only by the Head Nurse and Nursing Supervisor (if one) of the Emergency Unit.

As you are answering the questions in the SRN/HN SUPPLEMENT, you will find that they are designed to complement and extend the interview and questionnaire which you have completed. The questions cover certain aspects of work relations and work relations with the outside community, work activities and procedures, and some other aspects that were not covered in your interview or questionnaire. Most questions can be answered by checking (✓) one of the alternatives presented. If you do not find the exact alternative you desire, please check the one that comes closest or write your own answer. Thank you very much for your help; we appreciate your cooperation.

---

1. What is your current position in this Emergency Unit? (Please write in your official title)
VI:17
   My current title is: _____

2. How long have you held this particular position? (Check one)
VI:18
   ___ (1) Less than one year
   ___ (2) One year or more but less than two years
   ___ (3) Two years or more but less than four years
   ___ (4) Four years or more but less than ten years
   ___ (5) Ten years or more

ABOUT SOME ASPECTS OF WORK RELATIONS

3. In general, how well-established are the emergency unit rules and procedures regarding its work-related contacts with other departments and units of the hospital? (Check one)
VI:19
   ___ (1) The emergency unit's rules and procedures are extremely well-established
   ___ (2) Very well-established
   ___ (3) Fairly well-established
   ___ (4) Not so well-established
   ___ (5) Its rules and procedures are not at all well-established

4. On the whole, to what extent do these other departments and units of the hospital understand and appreciate the work problems and needs of the emergency unit staff? (Check one)
VI:20
   ___ (1) They have an excellent understanding
   ___ (2) A very good understanding
   ___ (3) A good understanding
   ___ (4) A fair understanding
   ___ (5) They have a rather poor understanding

EU Supervisory/Head Nurses' Questionnaire

5. In your view, about how many people in the rest of the hospital with whom you have relatively frequent work contacts do their jobs properly and efficiently? (Check one)

VI:21
- (1) All of them do their jobs properly and efficiently
- (2) Nearly all of them do
- (3) The large majority of them do
- (4) A little over half of them do their jobs properly and efficiently
- (5) About half of them do
- (6) Less than half of them do
- (7) Only a few of them do

6. On the whole, to what extent does Hospital Administration understand and appreciate the work problems and needs of the emergency unit staff? (Check one)

VI:22
- (1) They have an excellent understanding
- (2) A very good understanding
- (3) A good understanding
- (4) A fair understanding
- (5) They have a rather poor understanding

ABOUT WORK RELATIONS WITH THE OUTSIDE COMMUNITY

7. Considering all of the work-related contacts that the staff of the emergency unit have with each of the following, how satisfactory would you say are their contacts from the standpoint of accomplishing the work of the emergency unit? (Check one for each line)

These Contacts Are:

Contacts With:	Completely satisfactory (1)	Very satisfactory (2)	Fairly satisfactory (3)	Not so satisfactory (4)	Not satisfactory at all (5)	We have no contacts with this personnel (0)
VI:23 Sheriff's department personnel	☐	☐	☐	☐	☐	☐
VI:24 Police department personnel	☐	☐	☐	☐	☐	☐
VI:25 Fire department personnel	☐	☐	☐	☐	☐	☐
VI:26 Private ambulance services personnel	☐	☐	☐	☐	☐	☐
VI:27 Public safety department personnel	☐	☐	☐	☐	☐	☐
VI:28 Local health department personnel	☐	☐	☐	☐	☐	☐
VI:29 Coroner or medical examiner(s)	☐	☐	☐	☐	☐	☐
VI:30 Health Systems Agency (HSA) personnel	☐	☐	☐	☐	☐	☐

8. From the point of view of being able to do your work properly, on the whole, how adequate is the information that you have about the requirements and workings of these outside health agencies and regulatory bodies? (Check one)

VI:31
- (1) Completely adequate
- (2) Very adequate
- (3) Fairly adequate
- (4) Not so adequate
- (5) Not adequate at all

9. At the present time, to what extent is this hospital or emergency unit collaborating with other hospitals, emergency units, or other relevant service agencies for the following purposes? (Check one for each line)

It is Collaborating:

Purpose:	To a very great extent (1)	To a great extent (2)	To a fair extent (3)	To a small extent (4)	To a very small extent or not at all (5)
VI:32 To provide better or less costly emergency medical services to the community	☐	☐	☐	☐	☐
VI:33 To facilitate or improve the work of this emergency unit	☐	☐	☐	☐	☐
VI:34 To share useful information about the emergency medical needs of the community	☐	☐	☐	☐	☐
VI:35 To establish or maintain special emergency care facilities or a regional system	☐	☐	☐	☐	☐
VI:36 To train emergency medical technicians or other emergency service personnel	☐	☐	☐	☐	☐

10. To what extent are you able to get sufficient information about the emergency care needs of the community when desired? (Check one)

VI:37
- (1) To a very great extent
- (2) To a great extent
- (3) To a fair extent
- (4) To a small extent
- (5) To a very small extent or not at all

EU Supervisory/Head Nurses' Questionnaire

ABOUT WORK ACTIVITIES AND PROCEDURES

11. Considering the responsibilities and demands of your work in the Emergency Unit, how do you feel about the authority given to you to do your job? (Check one)

VI:38
___ (1) I probably have more than sufficient authority
___ (2) About the right amount of authority
___ (3) Somewhat less authority than I need
___ (4) Much less authority than I need

Appropriateness of Procedures

12. Please think of the various medical treatment and nursing care procedures used in this emergency unit. On the whole, are most of them appropriate from the standpoint of enabling the staff to provide care of the highest quality possible? (Check one)

VI:39
___ (1) All or almost all of the medical and nursing procedures used in this unit are very appropriate
___ (2) The large majority of them are
___ (3) The majority of them are
___ (4) About half of them are
___ (5) Fewer than half of them are very appropriate

13. Again, thinking of the same procedures, are most of them appropriate from the standpoint of enabling the staff to provide care at the lowest cost possible? (Check one)

VI:40
___ (1) All or almost all of them are very appropriate
___ (2) The large majority of them are
___ (3) The majority of them are
___ (4) About half of them are
___ (5) Fewer than half of them are very appropriate

14. Lastly, are most of these same procedures appropriate from the standpoint of enabling the staff to provide care as promptly as it should be provided? (Check one)

VI:41
___ (1) All or almost all of them are very appropriate
___ (2) The large majority of them are
___ (3) The majority of them are
___ (4) About half of them are
___ (5) Fewer than half of them are very appropriate

15. In emergency units like this, work problems may be handled in a number of different ways, some of which may be used more than others. Listed below are some ways that are perhaps being used here. Please rank them from the one that is generally used the most to the one that is used the least in this emergency unit. (Place 1 in front of the way that is most used, 2 in front of the next most used way, etc...., and 5 in front of the least used way.)

Rank →

VI:42 ___ Careful and precise timing and scheduling of tasks and work activities

VI:43 ___ Correcting immediately any departures from the proper way of doing things

VI:44 ___ Improving the staff's level of understanding of the work requirements of the unit so people can handle problems in a preventive way by anticipating them before they arise

VI:45 ___ Trying to find better ways of doing things even when things operate smoothly and without problems

VI:46 ___ Making sure that existing rules and regulations are followed by all concerned

16. Sometimes policies or procedures are established to regulate some of the activities performed in emergency units. For which of the following activities, if any, does this emergency unit have a written policy (or procedure) readily accessible to the professional staff here? (Please check all those for which there is a written policy or procedure)

Check as many as applicable:

VI:47 ___ Procedures for receiving and registering the patients visiting this emergency unit

VI:48 ___ Procedures (or triage protocols) for the initial screening of patients

VI:49 ___ Rules and procedures for examining and testing the patients

VI:50 ___ Procedures for preparing patients for discharge (including patient teaching and instruction for follow-up care)

VI:51 ___ Rules and procedures concerning patient disposition by the emergency unit

VI:52 ___ Procedures for notifying the patient's personal physician

VI:53 ___ Procedures for communicating with authorities (police, health authorities, etc.)

VI:54 ___ Procedures for communicating with other community emergency facilities (ambulance, poison center, etc.)

VI:55 ___ EMS contingency plans for disasters

EU Supervisory/Head Nurses' Questionnaire

- 6 -

17. In this institution at the present time, how is overall responsibility for each of the following kinds of decisions (or activities) divided between the emergency unit staff and other relevant groups or individuals in the hospital? (Check one for each line)

Overall Responsibility:

Responsibility For:	Belongs exclusively to emergency unit staff (1)	Belongs mainly to emergency unit staff (2)	Is shared about equally between emergency unit staff and other hospital staff (3)	Belongs mainly to people outside the emergency unit (4)	Belongs exclusively to people outside the emergency unit (5)
VI:56 Determining the priorities and goals of the emergency unit	☐	☐	☐	☐	☐
VI:57 Determining the emergency unit's operating budget	☐	☐	☐	☐	☐
VI:58 Establishing rules or procedures for patient care in the emergency unit	☐	☐	☐	☐	☐
VI:59 Deciding what tasks the different personnel in the emergency unit will perform or how their work roles are defined	☐	☐	☐	☐	☐
VI:60 Evaluating the work of the emergency unit	☐	☐	☐	☐	☐

18. Of the following statements, which one would you say most accurately
VI:61 reflects the principles or policy governing medical staffing of the Emergency Unit at the present time? (Check one)

___ (1) The unit is staffed for "peak patient load"
___ (2) It is staffed for an "above average" patient volume but not for "peak load"
___ (3) The unit is staffed for an "average" level of patient volume

19. And, which of the following statements most accurately reflects the principles
VI:62 or policy governing the non-medical staffing (i.e., nursing personnel, etc.) of the Emergency Unit? (Check one)

___ (1) The unit is staffed for "peak patient load"
___ (2) It is staffed for an "above average" patient volume but not for "peak load"
___ (3) The unit is staffed for an "average" level of patient volume

- 7 -

SOME FINAL QUESTIONS

20. In your judgment, about what percent of the patients visiting this emer-
VI:63-64 gency unit over the past four weeks were "true emergencies?" (Please write in %) _____ %

21. Over the past four weeks, about what percent of this emergency
VI:65-66 unit's patients were sent from the emergency unit to one of this hospital's intensive care units (ICU, CCU, or other critical care unit) or to the operating room of this hospital? (Write in %) _____ %

22. Considering both their quantity and quality (or adequacy), how stable over time would you say are the resources available to the emergency unit? (Check one for each line)

These Resources Are:

Resources:	Extremely stable (1)	Very stable (2)	Fairly stable (3)	Not so stable (4)	Not stable at all (5)	I can't judge (8)
VI:67 Medical staffing of the emergency unit	☐	☐	☐	☐	☐	
VI:68 RN staffing of the emergency unit	☐	☐	☐	☐	☐	
VI:69 Other staffing of the emergency unit	☐	☐	☐	☐	☐	
VI:70 The amount of total funds (total budget excluding capital funds) allocated to the emergency unit by the hospital	☐	☐	☐	☐	☐	
VI:71 The information received by emergency unit staff from other parts of the hospital	☐	☐	☐	☐	☐	

EU Supervisory/Head Nurses' Questionnaire

23. Based on your own knowledge and observations, how would you characterize the medical leadership of this emergency unit? (Check one)
VI:72

___ (1) The medical leadership is extremely effective
___ (2) Very effective
___ (3) Fairly effective
___ (4) Not so effective
___ (5) Not effective at all

24. At the present time, who would you say are the TWO or THREE most influential individuals in this hospital concerning the emergency unit's situation and operation? (Please enter the name and position or title of each of these individuals)

Name	Position or Title

VI:73 a. _____ _____

VI:74 b. _____ _____

VI:75 c. _____ _____

THANK YOU VERY MUCH. WE APPRECIATE YOUR COOPERATION.

Selected Hospital Physicians' Interview

The University of Michigan
Institute for Social Research

Study 462312
Fall 1977

HOSPITAL EMERGENCY SERVICES STUDY

FORM 4: INTERVIEW FOR SELECTED PHYSICIANS IN THE HOSPITAL
(OUTSIDE THE EMERGENCY UNIT)

Interviewer: _____
Interview No.: _____
Date: _____

Study 462312
Fall 1977

FORM 4: INTERVIEW FOR SELECTED PHYSICIANS IN THE HOSPITAL
(OUTSIDE THE EMERGENCY UNIT)

SOME GENERAL QUESTIONS ABOUT THE EMERGENCY UNIT

First, I would like to ask some general questions about the Emergency Unit (i.e., The Emergency Room or Department) here.

1. At the present time, what are the TWO or THREE most important areas, or respects, in which you consider the Emergency Unit of this hospital to be particularly strong or especially outstanding?

a. _____
I:17-18

b. _____
I:19-20

c. _____
I:21-22

Selected Hospital Physicians' Interview

- 2 -

2. Next, what sorts of problems does the Emergency Unit of the hospital face at the present time? What would you say are the major problems or key issues?

a.
I:23-
24 _____
_____
_____
_____

b.
I:25-
26 _____
_____
_____
_____

c.
I:27-
28 _____
_____
_____
_____

3. Is there anything about this hospital (e.g., its policies, financial situation,
I:29 staffing arrangements, and the like) that tends to create problems or difficulties for the Emergency Unit?

```
┌─────────┐      ┌─────────┐      ┌─────────┐
│ 1. YES  │      │  2. NO  │      │ 8. DON'T│
└────┬────┘      └────┬────┘      │   KNOW  │
     │                │           └────┬────┘
     ▼                └──────────┬─────┘
                                 ▼
                          GO TO Q.4 (NEXT PAGE)
```

3a. What kinds of things create problems or difficulties?

1.
I:30-
31 _____

2.
I:32-
33 _____

3.
I:34-
35 _____

- 3 -

4. The next question concerns the priorities and goals of the Emergency Unit. I'm going to read a list of seven possible priorities. Then, I would like to ask you which three of these priorities are most emphasized by the Emergency Unit here?

(INTERVIEWER: REPEAT LIST AS NECESSARY)

1. Maintaining a good reputation in the community
2. Improving working conditions for the staff
3. Minimizing patient waiting time
4. Keeping the costs of the emergency service down
5. Maintaining high standards of patient care
6. Providing comprehensive emergency services
7. Maintaining a high level of patient satisfaction

4a. First, which one of these priorities, would you say, is emphasized the
I:36 most?

_____ (PRIORITY NUMBER)

4b. And, which is the next most emphasized priority?
I:37

_____ (PRIORITY NUMBER)

4c. Finally, which priority is the third most emphasized?
I:38

_____ (PRIORITY NUMBER)

Selected Hospital Physicians' Interview

ABOUT WORK CONTACTS AND WORK RELATIONS WITH THE EMERGENCY UNIT

5. Hospital emergency units often have to work closely with other services or departments in order to accomplish their work. In this hospital, with which departments or services, would you say, does the Emergency Unit work most closely?

a. _____
I:39
b. _____
I:40
c. _____
I:41
d. _____
I:42

6. Ordinarily, how frequent are your work contacts with the Emergency Unit?
I:43
_____
_____
_____

6a. Briefly, what is the nature of these contacts?
I:44-45
_____
_____
_____

6b. From your point of view, how satisfactory are your work contacts with the Emergency Unit?
I:46
_____
_____
_____
_____

7. In general, to what extent do you feel that you and your associates can rely on people working in the Emergency Unit to do their jobs right? Would you say -- to a very great extent, a great extent, a fair extent, a small extent, or not at all?
I:47-48

| 1. TO A VERY GREAT EXTENT | 2. TO A GREAT EXTENT | 3. TO A FAIR EXTENT | 4. TO A SMALL EXTENT | 5. TO A VERY SMALL EXTENT OR NOT AT ALL |

8. Overall, how realistic are the expectations of the people who work in the Emergency Unit concerning the kinds of services, assistance, or support that you or your associates can provide? Would you say their expectations are -- extremely realistic, very realistic, fairly realistic, or not so realistic?
I:49-50

| 1. EXTREMELY REALISTIC | 2. VERY REALISTIC | 3. FAIRLY REALISTIC | 4. NOT SO REALISTIC |

9. All things considered, how much tension or friction, would you say, is there between the people working in the Emergency Unit, on the one hand, and you or your associates on the other? Is there -- a high level of tension, a moderate level, a low level, a very low level of tension, or no tension at all?
I:51-52

| 1. A HIGH LEVEL OF TENSION | 2. A MODERATE LEVEL | 3. A LOW LEVEL | 4. A VERY LOW LEVEL | 5. NO TENSION AT ALL |

- 453 -

Selected Hospital Physicians' Interview

ABOUT THE RESOURCES AND LEADERSHIP OF THE EMERGENCY UNIT

10. Compared to most other departments in the hospital, how likely is the Emergency
I:53- Unit to obtain the resources that it requires? (I mean staffing, financial, and
54 technical resources.)

_____
_____
_____
_____
_____
_____

11. Overall, considering what the Emergency Unit needs to provide high quality care
I:55- to its patients at reasonable cost, how sufficient would you say is its medical
56 staff in terms of available manpower?

_____
_____
_____
_____
_____
_____
_____

12. Based on your own knowledge and observations, how would you characterize the
I:57- current medical leadership of the Emergency Unit here? Would you say its
58 medical leadership is -- extremely effective, very effective, fairly effective,
or not so effective?

| 1. EXTREMELY EFFECTIVE | 2. VERY EFFECTIVE | 3. FAIRLY EFFECTIVE | 4. NOT SO EFFECTIVE | 5. NOT EFFECTIVE AT ALL | 8. I CAN'T JUDGE |

13. How about the nursing leadership in the Emergency Unit? Is it extremely effective,
I:59- very effective, fairly effective, or not so effective?
60

| 1. EXTREMELY EFFECTIVE | 2. VERY EFFECTIVE | 3. FAIRLY EFFECTIVE | 4. NOT SO EFFECTIVE | 5. NOT EFFECTIVE AT ALL | 8. I CAN'T JUDGE |

14. And, how would you characterize the administrative leadership of the Emergency
I:61- Unit provided by Hospital Administration here? Is it extremely effective, very
62 effective, fairly effective, or not so effective?

| 1. EXTREMELY EFFECTIVE | 2. VERY EFFECTIVE | 3. FAIRLY EFFECTIVE | 4. NOT SO EFFECTIVE | 5. NOT EFFECTIVE AT ALL | 8. I CAN'T JUDGE |

Selected Hospital Physicians' Interview

- 8 -

ABOUT PATIENT CARE IN THE EMERGENCY UNIT

15. On the basis of your experience and information, how would you rate the quality of nursing care that patients generally receive in this Emergency Unit? Would you rate it -- excellent, very good, good, fair, or rather poor?
I:63

| 1. EXCELLENT | 2. VERY GOOD | 3. GOOD | 4. FAIR | 5. RATHER POOR |

16. And how about the quality of medical care that patients generally receive in this Emergency Unit? Would you rate it -- excellent, very good, good, fair, or rather poor?
I:64

| 1. EXCELLENT | 2. VERY GOOD | 3. GOOD | 4. FAIR | 5. RATHER POOR |

17. Considering next the emergency units of all other hospitals with which you are familiar, how would you evaluate the overall quality of patient care provided in this Emergency Unit? Overall, is the quality of patient care -- much better, generally better, about the same, somewhat poorer, or generally poorer compared to these other facilities?
I:65-66

| 1. MUCH BETTER | 2. GENERALLY BETTER | 3. ABOUT THE SAME | 4. SOMEWHAT POORER | 5. GENERALLY POORER |

- 9 -

18. Please think of all the patients visiting this Emergency Unit who have come to your attention in the past six months or so. About what percent of them would you estimate should have gone to a private physician or had a problem that could have been handled in a doctor's office instead of the Emergency Unit?
I:67-68

_____ (PERCENT)

19. Next please think of those patients visiting the Emergency Unit over the past six months who required immediate hospitalization here for their medical treatment.

9a. Overall, how well were these patients managed in the Emergency Unit (prior to hospitalization)?
I:69-70

_____
_____
_____
_____
_____

9b. And, how well were they managed during their hospitalization here?
I:71-72

_____
_____
_____
_____
_____

Selected Hospital Physicians' Interview

- 10 -

20. Of all the patients visiting the Emergency Unit over the past six months or so, we would like to focus briefly on three particular sub-groups. They are:

"Lacerations of the Face or Neck involving more than skin";

"Drug Abuse Cases"; and,

"Fractures or Dislocations"

On the basis of your experience and information, how well would you say were the patients in each of these groups managed from a medical standpoint?

20a. First, how about patients with lacerations of the face or neck involving
I:73 more than skin? Were they managed -- extremely well, very well, fairly well, or not so well?

| 1. EXTREMELY WELL | 2. VERY WELL | 3. FAIRLY WELL | 4. NOT SO WELL | 8. I DON'T KNOW |

20b. Next, how well managed were drug abuse cases? Were they managed -- extremely
I:74 well, very well, fairly well, or not so well?

| 1. EXTREMELY WELL | 2. VERY WELL | 3. FAIRLY WELL | 4. NOT SO WELL | 8. I DON'T KNOW |

20c. Finally, what about the patients with fractures or dislocations? How well
I:75 managed were they? Were they managed -- extremely well, very well, fairly well, or not so well?

| 1. EXTREMELY WELL | 2. VERY WELL | 3. FAIRLY WELL | 4. NOT SO WELL | 8. I DON'T KNOW |

- 11 -

21. At the present time, is there any committee in this hospital for monitoring the
I:76 quality of work or performance of the Emergency Unit?

| 1. YES | 2. NO | 8. DON'T KNOW |

→ GO TO Q.22 (NEXT PAGE)

21a. What is the name of this committee?
I:77
_____

21b. Currently, do you happen to be a member of this committee?
I:78

| 1. YES | 2. NO |

21c. How active, would you say, is this committee?
I:79
_____
_____
_____
_____
_____
_____
_____
_____

Selected Hospital Physicians' Interview

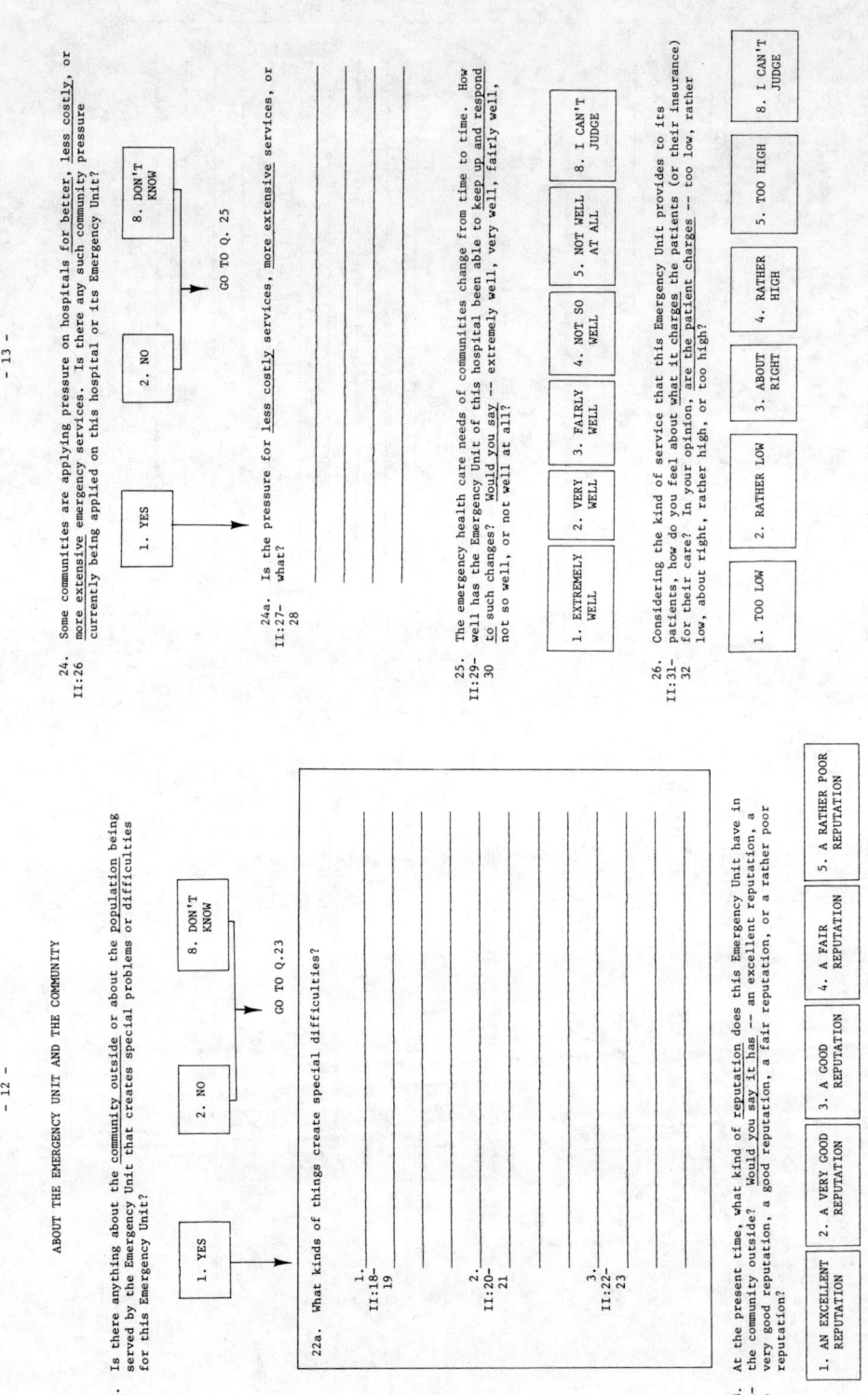

ABOUT THE EMERGENCY UNIT AND THE COMMUNITY

22. Is there anything about the community outside or about the population being served by the Emergency Unit that creates special problems or difficulties for this Emergency Unit?

II:17

| 1. YES | 2. NO | 8. DON'T KNOW |

GO TO Q.23

22a. What kinds of things create special difficulties?

1.
II:18-19

2.
II:20-21

3.
II:22-23

23. At the present time, what kind of reputation does this Emergency Unit have in the community outside? Would you say it has -- an excellent reputation, a very good reputation, a good reputation, a fair reputation, or a rather poor reputation?

II:24-25

| 1. AN EXCELLENT REPUTATION | 2. A VERY GOOD REPUTATION | 3. A GOOD REPUTATION | 4. A FAIR REPUTATION | 5. A RATHER POOR REPUTATION |

24. Some communities are applying pressure on hospitals for better, less costly, or more extensive emergency services. Is there any such community pressure currently being applied on this hospital or its Emergency Unit?

II:26

| 1. YES | 2. NO | 8. DON'T KNOW |

GO TO Q. 25

24a. Is the pressure for less costly services, more extensive services, or what?

II:27-28

25. The emergency health care needs of communities change from time to time. How well has the Emergency Unit of this hospital been able to keep up and respond to such changes? Would you say -- extremely well, very well, fairly well, not so well, or not well at all?

II:29-30

| 1. EXTREMELY WELL | 2. VERY WELL | 3. FAIRLY WELL | 4. NOT SO WELL | 5. NOT WELL AT ALL | 8. I CAN'T JUDGE |

26. Considering the kind of service that this Emergency Unit provides to its patients, how do you feel about what it charges the patients (or their insurance) for their care? In your opinion, are the patient charges -- too low, rather low, about right, rather high, or too high?

II:31-32

| 1. TOO LOW | 2. RATHER LOW | 3. ABOUT RIGHT | 4. RATHER HIGH | 5. TOO HIGH | 8. I CAN'T JUDGE |

Selected Hospital Physicians' Interview

- 14 -

Finally, a few background items.

27. How long have you been practicing medicine?
II:33-34
_____ (YEARS)

28. Professionally, what is your major field of interest or specialty within medicine?
II:35
_____ (MAJOR FIELD OR SPECIALTY)

29. How long have you been associated with this hospital?
II:36-37
_____ (YEARS)

30. Are you on the staff of any other hospitals at the present time?
II:38

1. YES   2. NO

31. What is your present position here?
II:39
_____ (PRESENT POSITION)

32. How long have you been associated with your present service or department here?
II:40-41
_____ (YEARS)

- 15 -

33. In the past six weeks, have you personally worked in the Emergency Unit here, either on a rotation basis or "on call"?
II:42

1. YES, BOTH ON ROTATION AND ON CALL
2. YES, ON ROTATION (ONLY)
3. YES, ON CALL (ONLY)
4. YES, ON SOME OTHER BASIS
5. NO

34. We have now completed your interview. Is there anything else besides what we have covered that you would like to comment on? Anything that might help us better understand the situation of this Emergency Unit?
II:43-44

_____
_____
_____
_____
_____
_____
_____
_____
_____
_____

INTERVIEWER READ TO R:

We are done. Thank you very much. We greatly appreciate your help and cooperation.

Community Respondents' Interview

The University of Michigan Study 462312
Institute for Social Research Fall 1977

HOSPITAL EMERGENCY SERVICES STUDY

FORM 5: INTERVIEW WITH RESPONDENTS FROM THE COMMUNITY

Interviewer: _____
Interview No.: _____
Date: _____

Study 462312 Fall 1977

FORM 5: INTERVIEW WITH RESPONDENTS FROM THE COMMUNITY

ABOUT WORK CONTACTS AND WORK RELATIONS

First, I have some questions about contacts with the Emergency Unit (i.e., Emergency Room or Department) of this hospital.

1. In the past six months or so, have you or your associates had any work contacts with personnel from the Emergency Unit of this hospital?
I:17

| 1. YES | 2. NO | 8. DON'T KNOW |

→ GO TO Q.3 (NEXT PAGE)

2. How frequent were these work contacts?
I:18-19
_____
_____
_____

2a. Would you briefly describe the nature of these contacts?
I:20-21
_____
_____
_____

2b. Overall, how satisfactory, would you say, were these contacts from your point of view?
I:22-23
_____
_____
_____

Community Respondents' Interview

- 2 -

3. To what extent, if any, does the work that you or your associates are doing affect the work of this Emergency Unit?
I:24-25

_____
_____
_____
_____

4. And to what extent, if any, does the work of this Emergency Unit affect the work that you or your associates are doing?
I:26-27

_____
_____
_____
_____

5. Considering the expectations that you and your associates may have of this Emergency Unit in connection with your work contacts, how well are these expectations being met by the Emergency Unit?
I:28-29

_____
_____
_____
_____

- 3 -

6. All things considered, how realistic are the expectations of the people who work in this Emergency Unit concerning any relevant services or support that you and your associates can provide? Are their expectations -- extremely realistic, very realistic, fairly realistic, or not so realistic?
I:30-31

| 1. EXTREMELY REALISTIC | 2. VERY REALISTIC | 3. FAIRLY REALISTIC | 4. NOT SO REALISTIC | 5. NOT REALISTIC AT ALL |

7. Generally, in their work relations with you and your associates, to what extent do you feel that the people who work in this Emergency Unit take into account your own work problems and needs? Would you say -- to a very great extent, a great extent, a fair extent, a small extent, or not at all?
I:32-33

| 1. TO A VERY GREAT EXTENT | 2. A GREAT EXTENT | 3. A FAIR EXTENT | 4. A SMALL EXTENT | 5. A VERY SMALL EXTENT OR NOT AT ALL |

8. All things considered, how much tension or friction would you say is there between the people working in this Emergency Unit, on the one hand, and you or your associates, on the other? Is there -- a high level of tension, a moderate level, a low level, a very low level of tension, or no tension at all?
I:34-35

| 1. A HIGH OR VERY HIGH LEVEL OF TENSION | 2. A MODERATE LEVEL | 3. A LOW LEVEL | 4. A VERY LOW LEVEL | 5. NO TENSION AT ALL |

Community Respondents' Interview

- 4 -

9. As far as you can tell from your work contacts with them, how well do the people who work in this Emergency Unit really seem to know what they are doing?

I:36-
37

_____

_____

_____

_____

_____

_____

_____

- 5 -

ABOUT THE EMERGENCY UNIT OVERALL

10. At the present time, from what you are able to tell, what are the TWO or THREE most important areas, or respects, in which you consider this Emergency Unit to be particularly strong or especially outstanding?

a. _____

I:38-
39 _____

_____

b. _____

I:40-
41 _____

_____

c. _____

I:42-
43 _____

_____

11. And, what are the TWO or THREE most important areas, or respects, in which you consider this Emergency Unit to be especially weak or to require the most improvement?

a. _____

I:44-
45 _____

b. _____

I:46-
47 _____

c. _____

I:48-
49 _____

Community Respondents' Interview

- 6 -

12. As far as you are able to tell, what are some of the priorities or goals that this Emergency Unit seems to emphasize at the present time?

a.
I:50 _____

b.
I:51 _____

c.
I:52 _____

13. Overall, from your point of view, what kind of a job is this Emergency Unit
I:53- doing at the present time?
54
_____
_____
_____
_____
_____
_____
_____

- 7 -

ABOUT PATIENT CARE IN THIS EMERGENCY UNIT

14. On the basis of your experience and information, how would you rate the overall
I:55- quality of patient care that patients generally receive in this Emergency Unit?
56   Would you rate it -- excellent, very good, good, fair, or rather poor?

| 1. EXCELLENT | 2. VERY GOOD | 3. GOOD | 4. FAIR | 5. RATHER POOR |

15. Considering the emergency units of all other hospitals with which you are familiar,
I:57- how would you evaluate the overall quality of patient care provided by this parti-
58   cular Emergency Unit? Would you say the quality of care in this Emergency Unit
       is -- much better, generally better, about the same, somewhat poorer, or generally
       poorer compared to most other emergency units?

| 1. IT IS MUCH BETTER | 2. GENERALLY BETTER | 3. ABOUT THE SAME | 4. SOMEWHAT POORER | 5. IT IS GENERALLY POORER |

16. Considering the kind of service that this Emergency Unit provides to its patients,
I:59- how do you feel about what it charges the patients (or their insurance) for their
60   care? Would you say patient charges are -- too low, rather low, about right,
       rather high, or very high?

| 1. TOO LOW | 2. RATHER LOW | 3. ABOUT RIGHT | 4. RATHER HIGH | 5. VERY HIGH |

Community Respondents' Interview

- 8 -

ABOUT THE COMMUNITY AND THIS EMERGENCY UNIT

17. Overall, how well are the emergency medical needs of this community taken care
I:61- of at the present time by the various emergency medical services available in
62   the community?

_____
_____
_____
_____
_____
_____
_____

18. At the present time, is there any BLS (Basic Life Support) or ALS (Advanced Life
I:63 Support) "system" functioning in this community?

    ┌────────┐   ┌────────┐   ┌──────────────┐
    │ 1. YES │   │ 2. NO │   │ 8. DON'T KNOW│
    └────┬───┘   └────┬───┘   └──────┬───────┘
         │   │   │
         ▼   └──→ GO TO Q.19 (NEXT PAGE) ←─┘

18a. What kind of system would this be?
I:64-
65
_____
_____
_____
_____
_____
_____
_____

- 9 -

19. Is there anything about the community here or about the population being served
I:66 by this particular Emergency Unit that tends to create problems or difficulties
     for this Emergency Unit?

    ┌────────┐   ┌────────┐   ┌──────────────┐
    │ 1. YES │   │ 2. NO │   │ 8. DON'T KNOW│
    └────┬───┘   └────┬───┘   └──────┬───────┘
         │   │   │
         ▼   └──→ GO TO Q.20 ←─┘

19a. What kinds of things create problems or difficulties?

     1. _____
     I:67-
     68 _____

     2. _____
     I:69-
     70 _____

20. At the present time, what kind of reputation does this Emergency Unit have in
I:71- the community, generally speaking? Does it have -- an excellent reputation,
72   a very good reputation, a good reputation, a fair reputation, or a rather poor
      reputation?

┌──────────────┬──────────────┬──────────────┬──────────────┬──────────────┐
│ 1. AN   │ 2. A VERY   │ 3. A GOOD   │ 4. A FAIR   │ 5. A RATHER │
│ EXCELLENT   │ GOOD   │ REPUTATION   │ REPUTATION   │ POOR   │
│ REPUTATION   │ REPUTATION   │   │   │ REPUTATION   │
│ IN THE   │   │   │   │ IN THE   │
│ COMMUNITY   │   │   │   │ COMMUNITY   │
└──────────────┴──────────────┴──────────────┴──────────────┴──────────────┘

Community Respondents' Interview

21. On the whole, how adequately would you say is this Emergency Unit meeting current community expectations regarding the services it provides? Do you think it is meeting community expectations extremely adequately, very adequately, fairly adequately, or not so adequately?
II:17-18

| 1. EXTREMELY ADEQUATELY | 2. VERY ADEQUATELY | 3. FAIRLY ADEQUATELY | 4. NOT SO ADEQUATELY | 5. NOT ADEQUATELY AT ALL |

22. All things considered, how realistic are the community's expectations regarding the services that this Emergency Unit can and cannot provide?
II:19-20

_____
_____
_____
_____
_____

23. As far as you can tell, do most of the people in this community seem to have adequate information about the services which this Emergency Unit can and cannot provide? Would you say that the information most people seem to have is -- completely adequate, very adequate, fairly adequate, not so adequate, or not adequate at all?
II:21-22

| 1. COMPLETELY ADEQUATE | 2. VERY ADEQUATE | 3. FAIRLY ADEQUATE | 4. NOT SO ADEQUATE | 5. NOT ADEQUATE AT ALL |

24. Some communities are applying pressure on hospitals for better, less costly, or more extensive emergency services. To the best of your knowledge, is any such community pressure currently being applied on this hospital or its Emergency Unit?
II:23

| 1. YES | 2. NO | 8. DON'T KNOW |

       ↓   GO TO Q.25

24a. Is this pressure for less costly emergency services, more extensive services, or what?
II:24-25

_____
_____
_____
_____
_____
_____
_____

25. The health care needs of communities change from time to time. As far as you are able to tell, how well has the Emergency Unit of this hospital been able to keep up and respond to such changes? Would you say -- extremely well, very well, fairly well, not so well, or not well at all?
II:26-27

| 1. EXTREMELY WELL | 2. VERY WELL | 3. FAIRLY WELL | 4. NOT SO WELL | 5. NOT WELL AT ALL |

Community Respondents' Interview

- 12 -

26. To the best of your knowledge, at the present time is this hospital (or its Emergency Unit) collaborating with any other hospitals or any health agencies for the purpose of providing better, less costly, or more extensive emergency medical care to the community?
II:28-29

_____
_____
_____
_____
_____
_____
_____

27. We are about finished. Is there anything else besides what we have covered concerning the Emergency Unit that you would like to add? Anything that might help us better understand the situation of this Emergency Unit?

a.
II:30-31
_____
_____
_____
_____
_____

b.
II:32-33
_____
_____
_____
_____
_____

- 13 -

Finally, some background items.

28. How long have you been in contact with this particular hospital, or its emergency unit, on a working basis?
II:34-35

_____ (YEARS)

29. How long have you worked in this area or community?
II:36-37

_____ (YEARS)

30. What is the name of the organization or agency in which you are working at the present time?
II:38

_____ (NAME OF ORGANIZATION)

31. What is your present position in this organization?
II:39

_____ (PRESENT POSITION)

32. How long have you been in your present position?
II:40

_____ (YEARS)

Community Respondents' Interview

INTERVIEWER: BY OBSERVATION

33. R's sex:
II:42 ☐ 1. MALE   ☐ 2. FEMALE

34. R's race: _____
II:43

35. How well educated did the respondent appear to be?
II:44

☐ 1. EXTREMELY WELL EDUCATED   ☐ 2. VERY WELL EDUCATED   ☐ 3. WELL EDUCATED   ☐ 4. NOT SO WELL EDUCATED

INTERVIEWER READ TO R:

We are done. Thank you very much. We greatly appreciate your help and cooperation.

EU Licensed Practical Nurses' Interview

The University of Michigan
Institute for Social Research

Study 462312
Fall 1977

HOSPITAL EMERGENCY SERVICES STUDY

FORM 6: INTERVIEW FOR FULL-TIME LPN's (LICENSED PRACTICAL NURSES)
WORKING IN THE EMERGENCY UNIT

Interviewer: _____
Interview No.: _____
Date: _____

Study 462312   Fall 1977

FORM 6: INTERVIEW FOR FULL-TIME LPN's (LICENSED PRACTICAL NURSES) WORKING IN THE EMERGENCY UNIT

SOME QUESTIONS ABOUT THE EMERGENCY UNIT IN GENERAL

First, I would like to ask you some general questions about the Emergency Unit (i.e., the Emergency Room or Department) here.

1. On the whole, what do you think of this Emergency Unit as a place to work? Would you say it is an excellent place, a very good place, a good place, a fair place, or a rather poor place to work?

I:17-18

| 1. IT IS AN EXCELLENT PLACE TO WORK | 2. A VERY GOOD PLACE | 3. A GOOD PLACE | 4. A FAIR PLACE | 5. A RATHER POOR PLACE |

2. At the present time, what kind of reputation does this Emergency Unit have in the community outside? Would you say it has an excellent reputation, a very good reputation, a good reputation, a fair reputation, or a rather poor reputation?

I:19-20

| 1. AN EXCELLENT REPUTATION | 2. A VERY GOOD REPUTATION | 3. A GOOD REPUTATION | 4. A FAIR REPUTATION | 5. A RATHER POOR REPUTATION |

3. On the basis of your experience and information while working here, about what percent of the patients speak very well of this Emergency Unit?

I:21-22

_____ (PERCENT)

EU Licensed Practical Nurses' Interview

- 2 -

4. At the present time, what sorts of problems does the Emergency Unit of this hospital face? What would you say are the major problems?

a.
I:23-
24 _____
_____

b.
I:25-
26 _____
_____

c.
I:27-
28 _____
_____

- 3 -

ABOUT WORK RELATIONS

Now, I would like to ask you some questions about work relations among the people who work in the Emergency Unit.

5. On the whole, to what extent does the medical staff understand and appreciate
I:29- the work problems and needs of the nursing staff in this Emergency Unit?
30 Would you say the medical staff has -- an excellent understanding, a very good understanding, a good understanding, a fair understanding, or a rather poor understanding of the work problems and needs of the nursing staff?

| 1. THEY HAVE AN EXCELLENT UNDERSTANDING | 2. A VERY GOOD UNDERSTANDING | 3. A GOOD UNDERSTANDING |

| 4. A FAIR UNDERSTANDING | 5. THEY HAVE A RATHER POOR UNDERSTANDING |

6. And, to what extent does the nursing staff understand and appreciate the work
I:31- problems and needs of the medical staff in this Emergency Unit? Would you
32 say the nursing staff has -- an excellent understanding, a very good understanding, a good understanding, a fair understanding, or a rather poor understanding of the work problems and needs of the medical staff?

| 1. THEY HAVE AN EXCELLENT UNDERSTANDING | 2. A VERY GOOD UNDERSTANDING | 3. A GOOD UNDERSTANDING |

| 4. A FAIR UNDERSTANDING | 5. THEY HAVE A RATHER POOR UNDERSTANDING |

EU Licensed Practical Nurses' Interview

- 4 -

7. Ordinarily, to what extent does your own work here depend on direct contacts with the other personnel in the Emergency Unit? Does it depend on direct contacts with them -- to a very great extent, a great extent, a fair extent, a small extent, or not at all?
I:33-34

| 1. TO A VERY GREAT EXTENT | 2. A GREAT EXTENT | 3. A FAIR EXTENT | 4. A SMALL EXTENT | 5. TO A VERY SMALL EXTENT OR NOT AT ALL |

8. And how about personnel from other parts of the hospital outside the Emergency Unit? Would you say your work depends on direct contacts with them -- to a very great extent, a great extent, a fair extent, a small extent, or not at all?
I:35-36

| 1. TO A VERY GREAT EXTENT | 2. A GREAT EXTENT | 3. A FAIR EXTENT | 4. A SMALL EXTENT | 5. TO A VERY SMALL EXTENT OR NOT AT ALL |

9. Here in the Emergency Unit, to what extent do the different people who have to work together take into account each other's work problems and needs as they go about doing their own activities? Do they take into account each other's work problems and needs -- to a very great extent, a great extent, a fair extent, a small extent, or not at all?
I:37-38

| 1. TO A VERY GREAT EXTENT | 2. A GREAT EXTENT | 3. A FAIR EXTENT | 4. A SMALL EXTENT | 5. TO A VERY SMALL EXTENT OR NOT AT ALL |

10. In this Emergency Unit, to what extent do you feel that you can rely on others whose jobs are related to yours (or affect your work) to do their job right? Would you say you can rely on them -- to a very great extent, a great extent, a fair extent, a small extent, or not at all?
I:39-40

| 1. TO A VERY GREAT EXTENT | 2. A GREAT EXTENT | 3. A FAIR EXTENT | 4. A SMALL EXTENT | 5. TO A VERY SMALL EXTENT OR NOT AT ALL |

- 5 -

11. After problems arise in the work activities of people who have to work together, corrections often are tried or steps are taken to handle the problem. Generally, how effective are such corrective efforts in this Emergency Unit? Are they -- completely effective, very effective, fairly effective, or not effective at all?
I:41-42

| 1. COMPLETELY EFFECTIVE | 2. VERY EFFECTIVE | 3. FAIRLY EFFECTIVE | 4. NOT SO EFFECTIVE | 5. NOT EFFECTIVE AT ALL |

12. Considering the information you need to do your work here, how adequate for your work needs is the information that you normally receive from the people you work with in the Emergency Unit? Would you say the information you get is -- completely adequate, very adequate, fairly adequate, not so adequate, or not adequate at all?
I:43-44

| 1. COMPLETELY ADEQUATE | 2. VERY ADEQUATE | 3. FAIRLY ADEQUATE | 4. NOT SO ADEQUATE | 5. NOT ADEQUATE AT ALL |

13. To what extent do you find that you have to do things on your job that you feel should be the responsibility of other people in the Emergency Unit? Do you find you have to do such things -- to a very great extent, a great extent, a fair extent, a small extent, or not at all?
I:45-46

| 1. TO A VERY GREAT EXTENT | 2. A GREAT EXTENT | 3. A FAIR EXTENT | 4. A SMALL EXTENT | 5. TO A VERY SMALL EXTENT OR NOT AT ALL |

EU Licensed Practical Nurses' Interview

ABOUT THE PATIENTS AND PATIENT CARE

Now, I have some questions about the patients and patient care in this Emergency Unit.

14. Thinking of all the patients visiting this Emergency Unit over the past four weeks, about what percent of them would you say were "true emergencies"?
I:47-48

_____ (PERCENT)

15. Thinking of all the patients visiting this emergency unit over the past four weeks, about how long after arriving did most of them have to wait until they were seen by a doctor? (About how many minutes did most of them have to wait?)
I:49-50

_____ (MINUTES UNTIL SEEN BY A DOCTOR)

16. On the basis of your experience and information, how would you rate the quality of nursing care that patients generally receive in this Emergency Unit? Would you say the quality of nursing care is -- excellent, very good, good, fair, or rather poor?
I:51-52

| 1. EXCELLENT | 2. VERY GOOD | 3. GOOD | 4. FAIR | 5. RATHER POOR |

ABOUT TENSIONS AND PRESSURE AT WORK

Next, I have some questions about tensions and pressure among the people working here.

17. All things considered, how much tension or friction would you say is there between emergency unit staff and hospital staff outside the Emergency Unit? Would you say there is -- a high level of tension, a moderate level of tension, a low level of tension, a very low level of tension, or no tension at all?
I:53-54

| 1. A HIGH LEVEL OF TENSION | 2. A MODERATE LEVEL | 3. A LOW LEVEL | 4. A VERY LOW LEVEL | 5. NO TENSION AT ALL |

18. Next, what about tension between doctors in the Emergency Unit and nurses in the Emergency Unit? Is there -- a high level of tension between them, a moderate level of tension, a low level of tension, a very low level of tension, or no tension at all?
I:55-56

| 1. A HIGH LEVEL OF TENSION | 2. A MODERATE LEVEL | 3. A LOW LEVEL | 4. A VERY LOW LEVEL | 5. NO TENSION AT ALL |

19. And, what about tension between some nursing personnel in the Emergency Unit and other nursing personnel in the Emergency Unit? Is there -- a high level of tension between them, a moderate level of tension, a low level of tension, a very low level of tension, or no tension at all?
I:57-58

| 1. A HIGH LEVEL OF TENSION | 2. A MODERATE LEVEL | 3. A LOW LEVEL | 4. A VERY LOW LEVEL | 5. NO TENSION AT ALL |

EU Licensed Practical Nurses' Interview

- 470 -

- 8 -

20. Here at work, do you feel any pressure for better performance over and above
I:59 what you think is reasonable?

| 1. YES | 2. NO | 8. DON'T KNOW |

→ GO TO Q.21 (NEXT PAGE)

20a. How much pressure do you feel over and above what you think is
reasonable? Would you say -- a very small amount of pressure,
a small amount of pressure, a moderate amount of pressure, or
a great amount of pressure?

| 1. A VERY SMALL AMOUNT OF PRESSURE | 2. A SMALL AMOUNT OF PRESSURE | 3. A MODERATE AMOUNT OF PRESSURE | 4. A GREAT AMOUNT OF PRESSURE |

20b. What is the main source of this pressure?
I:61

☐ 1 MY SUPERIORS
☐ 2 MY CO-WORKERS
☐ 3 THE DOCTORS
☐ 4 THE WORKLOAD
☐ 5 "MYSELF"
☐ 6 POOR OR INADEQUATE PERFORMANCE BY OTHERS
☐ 7 THE PATIENTS OR THEIR RELATIVES
☐ 8 SOMETHING ELSE

- 9 -

ABOUT YOUR JOB

Now I would like to ask you some more questions about your job here.

21. How strongly identified with or how strongly committed do you feel you are to
I:62- this hospital? (I mean, personally how strongly do you feel that you belong
63 here?) Do you feel identified with this hospital -- extremely strongly, very
strongly, fairly strongly, not so strongly, or not at all strongly?

| 1. EXTREMELY STRONGLY | 2. VERY STRONGLY | 3. FAIRLY STRONGLY | 4. NOT SO STRONGLY | 5. NOT AT ALL STRONGLY |

22. And, what about the Emergency Unit? Do you feel identified with this Emergency
I:64- Unit -- extremely strongly, very strongly, fairly strongly, not so strongly, or
65 not at all strongly?

| 1. EXTREMELY STRONGLY | 2. VERY STRONGLY | 3. FAIRLY STRONGLY | 4. NOT SO STRONGLY | 5. NOT AT ALL STRONGLY |

23. Generally, how much variety would you say is there in the activities that you
I:66- perform on the job here in this Emergency Unit? Is there -- very considerable
67 variety, considerable variety, moderate variety, some variety, or very little
variety?

| 1. VERY CONSIDERABLE VARIETY | 2. CONSIDERABLE VARIETY | 3. MODERATE VARIETY | 4. SOME VARIETY | 5. LITTLE OR VERY LITTLE VARIETY |

EU Licensed Practical Nurses' Interview

24. Considering your work efforts and contributions here, how satisfied are you with
I:68- the financial or monetary rewards that you receive for your work in this Emergency
69 Unit? (I mean the wages and fringe benefits that you receive.) Are you --
completely satisfied, very satisfied, fairly satisfied, not so satisfied, or not
at all satisfied?

| 1. COMPLETELY SATISFIED | 2. VERY SATISFIED | 3. FAIRLY SATISFIED | 4. NOT SO SATISFIED | 5. NOT AT ALL SATISFIED |

25. And, how satisfied are you with all of the non-financial aspects of your job?
I:70- (I mean, aside from wages and fringe benefits, how satisfied are you with
71 working here?) Are you -- completely satisfied, very satisfied, fairly satisfied,
not so satisfied, or not at all satisfied?

| 1. COMPLETELY SATISFIED | 2. VERY SATISFIED | 3. FAIRLY SATISFIED | 4. NOT SO SATISFIED | 5. NOT AT ALL SATISFIED |

26. When you need help or advice from the doctors here in deciding what to do for
II:17- emergency patients, how do you feel about the help or advice that you can get
18 from them?

_____
_____
_____
_____
_____
_____
_____

27. When you need help or advice from the nurses in the Emergency Unit who supervise
II:19- your work, how do you feel about the help or advice that you can get?
20

_____
_____
_____
_____
_____
_____
_____

28. How frequently does the supervising nurse who is your immediate superior let
II:21- you know how well you are doing your job and whether or not you are doing it
22 properly? Would you say (she/he) lets you know -- about as frequently as she
should, more frequently than she should, somewhat less frequently than she should,
or much less frequently than she should?

| 1. MORE FREQUENTLY THAN SHE SHOULD | 2. ABOUT AS FREQUENTLY AS SHE SHOULD | 3. SOMEWHAT LESS FREQUENTLY THAN SHE SHOULD | 4. MUCH LESS FREQUENTLY THAN SHE SHOULD |

EU Licensed Practical Nurses' Interview

- 12 -

Finally, some background items.

29. How long have you been working in this hospital?
II:23-24
_____ (TOTAL NUMBER OF YEARS)

30. How long have you been working in the Emergency Unit here?
II:25-26
_____ (TOTAL NUMBER OF YEARS)

31. At the present time, are you working in the Emergency Unit on a regular basis?
II:27

| 1. YES | 2. NO |

32. Usually, about how many hours a week do you work in this Emergency Unit?
II:28-29
_____ (HOURS PER WEEK)

33. What shift are you working on at the present time?
II:30

| 1. DAY SHIFT | 2. AFTERNOON (EVENING) SHIFT | 3. NIGHT SHIFT | 4. I ROTATE |

- 13 -

34. Have you had any special training in emergency nursing?
II:31

| 1. YES | 2. NO |

35. How much formal education have you had?
II:32

| 1. SOME HIGH SCHOOL | 2. COMPLETED HIGH SCHOOL | 3. SOME COLLEGE | 4. COMPLETED COLLEGE |

36. How old are you?
II:33-34
_____ (YEARS)

37. What is your present marital status?
II:35

| 1. MARRIED | 2. NOT MARRIED |

INTERVIEWER OBSERVATION:

38. Respondent's sex?
II:36

| 1. FEMALE | 2. MALE |

EU Licensed Practical Nurses' Interview

39. We have now completed your interview. Is there anything besides what we have
II:37- covered that you would like to add? Anything which <u>might help us better understand</u>
38   the situation of this Emergency Unit?

_____
_____
_____
_____
_____
_____
_____
_____
_____
_____

INTERVIEWER READ TO R:

> We are done. Thank you very much. We greatly appreciate your cooperation.

Organizational & Administrative Records' Form

The University of Michigan
Institute for Social Research

Study 462312
Fall 1977

HOSPITAL EMERGENCY SERVICES STUDY

FORM 7: INFORMATION FROM ADMINISTRATIVE AND ORGANIZATIONAL RECORDS
(Staffing, Personnel, Census, and Financial Data)

Interviewer: _____
Interview No.: _____
Date: _____

Study 462312
Fall 1977

FORM 7: INFORMATION FROM ADMINISTRATIVE AND ORGANIZATIONAL RECORDS
(Staffing, Personnel, Census, and Financial Data)

SECTION I: THE EMERGENCY UNIT FACILITY

1. How many rooms are there in the Emergency Unit of this hospital?

   a. Number of <u>treatment</u> rooms: _____
   b. All other rooms: _____

2. How many beds are there <u>in</u> the emergency unit?

   Total number of beds: _____

3. Is the emergency unit located on the ground floor of the hospital?

   _____ YES   _____ NO

4. To what other departments or services is the emergency unit adjacent (physically contiguous)? Please list these departments or services:

   a. _____
   b. _____
   c. _____
   d. _____
   e. _____

Organizational & Administrative Records' Form

5. Does this hospital or emergency unit operate an ambulance service of its own? (Check one)

  _____ YES   _____ NO

Availability of Special Clinical Facilities and Medical Specialists

6. Listed below are a number of special emergency care facilities which may be operated by hospitals or other institutions as centers, units, or programs. Please indicate whether each of these facilities is available within the emergency unit of this hospital, within the hospital (but outside the emergency unit), or in the immediate geographical area. (Check one for each facility listed)

Special Clinical Facility:	Located within the emergency unit of this hospital (1)	Located within this hospital (but not as a part of the emergency unit) (2)	Available in the immediate area (but not in this hospital) (3)	Not available in the immediate area (4)
General or Special Trauma Center or Trauma Unit	☐	☐	☐	☐
Poison Control Center	☐	☐	☐	☐
Mental Health or Crisis Center	☐	☐	☐	☐
Substance Abuse Center, Unit, or Program	☐	☐	☐	☐
Burn Center or Burn Unit	☐	☐	☐	☐
Special Burn Program	☐	☐	☐	☐

7. Please indicate whether each of the following medical specialists is regularly available within the Emergency Unit here or available in the hospital on-call to the Emergency Unit. (Check one for each specialist listed)

Specialist:	Available within the emergency unit (1)	Available in the hospital, on call to the emergency unit (2)	Not available in the hospital on a regular basis (3)
Pediatrician	☐	☐	☐
Cardiologist	☐	☐	☐
Opthalmologist	☐	☐	☐
Psychiatrist	☐	☐	☐
Orthopedist	☐	☐	☐
Burn Medicine Physician	☐	☐	☐
Neurosurgeon	☐	☐	☐
Oral Surgeon	☐	☐	☐
Plastic Surgeon	☐	☐	☐
Obstetrician/Gynecologist	☐	☐	☐

Organizational & Administrative Records' Form

SECTION II: MEDICAL STAFFING OF THE HOSPITAL

8. How many doctors in each of the following groups are associated with this hospital at the present time?

	Total Number
Active Attending Physicians	_____
Associate Attending Physicians	_____
Courtesy Physicians	_____
Residents (if any)	_____
Interns (if any)	_____

9. How many of the attending physicians (both active and associate members) are board-certified or board-eligible at the present time?

_____ (number) are board-certified or board-eligible

10. Excluding interns and residents, how many physicians (if any) are currently employed on a salaried basis by this hospital?

Number employed on a salaried basis: _____

11. Please provide the following information about hospital employment for the periods indicated.

	Yearly For most recent fiscal year (year ended) mo. day yr.	Quarterly For most recent quarter (quarter ended) mo. day yr.	Monthly For most recent month for which data are available ( ) month
Total Number of Employees in the Hospital (including those in the Emergency Unit)[1]			
Total Number of Employees in the Emergency Unit[1]			

[1] In full-time equivalents, excluding physicians

SECTION III: STAFFING OF THE EMERGENCY UNIT

12. Is there an RN physically present in the emergency unit at all times (i.e., 24 hours a day, seven days a week)?

    YES _____   NO _____

13. Is there a doctor physically present or on-call to the emergency unit at all times during each of the shifts indicated? (Check one for each shift)

	A doctor is physically present in the emergency unit at all times	A doctor is on-call within 15 minutes (but not physically present) at all times	A doctor is on-call within 30 minutes at all times	A doctor is not always on-call within 30 minutes
Day Shift	☐	☐	☐	☐
Evening Shift	☐	☐	☐	☐
Night Shift	☐	☐	☐	☐

14. Please indicate the total number of hours worked in the Emergency Unit by members of each of the following groups during the most recent week for which data are available.

Group:	Total Number of Hours Worked in Emergency Unit During This Week (week ended: ___-___-___) mo. day yr.
All Full-time LPN's	_____
All Part-time LPN's	_____
All Nurses' Aides and Assistants	_____
All Technicians	_____
All Secretaries and Clerks	_____

15. Please provide the name and number of hours worked in the Emergency Unit for each RN (including the Supervising Nurse or Head Nurse) who worked there during the most recent week for which data are available. Include both full-time and part-time RN's.

Name	Total Number of Hours Worked in Emergency Unit During This Week (week ended: ___-___-___) mo. day yr.
1.	
2.	
3.	
4.	
5.	
6.	
7.	
8.	
9.	
10.	
11.	
12.	
13.	
14.	
15.	
16.	

Organizational & Administrative Records' Form

Organizational & Administrative Records' Form

- 8 -

16. Please provide the name and number of hours worked in the Emergency Unit for each member of the medical staff who worked there during the most recent week for which data are available. List every doctor, including residents and interns, if any, who worked in the Emergency Unit (other than on an "on-call" basis).

Name	Total Number of Hours Worked in Emergency Unit During This Week (week ended: ___/___/___ mo. day yr.)
1.	
2.	
3.	
4.	
5.	
6.	
7.	
8.	
9.	
10.	
11.	
12.	

- 9 -

SECTION IV: PATIENT CENSUS INFORMATION

17. The "census" information requested in this section pertains both to the emergency unit and to the entire hospital. In the table below, please provide the most accurate information available for each of the time periods indicated.

	For most recent fiscal year (year ended ___/___/___ mo. day yr.)	For most recent quarter (quarter ended ___/___/___ mo. day yr.)	For most recent month for which data are available (_____ month)
Total Patient Visits to the Emergency Unit (Emergency Room or Department) ONLY			
Total Outpatient Visits to any part of the hospital excluding Emergency Unit Visits			
Total In-patient Admissions to the Hospital[1]			
Total Patient Days[1] (In-patient)			
Average Number of Beds[2] in the Hospital set up and staffed for use			
Average Occupancy Rate (In-patient)			
Average In-patient Length of Stay			

[1] Excluding births
[2] Excluding bassinets

Organizational & Administrative Records' Form

18. What was the total number of patient visits to the Emergency Unit during the most recent week for which data are available?

    _____ Number of patient visits to the Emergency Unit for

    the week ending ___ - ___ - ___ .
                    mo.   day   yr.

19. During the most recent month for which data are available, how many patients visiting this Emergency Unit were brought in by ambulance or other emergency vehicle?

    _____ Number of patients who were brought in by emergency

    vehicle during the month ending ___ - ___ - ___ .
                                    mo.   day   yr.

20. The table below requests information concerning (1) the number of patient visits to the emergency unit that were scheduled in advance, (2) the number of patient visits to the emergency unit that were referrals or transfers from facilities outside this hospital, and (3) the number of visits to the emergency unit by patients sent there by other units of this hospital. In each case, please provide the information for the most recent quarter and for the most recent month for which this information is available.

Type of Emergency Unit Visit:	For most recent quarter (quarter ended ___-___-___) mo. day yr.	For most recent month for which data are available (_____) month
Number of patient visits to the Emergency Unit that were scheduled in advance		
Visits to Emergency Unit as a result of referral or transfer from other hospitals or outside facilities		
Visits to the Emergency Unit by patients from other parts of this hospital		
All other patient visits to the Emergency Unit during the period indicated		

21. The information requested in the following table concerns the number of patients visiting the emergency unit who were: (1) sent by the emergency unit to other parts of this hospital; (2) transferred by the emergency unit to facilities outside the hospital; and (3) handled by the emergency unit itself and discharged. Please provide this information for the most recent quarter and for the most recent month for which this information is available.

Total Number of Emergency Unit Patients Who Were:	For most recent quarter (quarter ended ___-___-___) mo. day yr.	For most recent month for which data are available (_____) month
Sent to the operating room of this hospital by the Emergency Unit		
Sent to an intensive care unit (e.g., ICU, CCU) of this hospital by the Emergency Unit		
Sent by the Emergency Unit to an in-patient service of this hospital other than an intensive care unit		
Transferred by the Emergency Unit to some other medical care facility outside this hospital		
Handled by the Emergency Unit itself and discharged directly by the Emergency Unit		

Organizational & Administrative Records' Form

- 12 -

22. Please provide, in the table below, information concerning the total number of deaths among patients who visited this Emergency Unit during the time periods indicated.

Total Number of Deaths During:

Total Number of Emergency Unit Patients Who:	Most recent fiscal year (year ended mo. day yr.)	Most recent quarter (quarter ended mo. day yr.)	Most recent month for which data are available (_____) month
Were dead on arrival (DOA) at the Emergency Unit			
Died while in the Emergency Unit			
Died after leaving the Emergency Unit (within 48 hours of their arrival)			

- 13 -

SECTION V: FINANCIAL DATA

23a. At the present time, what is the basic fee that this hospital charges for a patient visit to the Emergency Unit (exclusive of physician fees)?

Basic fee: $ _____ per visit

23b. What are the total "average charges per patient visit" to the Emergency Unit over and above the basic fee (exclusive of physician fees)?

Average total charges in addition to "basic fee": $ _____ per visit

23c. And, what is the basic physician fee charged for an average patient visit to the Emergency Unit?

Basic physician fee: $ _____ per visit

24a. At the present time, what is the TOTAL COST to this hospital of an average patient visit to the Emergency Unit (including both direct and indirect costs but exclusive of any physician fees)?

Average total cost to the hospital per emergency visit: $ _____

24b. Is this average TOTAL COST figure based on records or is it a best estimate? _____ Based on Records _____ Best Estimate

24c. Does this average TOTAL COST figure include costs for any of the following services? (Check one for each service listed)

Costs for:	Included	Not Included
X-ray		
EKG		
Laboratory		
Anesthesiology		
Social Services		
Respiratory Therapy		
Ambulance Service		

Organizational & Administrative Records' Form

25. Please provide the financial information requested below on the basis of records when possible. If data from records are not available, please consult with Hospital Administration, as necessary, and provide a best estimate.

	For most recent fiscal year (year ended __-__-__ mo. day yr.)	For most recent quarter ended (quarter ended __-__-__ mo. day yr.)	For most recent month for which data are available (_____ month)
Total Operating Budget (i.e., amount of funds budgeted) for the entire Hospital, excluding capital funds			
For payroll only:	$	$	$
All other:	$	$	$
Total Operating Budget (i.e., amount of funds budgeted) for the Emergency Unit, excluding capital funds			
For payroll only:	$	$	$
All other:	$	$	$
Total Actual Expenditures for and by the Emergency Unit			
For payroll only:	$	$	$
All other:	$	$	$
Total Revenues from Patient Visits to the Emergency Unit	$	$	$

25a. If any of these financial data are not based on records, please place an asterisk (*) next to each estimated figure given.

25b. In this hospital, is the Emergency Unit considered a separate "cost center"?

    _____ YES   _____ NO

26. Finally, please provide the information requested below about the number of budgeted positions, budgeted amounts, and corresponding actual expenditures for the Emergency Unit's personnel during the time periods indicated. (Include salaries, wages, and fringe benefits.)

BUDGET AND PAYROLL DATA FOR PEOPLE WHO WORKED IN THE EMERGENCY UNIT

	RN's (including supervising nurses), both full-time and part-time (1)	LPN's, full-time and part-time (2)	Technicians, full-time and part-time (3)	Interns and Residents, if any (4)	Other Physicians on Payroll, if any (5)	All other personnel on payroll (6)
A. MOST RECENT QUARTER (quarter ended __-__-__ mo. day yr.)						
Total Budgeted Positions (all shifts), FTE	(1) →	(2) →	(3) →	(4) →	(5) →	(6) →
Budgeted Amount for Payroll	$	$	$	$	$	$
Actual Payroll Expenditures	$	$	$	$	$	$
B. MOST RECENT MONTH (_____ month)						
Total Budgeted Positions (all shifts), FTE	(1) →	(2) →	(3) →	(4) →	(5) →	(6) →
Budgeted Amount for Payroll	$	$	$	$	$	$
Actual Payroll Expenditures	$	$	$	$	$	$

THANK YOU VERY MUCH. WE APPRECIATE YOUR COOPERATION.

EU Patients' Questionnaire

The University of Michigan
Institute for Social Research

Fall 1977
Study 462312

QUESTIONNAIRE FOR RECENT EMERGENCY ROOM PATIENTS

HOSPITAL EMERGENCY SERVICES STUDY

QUESTIONNAIRE FOR PERSONS WHO HAVE RECENTLY VISITED
A HOSPITAL EMERGENCY ROOM FOR PATIENT CARE

I N T R O D U C T I O N

The questions we are asking are about the emergency room that you visited and about your experience there. We are interested in your personal opinions and reactions as one who was a patient in that particular emergency room. The questions cover a number of topics which are very important to our study. At the beginning, there are a few questions about how and why you visited the emergency room at that time. Then, there are questions about how the emergency room staff handled your problem, about the care that you received, and about the bill for your visit. And finally, there are some questions about yourself.

Most of the questions can be answered by checking (✓) one of the answers provided. If you do not find the exact answer that fits your case, check the one which comes closest or write the answer in your own words. The important thing is for you to answer each question the way you really feel -- the way you see it. If you are not able to answer a particular question, please skip to the next one.

******** Now for the Questions ********

THE FIRST FEW QUESTIONS ARE ABOUT GETTING TO THE EMERGENCY ROOM AND
THE REASONS FOR YOUR VISIT THERE

I:17 1. For this visit, how did you get to the emergency room? (Check one)

_____ (1) By police car or fire department vehicle
_____ (2) By ambulance or similar other emergency vehicle
_____ (3) By taxi-cab, bus, or other public transportation
_____ (4) I walked to the emergency room
_____ (5) I drove (myself)
_____ (6) A relative or friend drove me
_____ (7) Other (please describe): _____

I:18-19 2. About how long did you have to travel to reach the emergency room? (Please write in the approximate number of minutes)

It took about _____ minutes to get there

I:20 3. Was there a relative or friend with you (at any time) when you were in the emergency room? (Check one)

_____ (1) Yes _____ (2) No

Please Return Your Completed Questionnaire
Directly to the Research Staff by Mail,
Using the Stamped Envelope Provided

EU Patients' Questionnaire

- 2 -

4. Why did you go to this particular emergency room instead of some other
I:21- emergency room? What would you say was the main reason? (Check one)
22
_____ (1) I (or my family) had used this emergency room before
_____ (2) I thought this would be a good emergency room
_____ (3) I knew that the hospital is a good one
_____ (4) This emergency room was the nearest one to go to
_____ (5) This was the only available place to go for care
_____ (6) They just took me there
_____ (7) My visit there was scheduled in advance
_____ (8) My doctor told me to go there
_____ (9) I wanted to see a particular doctor who works there
_____ (10) I was sent there from another emergency room or hospital
_____ (11) Some other reason (please specify):

5. Did you know exactly what your problem was or what was wrong with you before
I:23 you arrived at the emergency room? (Check one)

_____ (1) Yes, I knew exactly what was wrong
_____ (2) I had a very good idea
_____ (3) I had a fair idea
_____ (4) I had only a vague idea
_____ (5) No, I did not know what was wrong

6. What was the main cause for your visit to the emergency room? (Check one)
I:24-
25
_____ (1) The main cause was a traffic accident
_____ (2) An accident at home
_____ (3) An accident at work
_____ (4) An accident at school
_____ (5) A recreational or sports-related accident (not at home or school)
_____ (6) An unexpected pain or sudden illness
_____ (7) A previous illness or an old injury that acted up
_____ (8) Return visit to the emergency room for "follow-up" care
_____ (9) Bad reaction to a drug
_____ (10) Something else was the main cause (please describe):

- 3 -

7. Please describe as clearly as you can the specific illness or injury that
I:26- was the reason for your visit to the emergency room. (Write in):
27

MORE ABOUT YOUR ILLNESS OR INJURY

8. Thinking back to your visit, how serious did you think was your illness or
I:28 injury when it became necessary for you to go to the emergency room for
treatment? (Check one)

_____ (1) I thought it was extremely serious
_____ (2) Very serious
_____ (3) Fairly serious
_____ (4) Not so serious
_____ (5) I thought it was not serious at all
_____ (8) I did not know

9. And, after you arrived at the emergency room, how serious did they tell you
I:29 was your illness or injury? (Check one)

_____ (1) They told me it was extremely serious
_____ (2) Very serious
_____ (3) Fairly serious
_____ (4) Not so serious
_____ (5) They told me it was not serious at all
_____ (0) They didn't tell me how serious it was

10. As far as you can tell now, how important was it to have received immediate
I:30 medical attention at that time? (Check one)

_____ (1) It was extremely important
_____ (2) It was very important
_____ (3) It was fairly important
_____ (4) It was not so important
_____ (5) It was not important at all
_____ (8) I don't know

EU Patients' Questionnaire

THE NEXT FEW QUESTIONS ARE ABOUT WHAT HAPPENED WHEN YOU ARRIVED AT THE EMERGENCY ROOM AND ABOUT THE DOCTORS AND NURSES WHO TOOK CARE OF YOU THERE

11. After arriving at the emergency room, about how long did you have to wait
I:31- until you were seen by a nurse or a doctor? (Please write in the approximate
32 number of minutes you had to wait)

I had to wait about _____ minutes

12. Did the staff of the emergency room try to make you as comfortable as possible
I:33 while you were waiting to be treated? (Check one)

___ (1) Yes, they did try to make me as comfortable as possible
___ (2) No, they did not try to make me as comfortable as possible

13. Considering how busy the emergency room doctors and nurses were when
I:34 you arrived there, would you say that they took care of you as soon as possible? (Check one)

___ (1) They took care of me as soon as possible
___ (2) They should have taken care of me a little sooner
___ (3) They should have taken care of me much sooner

14. How many different doctors took care of you while you were in the
I:35 emergency room? (Check one)

___ (0) No doctors at all; I was seen only by a nurse
___ (1) One doctor took care of me
___ (2) Two doctors took care of me
___ (3) Three or more doctors took care of me
___ (8) I don't know

15. Overall, how well would you say
I:36 did the doctor (or doctors) who treated you in the emergency room take care of you? (Check one)

___ (1) The doctor(doctors) took care of me extremely well
___ (2) Very well
___ (3) Fairly well
___ (4) Not so well
___ (5) Not well at all
___ (0) I did not see a doctor

16. And how about the nurse (or nurses)
I:37 who took care of you in the emergency room? Overall, how well did they take care of you? (Check one)

___ (1) The nurse(nurses) took care of me extremely well
___ (2) Very well
___ (3) Fairly well
___ (4) Not so well
___ (5) Not well at all
___ (0) I did not see a nurse

THE NEXT FEW QUESTIONS ARE ABOUT THE WAY IN WHICH THE EMERGENCY ROOM STAFF HANDLED YOUR PROBLEM AND ABOUT THE KIND OF CARE YOU RECEIVED

17. Thinking of the emergency room staff
I:38 who took care of you, overall, how considerate were they of you as a person? (Check one)

___ (1) Overall, they were extremely considerate
___ (2) They were very considerate
___ (3) They were fairly considerate
___ (4) They were not so considerate
___ (5) They were not considerate at all

18. In your opinion, did the staff who
I:39 took care of you in the emergency room ask you about your problem in as much detail as they should have? (Check one)

___ (1) Definitely yes
___ (2) Probably yes
___ (3) Probably no
___ (4) Definitely no
___ (8) I don't know
___ (0) There was no reason for them to ask

19. To what extent did the staff who
I:40 took care of you make an effort to really understand your problem? (Check one)

___ (1) To a very great extent
___ (2) To a great extent
___ (3) To a fair extent
___ (4) To a small extent
___ (5) To a very small extent or not at all
___ (0) There was no need for them to make such an effort

20. On the whole, were you satisfied
I:41 with the way the emergency room staff explained to you how your problem should be handled? (Check one)

___ (1) I was extremely satisfied
___ (2) Very satisfied
___ (3) Fairly satisfied
___ (4) Not so satisfied
___ (5) I was not satisfied at all

21. Again thinking of the staff who
I:42 took care of you in the emergency room, to what extent did they really seem to know what they were doing? (Check one)

___ (1) To a very great extent
___ (2) To a great extent
___ (3) To a fair extent
___ (4) To a small extent
___ (5) To a very small extent
___ (8) I can't judge

22. And, how smoothly did the staff
I:43 seem to work together while you were there? (Check one)

___ (1) They seemed to work together extremely smoothly
___ (2) Very smoothly
___ (3) Fairly smoothly
___ (4) Not so smoothly
___ (5) Not smoothly at all

EU Patients' Questionnaire

- 6 -

23. All in all, about how much time did you spend in the emergency room during your visit? In other words, how long did your visit last from the time you arrived there until you were discharged from the emergency room? (Check one):
I:44-45

_____ (1) I spent a total of about 15 minutes in the emergency room
_____ (2) About 30 minutes
_____ (3) About 45 minutes
_____ (4) About one hour
_____ (5) About 1 hour and 15 minutes (75 minutes)
_____ (6) About 1 hour and 30 minutes (90 minutes)
_____ (7) About 2 hours
_____ (8) About 2 hours and 30 minutes
_____ (9) About 3 hours
_____ (10) I spent a total of more than 3 hours in the emergency room

24. During your visit, did they seem to have enough doctors on hand to take care of all the patients in the emergency room within a reasonable amount of time? (Check one)
I:46

_____ (1) They seemed to have more than enough doctors
_____ (2) They seemed to have enough doctors
_____ (3) They seemed to have not enough doctors
_____ (8) I couldn't tell

25. All things considered, how satisfied are you with the care that was given to you in the emergency room during this visit? (Check one)
I:47

_____ (1) I am completely satisfied
_____ (2) Very satisfied
_____ (3) Fairly satisfied
_____ (4) Not so satisfied
_____ (5) I am not satisfied at all

26. Compared to what you might have expected before you got there, how good a job did the emergency room staff do for you? (Check one)
I:48

_____ (1) Overall, they did a much better job than I had expected
_____ (2) They did a better job than I had expected
_____ (3) About as good a job as I had expected
_____ (4) A poorer job than I had expected
_____ (5) Overall, they did a much poorer job than I had expected
_____ (8) I didn't know what to expect

- 7 -

27. Thinking back to your visit, what parts or aspects of your experience in the emergency room did you find the most satisfactory? (Please describe):

a.
I:49-50 _____
_____
_____

b.
I:51-52 _____
_____
_____

28. And, what parts or aspects of your experience in the emergency room did you find least satisfactory? (Please describe):

a.
I:53-54 _____
_____
_____

b.
I:55-56 _____
_____
_____

EU Patients' Questionnaire

- 8 -

29. In your opinion, are there any things the emergency room staff could have
I:57   done, but did not do, to give you better care? (Check one)

_____ (1) Yes   _____ (2) No   _____ (8) I don't know

                                        (If you answer "no"
                                        or "I don't know")
                                        GO TO QUESTION 30

29a. If yes, please describe what they could have done:
I:58- _____
  59   _____
       _____
       _____
       _____

30. Thinking of all the things that the staff did when taking care of you, are there
I:60   any things that they did but should not have done in your case? (Check one)

_____ (1) Yes   _____ (2) No   _____ (8) I don't know

                                        GO TO QUESTION 31
                                        (PAGE 9)

30a. If yes, please describe what they should not have done:
I:61- _____
  62   _____
       _____
       _____
       _____

- 9 -

SOME ADDITIONAL QUESTIONS ABOUT THE EMERGENCY ROOM AND YOUR VISIT

31. During your visit, did the emergency room staff seem to have everything they
I:63   needed to take care of you as quickly as possible? (Check one)

_____ (1) Yes   _____ (2) No   _____ (8) I don't know

32. All other things aside, how satisfactory would you say was the physical plant
I:64   and layout of the emergency room that you visited? (Check one)

_____ (1) The physical plant and layout was
           extremely satisfactory
_____ (2) Very satisfactory
_____ (3) Fairly satisfactory
_____ (4) Not so satisfactory
_____ (5) The physical plant and layout was
           not satisfactory at all

33. If you (or a member of your family) had a similar illness or injury in the
I:65   future, is there any reason why you might prefer to go to another emergency
       room instead of the one you visited this time? (Check one)

_____ (1) Yes   _____ (2) No

                                        GO TO QUESTION 34
                                        (PAGE 10)

33a. If yes, why would you prefer to go to a different emergency room?
I:66- _____
  67   _____
       _____
       _____
       _____

EU Patients' Questionnaire

- 10 -

34. During the first week after you returned home following your visit to the emergency room, did you have any difficulties or complications related to
I:68 the problem for which you had gone there in the first place? (Check one)

___ (1) Yes

___ (2) No ──► GO TO QUESTION 35

34a. If yes, please describe these difficulties:
I:69-
70
_____
_____
_____
_____
_____

AND NOW, A QUESTION ABOUT THE HOSPITAL WHICH RUNS
THE EMERGENCY ROOM THAT YOU VISITED

35. Thinking of this particular hospital, what kind of reputation does it have in the
I:71 community? (Check one)

___ (1) This hospital has an excellent reputation
___ (2) A very good reputation
___ (3) A good reputation
___ (4) A fair reputation
___ (5) This hospital has a rather poor reputation
___ (8) I don't know

- 11 -

THE NEXT FEW QUESTIONS ARE ABOUT SOME THINGS THAT MIGHT HAVE HAPPENED
DURING YOUR VISIT TO THE EMERGENCY ROOM

36. On the day of your visit, were they able to treat you in this emergency room
II:17 and then send you directly home or back to work? (Check one)

___ (1) Yes

___ (2) No ──► GO TO QUESTION 37

36a. At the time they discharged you from the emergency room, did they
II:18 advise you to come back or to go somewhere else for follow-up care
at a later date? (Check one)

___ (1) Yes, they told me to come back to the same
        emergency room
___ (2) Yes, they told me to come back to the same hospital,
        but not to the emergency room
___ (3) Yes, they told me to go to my own doctor or a
        private physician
___ (4) Yes, they told me to go to some other care facility
___ (0) No, they did not advise follow-up care

36b. By the time they discharged you from the emergency room, had they
II:19 given you enough information (or instructions) to take care of
yourself after returning home? (Check one)

___ (1) Yes   ___ (2) No

37. During this visit, were you sent from the emergency room to an operating room
II:20 of the hospital for surgery? (Check one)

___ (1) Yes   ___ (2) No

EU Patients' Questionnaire

- 12 -

38. During this visit, were you admitted to the hospital as an in-patient? In other words, did you have to stay in the hospital as a patient more than one day? (Check one)
II:21

 _____ (1) Yes   _____ (2) No

39. On the day of your visit, did they happen to send you directly from the emergency room to some other place outside the hospital for treatment? (Check one)
II:22

 _____ (1) Yes   _____ (2) No → GO TO QUESTION 40 (PAGE 13)

> 39a. If yes, where did they send you? (Check one)
> II:23
>
> _____ (1) To another hospital
> _____ (2) To a doctor's office
> _____ (3) To some other care facility
>
> 39b. How satisfied are you with the treatment you received at this other place where they sent you? (Check one)
> II:24
>
> _____ (1) Extremely satisfied
> _____ (2) Very satisfied
> _____ (3) Fairly satisfied
> _____ (4) Not so satisfied
> _____ (5) Not satisfied at all

- 13 -

> THE NEXT FEW QUESTIONS REFER TO WHAT YOU OR YOUR INSURANCE COMPANY WERE CHARGED FOR YOUR VISIT TO THE EMERGENCY ROOM

40. Do you know what the charges were for your emergency visit? (Check one)
II:25

 _____ (1) Yes   _____ (2) No → GO TO QUESTION 41

> 40a. What was the total amount charged for your visit? In other words, how much was the total bill? (Please write in)
> II:26-28
>
> Total charges for my visit were: $ _____
>
> 40b. How do you feel about the charges for your visit? (Check one)
> II:29
>
> _____ (1) The charges were too low considering the service I received
> _____ (2) They were rather low
> _____ (3) They were about right
> _____ (4) They were rather high
> _____ (5) They were too high
> _____ (6) The charges were extremely high considering the service I received

41. Did you or your family have health insurance coverage at the time of your emergency visit? (Check one)
II:30

 _____ (1) Yes   _____ (2) No → GO TO QUESTION 42 (PAGE 14)

> 41a. What kind(s) of health insurance did you have? (Please check each kind of insurance that you had)
> II:31
>
> _____ (1) Blue Cross/Blue Shield
> _____ (2) Medicare
> _____ (3) Medicaid
> _____ (4) Private or commercial health insurance
> _____ (5) Other (please specify): _____

EU Patients' Questionnaire

42. Whether or not you had any insurance coverage, did you pay (or will you be paying) any part of the bill for your visit yourself? (Check one)
II:32

___ (1) Yes   ___ (2) No   ___ (8) I don't know

                                        GO TO QUESTION 43

42a. How much of the bill will you be paying yourself? (Check one)
II:33
___ (1) All of it
___ (2) Most of it
___ (3) About half of it
___ (4) Less than half of it
___ (8) I don't know

42b. How are you handling your share of the bill? (Check one)
II:34
___ (1) From savings
___ (2) By borrowing money
___ (3) Paying the hospital in installments
___ (4) Some other way

FINALLY, A FEW QUESTIONS ABOUT YOURSELF

To help us understand how different persons look at their emergency room experience, we need some background information about such things as their age, education, sex, and family income. The way people feel and react may be different because of their personal characteristics. This is why it is important to ask you these questions about yourself. Your answers to these and all of the previous questions will be treated with the strictest confidentiality.

43. At the present time, are you a student? (Check one)
II:35
___ (1) Yes, I am a high school or a vocational school student
___ (2) Yes, I am a college student
___ (3) No, I am not a student

44. How much formal education have you had? (Check the highest completed)
II:36
___ (1) Grade school education only
___ (2) Some high school
___ (3) Completed high school
___ (4) Some college
___ (5) Completed college
___ (6) Completed more than four years of college
___ (7) Other (please write in): _____

45. At the present time, are you married? (Check one)
II:37
___ (1) Yes   ___ (2) No

46. What is your sex? (Check one)
II:38
___ (1) Male   ___ (2) Female

47. What is your race? (Check one)
II:39
___ (1) White
___ (2) Black
___ (3) Other

48. How old are you? (Write in number of years)
II:40-41
_____ Years old

49. At the present time, are you employed? (Check one)
II:42
___ (1) Yes   ___ (2) No

50. What was your total family income before taxes in 1976? (Check one)
II:43
___ (1) Less than $2,000
___ (2) $2,000 - $3,999
___ (3) $4,000 - $5,999
___ (4) $6,000 - $8,999
___ (5) $9,000 - $11,999
___ (6) $12,000 - $14,999
___ (7) $15,000 - $19,999
___ (8) $20,000 - $29,999
___ (9) $30,000 or more

51. How long have you lived in the community in which you now live? (Check one)
II:44
___ (1) Less than one year
___ (2) One or two years
___ (3) Three or four years
___ (4) Five to ten years
___ (5) More than ten years

EU Patients' Questionnaire

- 16 -

52. In the 12-month period before this particular visit, have you or any other member of your family gone to this same emergency room for care? (Check one)
II:45
_____ (1) Yes _____ (2) No

53. And what about the past two years before this visit, have you or any other member of your family gone to this emergency room for care? (Check one)
II:46
_____ (1) Yes _____ (2) No

54. When you or a member of your family needs medical attention, where do you usually go for care? (Check one)
II:47
_____ (1) To our regular family doctor
_____ (2) To a private doctor's office but not a regular family doctor
_____ (3) To a clinic which is not located in a hospital
_____ (4) To a hospital clinic (or outpatient department)
_____ (5) To a hospital emergency room
_____ (6) To some other care facility

THANK YOU VERY MUCH FOR YOUR COOPERATION. THESE ARE ALL THE QUESTIONS THAT WE NEEDED TO ASK. IF THERE IS ANYTHING ELSE THAT YOU WOULD LIKE TO ADD ABOUT YOUR VISIT TO THE EMERGENCY ROOM, PLEASE FEEL FREE TO DO SO IN THE SPACE BELOW:

_____
_____
_____
_____
_____
_____
_____

Again, many thanks for your help in our study. Please put your completed questionnaire in the envelope that we sent you and mail it to us. As soon as we receive it, we will ask the University to send you the $10.00 which we promised.